NOT
ANA
ANE 19
ANTI 20
 Aminoglycosides, Antifungals, Antimalarials, Antimyco-
 bacterials, Antiparasitics, Antivirals, Carbapenems, Cephalosporins,
 Macrolides, Penicillins, Quinolones, Sulfas, Tetracyclines, Other
CARDIOVASCULAR – ACE inhibitors, Angiotensin Receptor Blockers, Anti-   35
 adrenergic agents, Antidysrhythmics, Antihyperlipidemic agents, Antihy-
 pertensives, Antiplatelet drugs, Beta blockers, Calcium channel blockers,
 Diuretics, Nitrates, Pressors, Thrombolytics, Volume expanders, Other
CONTRAST MEDIA – MRI, Radiography, and Ultrasound contrast   51
DERMATOLOGY – Acne, Actinic Keratosis, Antibacterials, Antifungals,   51
 Antiparasitics, Antipsoriatics, Antivirals, Corticosteroids, Hemorrhoid care
ENDOCRINE & METABOLIC – Androgens / Anabolic Steroids, Bisphospho-   58
 nates, Corticosteroids, Diabetes-related agents, Gout-Related, Minerals,
 Nutritionals, Thyroid agents, Vitamins, Other
ENT - Antihistamines, Antitussives, Decongestants, Ear preparations, ENT   69
 Combinations, Mouth and Lip preparations, Nasal preparations
GASTROENTEROLOGY - Antidiarrheals, Antiemetics, Antiulcer, Laxatives   74
HEMATOLOGY – Anticoagulants, Other   82
HERBAL & ALTERNATIVE THERAPIES   84
IMMUNOLOGY – Immunizations, Immunoglobulins, Immunosuppresion   89
NEUROLOGY – Alzheimer's, Anticonvulsants, Migraine, Parkinsons, Other   92
OBSTETRICS & GYNECOLOGY – Contraceptives, Estrogens, GnRH   97
 Agonists, Hormone Replacement combos, Labor induction / Cervical
 ripening, Ovulation Stimulants, Progestins, Selective Estrogen Receptor
 Modulators, Tocolytics, Uterotonics, Vaginitisl preparations, Other
ONCOLOGY   103
OPHTHALMOLOGY – Antiallergy, Antibacterials, Antivirals, Corticosteroids,   104
 Glaucoma agents, Mydriatics/Cycloplegics, NSAIDs, Other
PSYCHIATRY – Antidepressants, Antimanics, Antipsychotics, Anxiolytics/   108
 Hypnotics - Benzodiazepines, Anxiolytics/Hypnotics - Other, Drug
 dependence therapy, Stimulants / ADHD / Anorexiants, Other
PULMONARY – Beta agonists, Combinations, Inhaled steroids, Leukotriene   116
 inhibitors, Other
TOXICOLOGY   119
UROLOGY – Benign prostatic hyperplasia, Bladder agents, Erectile   121
 dysfunction, Nephrolithiasis
INDEX   123
EMERGENCY DRUGS , CARDIAC DYSRHYTHMIAS, ORDERING INFO   141

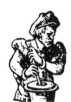

FOR TARASCON BOOKS/SOFTWARE, VISIT **WWW.TARASCON.COM**

Tarascon Pocket Pharmacopoeia®
- Classic Shirt-Pocket Edition
- Deluxe Labcoat Pocket Edition
- PDA software for Palm OS® or Pocket PC®

Other Tarascon Pocketbooks
- Tarascon Primary Care Pocketbook
- Tarascon Internal Medicine & Critical Care Pocketbook
- Tarascon Pocket Orthopaedica®
- Tarascon Adult Emergency Pocketbook
- Tarascon Pediatric Emergency Pocketbook & software
- How to be a Truly Excellent Junior Medical Student

See faxable order form on page 144

"It's not how much you know, it's how fast you can find the answer."®

Important Caution – Please Read This! The information in the *Pocket Pharmacopoeia* is compiled from sources believed to be reliable, and exhaustive efforts have been put forth to make the book as accurate as possible. The *Pocket Pharmacopoeia* is edited by a panel of drug information experts with extensive peer review and input from more than 50 practicing clinicians of multiple specialties. Our goal is to provide health professionals focused, core prescribing information in a convenient, organized, and concise fashion. We include FDA-approved dosing indications and those off-label uses that have a reasonable basis to support their use. *However the accuracy and completeness of this work cannot be guaranteed.* Despite our best efforts this book may contain typographical errors and omissions. The *Pocket Pharmacopoeia* is intended as a quick and convenient reminder of information you have already learned elsewhere. The contents are to be used as a guide only, and health care professionals should use sound clinical judgment and individualize therapy to each specific patient care situation. This book is not meant to be a replacement for training, experience, continuing medical education, studying the latest drug prescribing literature, raw intelligence, good hair, or common sense. This book is sold without warranties of any kind, express or implied, and the publisher and editors disclaim any liability, loss, or damage caused by the contents. *If you do not wish to be bound by the foregoing cautions and conditions, you may return your undamaged and unexpired book to our office for a full refund.* Tarascon Publishing is independent from and has no affiliation with pharmaceutical companies. Although drug companies purchase and distribute our books as promotional items, the Tarascon editorial staff alone determine all book content.

Tarascon Pocket Pharmacopoeia® 2006 Classic Edition

D2

HOW TO USE THE TARASCON POCKET PHARMACOPOEIA®

The *Tarascon Pocket Pharmacopoeia* arranges drugs by clinical class with a comprehensive index in the back. Trade names are italicized and capitalized. Drug doses shown in mg/kg are generally intended for children, while fixed doses represent typical adult recommendations. Brackets indicate currently available formulations, although not all pharmacies stock all formulations. The availability of generic, over-the-counter, and scored formulations are mentioned. Codes are as follows:

▶ **METABOLISM & EXCRETION**: **L** = primarily liver, **K** = primarily kidney, **LK** = both, but liver > kidney, **KL** = both, but kidney > liver, **LO** = liver & onions

♀ **SAFETY IN PREGNANCY**: **A** = Safety established using human studies, **B** = Presumed safety based on animal studies, **C** = Uncertain safety; no human studies and animal studies show an adverse effect, **D** = Unsafe - evidence of risk that may in certain clinical circumstances be justifiable, **X** = Highly unsafe - risk of use outweighs any possible benefit. For drugs which have not been assigned a category: **+** Generally accepted as safe, **?** Safety unknown or controversial, **-** Generally regarded as unsafe.

▶ **SAFETY IN LACTATION**: **+** Generally accepted as safe, **?** Safety unknown or controversial, **-** Generally regarded as unsafe. Many of our "+" listings are from the *American Academy of Pediatrics* website (www.aap.org/policy/0063.html), and may differ from those recommended by the manufacturer.

© **DEA CONTROLLED SUBSTANCES**: **I** = High abuse potential, no accepted use (eg, heroin, marijuana), **II** = High abuse potential and severe dependence liability (eg, morphine, codeine, hydromorphone, cocaine, amphetamines, methylphenidate, secobarbital). Some states require triplicates. **III** = Moderate dependence liability (eg, *Tylenol #3, Vicodin*), **IV** = Limited dependence liability (benzodiazepines, propoxyphene, phentermine), **V** = Limited abuse potential (eg, *Lomotil*).

$ **RELATIVE COST**: Cost codes used are "per month" of maintenance therapy (eg, antihypertensives) or "per course" of short-term therapy (eg, antibiotics). Codes are calculated using average wholesale prices (at press time in US dollars) for the most common indication and route of each drug at a typical adult dosage. For maintenance therapy, costs are calculated based upon a 30 day supply or the quantity that might typically be used in a given month. For short-term therapy (ie, 10 days or

Code	Cost
$	< $25
$$	$25 to $49
$$$	$50 to $99
$$$$	$100 to $199
$$$$$	≥ $200

less), costs are calculated on a single treatment course. When multiple forms are available (eg, generics), these codes reflect the least expensive generally available product. When drugs don't neatly fit into the classification scheme above, we have assigned codes based upon the relative cost of other similar drugs. *These codes should be used as a rough guide only*, as (1) they reflect cost, not charges, (2) pricing often varies substantially from location to location and time to time, and (3) HMOs, Medicaid, and buying groups often negotiate substantially different pricing. Your mileage may vary. Check with your local pharmacy if you have any question.

🍁 **CANADIAN TRADE NAMES**: Unique common Canadian trade names not used in the US are listed after a maple leaf symbol. Trade names used in both nations or only in the US are displayed without such notation.

PAGE INDEX FOR TABLES*		
General	ACE inhibitors 36	**Immunology**
Therapeutic drug levels 5	Statins, LDL goals 41	Peds immunizations 90
Outpatient peds drugs 6	Cardiac parameters 48	Tetanus 91
Peds vitals & drugs 7	Thrombolysis in MI 50	**Neurology**
Conversions 7	**Dermatology**	Dermatomes 94
Formulas, websites 9	Topical Steroids 55	Nerve roots, LS spine 94
QT interval drugs 9	**Endocrine**	Coma scale 94
Adult emerg drugs 141	Corticosteroids 59	**OB/GYN**
Cardiac protocols 142	Diabetes numbers 60	Oral contraceptives 98
Analgesics Nonsteroidals 13	Insulin 62	Emerg contraception 99
Fentanyl transdermal 14	IV solutions 64	Drugs in pregnancy 101
Opioid equivalency 15	Fluoride dose 64	APGAR score 101
Antimicrobials	Potassium forms 65	**Psychiatry**
Bacterial pathogens 28	Peds rehydration 66	Body mass index 116
Cephalosporins 29	**ENT** ENT combinations 70	**Pulmonary**
STDs/Vaginitis 30	**Gastroenterology**	Inhaler colors 117
Penicillins 31	H pylori Rx 78	Peak flow by age 117
SBE prophylaxis 32	**Hematology**	Inhaled steroids 118
Quinolones 34	Heparin dosing 82	**Toxicology**
Cardiovascular	Anticoagulation goals 83	Antidotes 120

*Please see the *Deluxe Edition* of the *Tarascon Pocket Pharmacopoeia* for extra large format tables as follows. General: P450 Enzymes. CV: CAD 10-year risk, HTN risk stratification & treatment. Heme: Warfarin interactions. Ophth: Visual acuity screen.

ABBREVIATIONS IN TEXT			
AAP - American Academy of Pediatrics	d - day	IV - intravenous	prn - as needed
ac - before meals	D5W - 5% dextrose	JRA - juvenile rheumatoid arthritis	q - every
ADHD - attention deficit & hyperactivity disorder	DPI - dry powder inhaler	kg - kilogram	qd - once daily
	elem - elemental	LFTs - liver fxn tests	qhs - at bedtime
AHA - American Heart Association	ET - endotracheal	LV - left ventricular	qid - four times/day
	EPS - extrapyramidal symptoms	mcg - microgram	qod - every other day
ANC - absolute neutrophil count	g - gram	MDI - metered dose inhaler	q pm - every evening
ASA - aspirin	gtts - drops	mEq - milliequivalent	RA - rheumatoid arthritis
bid - twice per day	GERD - gastroesophageal reflux dz	mg - milligram	SC - subcutaneous
BP - blood pressure	GU - genitourinary	MI - myocardial infarction	soln - solution
BPH - benign prostatic hypertrophy	h - hour	min - minute	supp - suppository
CAD - coronary artery disease	HAART - highly active antiretroviral therapy	mL - milliliter	susp - suspension
		mo - months old	tab - tablet
cap - capsule	HCTZ - hydrochlorothiazide	ng - nanogram	TB - tuberculosis
CMV - cytomegalovirus	HRT - hormone replacement therapy	NHLBI – National Heart, Lung, and Blood Institute	TCAs - tricyclic antidepressants
CNS - central nervous system	HSV - herpes simplex virus	NS - normal saline	TIA - transient ischemic attack
COPD - chronic obstructive pulmonary disease	HTN - hypertension	NYHA - New York Heart Association	tid - 3 times/day
	IM - intramuscular	N/V -nausea/vomiting	tiw - 3 times/week
CPZ - chlorpromazine	INR - international normalized ratio	OA - osteoarthritis	TNF - tumor necrosis factor
CrCl - creatinine clearance	IU - international units	pc - after meals	UC - ulcerative colitis
		PO - by mouth	UTI - urinary tract infection
		PR - by rectum	wk - week
			yo - years old

THERAPEUTIC DRUG LEVELS

Drug	Level	Optimal Timing
amikacin peak	20-35 mcg/ml	30 minutes after infusion
amikacin trough	<5 mcg/ml	Just prior to next dose
carbamazepine trough	4-12 mcg/ml	Just prior to next dose
cyclosporine trough	50-300 ng/ml	Just prior to next dose
digoxin	0.8-2.0 ng/ml	Just prior to next dose
ethosuximide trough	40-100 mcg/ml	Just prior to next dose
gentamicin peak	5-10 mcg/ml	30 minutes after infusion
gentamicin trough	<2 mcg/ml	Just prior to next dose
lidocaine	1.5-5 mcg/ml	12-24 hours after start of infusion
lithium trough	0.6-1.2 meq/l	Just prior to first morning dose
NAPA	10-30 mcg/ml	Just prior to next procainamide dose
phenobarbital trough	15-40 mcg/ml	Just prior to next dose
phenytoin trough	10-20 mcg/ml	Just prior to next dose
primidone trough	5-12 mcg/ml	Just prior to next dose
procainamide	4-10 mcg/ml	Just prior to next dose
quinidine	2-5 mcg/ml	Just prior to next dose
theophylline	5-15 mcg/ml	8-12 hrs after once daily dose
tobramycin peak	5-10 mcg/ml	30 minutes after infusion
tobramycin trough	<2 mcg/ml	Just prior to next dose
valproate trough (epilepsy)	50-100 mcg/ml	Just prior to next dose
valproate trough (mania)	45-125 mcg/ml	Just prior to next dose
vancomycin trough	5-10 mcg/ml	Just prior to next dose

Tarascon Pocket Pharmacopoeia®
Deluxe PDA Edition

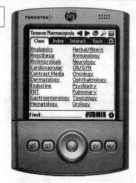

Features
- Palm OS® and Pocket PC® versions
- Meticulously peer-reviewed drug information
- Multiple drug interaction checking
- Continuous internet auto-updates
- Extended memory card support
- Multiple tables & formulas
- Complete customer privacy

Download a FREE 30-day trial version at www.tarascon.com

Subscriptions thereafter priced at $2.29/month

Tarascon Publishing is proud to partner with the following organizations in bringing you the top-quality PDA edition of the *Pocket Pharmacopoeia*: USBMIS, Inc (software production and support), Drugstore.com (exact drug pricing information), and NeedyMeds.com (patient assistance program data).

PEDIATRIC DRUGS		*Age*	*2m*	*4m*	*6m*	*9m*	*12m*	*15m*	*2y*	*3y*	*5y*
		Kg	5	6½	8	9	10	11	13	15	19
		Lbs	11	15	17	20	22	24	28	33	42
med	***strength***	***freq***	***teaspoons of liquid per dose** (1 tsp= 5 ml)*								
Tylenol (mg)		q4h	80	80	120	120	160	160	200	240	280
Tylenol (tsp)	160/t	q4h	½	½	¾	¾	1	1	1¼	1½	1¾
ibuprofen (mg)		q6h	-	-	75†	75†	100	100	125	150	175
ibuprofen (tsp)	100/t	q6h	-	-	¾†	¾†	1	1	1¼	1½	1¾
amoxicillin or	125/t	bid	1	1¼	1½	1¾	1¾	2	2¼	2¾	3½
Augmentin	200/t	bid	½	¾	1	1	1¼	1¼	1½	1¾	2¼
(not otitis media)	250/t	bid	½	½	¾	¾	1	1	1¼	1¼	1¾
	400/t	bid	¼	½	½	½	¾	¾	¾	1	1
amoxicillin,	200/t	bid	1	1¼	1¾	2	2	2¼	2¾	3	4
(otitis media)‡	250/t	bid	¾	1¼	1½	1½	1¾	1¾	2¼	2½	3¼
	400/t	bid	½	¾	¾	1	1	1¼	1½	1½	2
Augmentin ES‡	600/t	bid	⅜	½	½	¾	¾	¾	1	1¼	1½
azithromycin*§	100/t	qd	¼†	½†	½	½	½	½	¾	¾	1
(5-day Rx)	200/t	qd	--	¼†	¼	¼	¼	¼	½	½	½
Bactrim/Septra	---	bid	½	¾	1	1	1	1¼	1½	1½	2
cefaclor*	125/t	bid	1	1	1¼	1½	1½	1¾	2	2½	3
"	250/t	bid	½	½	¾	¾	¾	1	1	1¼	1½
cefadroxil	125/t	bid	½	¾	1	1	1¼	1¼	1½	1¾	2¼
"	250/t	bid	¼	½	½	½	¾	¾	¾	1	1
cefdinir	125/t	qd	--	¾†	1	1	1	1¼	1½	1¾	2
cefixime	100/t	qd	½	½	¾	¾	¾	1	1	1¼	1½
cefprozil*	125/t	bid	--	¾†	1	1	1¼	1½	1½	2	2¼
"	250/t	bid	--	½†	½	½	¾	¾	¾	1	1¼
cefuroxime	125/t	bid	--	¾	¾	1	1	1	1½	1¾	2¼
cephalexin	125/t	qid	--	½	¾	¾	1	1	1¼	1½	1¾
"	250/t	qid	--	¼	¼	½	½	½	¾	¾	1
clarithromycin	125/t	bid	½†	½†	½	½	¾	¾	¾	1	1¼
"	250/t	bid	--	--	--	¼	½	½	½	½	¾
dicloxacillin	62½/t	qid	½	¾	1	1	1¼	1¼	1½	1¾	2
loracarbef*	100/t	bid	--	1†	1¼	1½	1½	1¾	2	2¼	3
nitrofurantoin	25/t	qid	¼	½	½	½	½	¾	¾	¾	1
Pediazole	---	tid	½	½	¾	¾	1	1	1	1¼	1½
penicillin V**	250/t	bid-tid	--	1	1	1	1	1	1	1	1
cetirizine	5/t	qd	-	-	½	½	½	½	½	½	½
Benadryl	12.5/t	q6h	½	½	¾	¾	1	1	1¼	1½	2
prednisolone	15/t	qd	¼	½	½	¾	¾	¾	1	1	1¼
prednisone	5/t	qd	1	1¼	1½	1¾	2	2¼	2½	3	3¾
Robitussin	---	q4h	-	-	¼†	¼†	½	½	¾	¾	1
Tylenol w/ codeine		q4h	-	-	-	-	-	-	-	1	1

* Dose shown is for otitis media only; see dosing in text for alternative indications.
† Dosing at this age/weight not recommended by manufacturer.
‡ AAP now recommends high dose (80-90 mg/kg/d) for all otitis media in children; with Augmentin used as ES only.
§Give a double dose of azithromycin the first day.
**AHA dosing for streptococcal pharyngitis. Treat for 10 days.

PEDIATRIC VITAL SIGNS AND INTRAVENOUS DRUGS

Age		Pre-matr	New-born	2m	4m	6m	9m	12m	15m	2y	3y	5y
Weight	(Kg)	2	3½	5	6½	8	9	10	11	13	15	19
	(Lbs)	4½	7½	11	15	17	20	22	24	28	33	42
Maint fluids	(ml/kg)	8	14	20	26	32	36	40	42	46	50	58
ET tube	(mm)	2½	3/3½	3½	3½	3½	4	4	4½	4½	4½	5
Defib	(Joules)	4	7	10	13	16	18	20	22	26	30	38
Systolic BP	(high)	80	80	85	90	95	100	103	104	106	109	114
	(low)	40	60	70	70	70	70	70	70	70	75	80
Pulse rate	(high)	145	145	180	180	180	160	160	160	150	150	135
	(low)	100	100	110	110	110	100	100	100	90	90	65
Resp rate	(high)	60	60	50	50	50	46	46	30	30	25	25
	(low)	35	30	30	24	24	20	20	20	20	20	20
adenosine	(mg)	0.2	0.3	0.5	0.6	0.8	0.9	1	1.1	1.3	1.5	1.9
atropine	(mg)	0.1	0.1	0.1	0.13	0.16	0.18	0.2	0.22	0.26	0.30	0.38
Benadryl	(mg)	-	-	5	6½	8	9	10	11	13	15	19
bicarbonate	(meq)	2	3½	5	6½	8	9	10	11	13	15	19
dextrose	(g)	1	2	5	6½	8	9	10	11	13	15	19
epinephrine	(mg)	.02	.04	.05	.07	.08	.09	0.1	0.11	0.13	0.15	0.19
lidocaine	(mg)	2	3½	5	6½	8	9	10	11	13	15	19
morphine	(mg)	0.2	0.3	0.5	0.6	0.8	0.9	1	1.1	1.3	1.5	1.9
mannitol	(g)	2	3½	5	6½	8	9	10	11	13	15	19
naloxone	(mg)	.02	.04	.05	.07	.08	.09	0.1	0.11	0.13	0.15	0.19
diazepam	(mg)	0.6	1	1.5	2	2.5	2.7	3	3.3	3.9	4.5	5
fosphenytoin*	(PE)	40	70	100	130	160	180	200	220	260	300	380
lorazepam	(mg)	0.2	0.35	0.5	0.65	0.8	0.9	1	1.1	1.3	1.5	1.9
phenobarb	(mg)	30	60	75	100	125	125	150	175	200	225	275
phenytoin*	(mg)	40	70	100	130	160	180	200	220	260	300	380
ampicillin	(mg)	100	175	250	325	400	450	500	550	650	750	1000
ceftriaxone	(mg)	-	-	250	325	400	450	500	550	650	750	1000
cefotaxime	(mg)	100	175	250	325	400	450	500	550	650	750	1000
gentamicin	(mg)	5	8	12	16	20	22	25	27	32	37	47

*Loading doses; fosphenytoin dosed in "phenytoin equivalents".

If you obtained your *Pocket Pharmacopoeia* from a bookstore, <u>please</u> send your address to info@tarascon.com. This allows you to be the first to hear of updates! (We don't sell or distribute our mailing lists, by the way.) The cover woodcut is *The Apothecary* by Jost Amman, Frankfurt, 1574. Several of you knew that it was HAL (the malicious computer in the epic movie *2001: A Space Odyssey*) who didn't quite finish his song about a super-sized bicycle. As he was being disconnected he intellectually regressed, ultimately singing part of "Daisy, Daisy, give me your answer, do." We will send a free copy of next year's edition to the first 25 who know what yelps in the presence of intruders and is gravid at birth.

CONVERSIONS		
Temperature:	*Liquid:*	*Weight:*
F = (1.8) C + 32	1 fluid ounce = 30ml	1 kilogram = 2.2 lbs
C = (F - 32)/(1.8)	1 teaspoon = 5ml	1 ounce = 30 g
	1 tablespoon = 15ml	1 grain = 65 mg

Alveolar-arterial oxygen gradient = A-a = 148 - 1.2(PaCO2) - PaO2
[normal = 10-20 mmHg, breathing room air at sea level]

Calculated osmolality = 2Na + glucose/18 + BUN/2.8 + ethanol/4.6
[norm 280-295 meq/L. Na in meq/L; all others in mg/dL]

Pediatric IV maintenance fluids (see table on page 7)
4 ml/kg/hr **or** 100 ml/kg/day for first 10 kg, plus
2 ml/kg/hr **or** 50 ml/kg/day for second 10 kg, plus
1 ml/kg/hr **or** 20 ml/kg/day for all further kg

$$mcg/kg/min = \frac{16.7 \times drug\ conc\ [mg/ml] \times infusion\ rate\ [ml/h]}{weight\ [kg]}$$

$$Infusion\ rate\ [ml/h] = \frac{desired\ mcg/kg/min \times weight\ [kg] \times 60}{drug\ concentration\ [mcg/ml]}$$

Fractional excretion of sodium =
[Pre-renal, etc <1%; ATN, etc >1%] $\left[\dfrac{urine\ Na\ /\ plasma\ Na}{urine\ creat\ /\ plasma\ creat} \right] \times 100\%$

Anion gap = Na – (Cl + HCO3)   [normal = 10-14 meq/L]

$$Creatinine\ clearance = \frac{(lean\ kg)(140 - age)(0.85\ if\ female)}{(72)(stable\ creatinine\ [mg/dL])}$$
[normal >80]

Glomerular filtration rate using MDRD equation (ml/min/1.73 m^2)
= 186 x (creatinine)$^{-1.154}$ x (age)$^{-0.203}$ x (0.742 if ♀) x (1.210 if African American)

Body surface area (BSA) = square root of: $\left[\dfrac{height\ (cm) \times weight\ (kg)}{3600} \right]$
[in m^2]

DRUG THERAPY REFERENCE WEBSITES (selected)

Professional societies or governmental agencies with drug therapy guidelines		
AHRQ	Agency for Healthcare Research and Quality	www.ahcpr.gov
AAP	American Academy of Pediatrics	www.aap.org
ACC	American College of Cardiology	www.acc.org
ACCP	American College of Chest Physicians	www.chestnet.org
ACCP	American College of Clinical Pharmacy	www.accp.com
AHA	American Heart Association	www.americanheart.org
ADA	American Diabetes Association	www.diabetes.org
AMA	American Medical Association	www.ama-assn.org
ATS	American Thoracic Society	www.thoracic.org
ASHP	Amer. Society Health-Systems Pharmacists	www.ashp.org
CDC	Centers for Disease Control & Prevention	www.cdc.gov
CDC	CDC bioterrorism and radiation exposures	www.bt.cdc.gov
IDSA	Infectious Diseases Society of America	www.idsociety.org
MHA	Malignant Hyperthermia Association	www.mhaus.org
NHLBI	National Heart, Lung, & Blood Institute	www.nhlbi.nih.gov
Other therapy reference sites		
Cochrane library		www.cochrane.org
Emergency Contraception Website		www.not-2-late.com
Immunization Action Coalition		www.immunize.org
Int'l Registry for Drug-Induced Arrhythmias		www.qtdrugs.org
Managing Contraception		www.managingcontraception.com
Nephrology Pharmacy Associates		www.nephrologypharmacy.com

SELECTED DRUGS THAT MAY PROLONG THE QT INTERVAL

alfuzosin	dofetilide*	indapamide*	pentamidine*†	sotalol*†
amiodarone*†	dolasetron	isradipine	phenothiazines‡¶	tacrolimus
arsenic trioxide*	droperidol*	levofloxacin*	pimozide*	tamoxifen
azithromycin*	erythromycin*†	lithium	polyethylene glycol	telithromycin
bepridil*†	flecainide	mefloquine	(PEG-salt solution)§	tizanidine
chloroquine*	foscarnet	methadone*†	procainamide*	vardenafil
cisapride*†	fosphenytoin	moexipril/HCTZ	quetiapine‡	venlafaxine
clarithromycin*	gatifloxacin*	moxifloxacin	quinidine*†	*Visicol*§
clozapine	gemifloxacin	nicardipine	quinine	voriconazole
cocaine*	haloperidol*†	octreotide	risperidone‡	ziprasidone‡
disopyramide*†	ibutilide*†	ondansetron	salmeterol	

This table may not include all drugs that prolong the QT interval or cause torsades. Risk of drug-induced QT prolongation may be increased in women, older age, ↓K, ↓Mg, bradycardia, starvation, & CNS injuries. Hepatorenal dysfunction & drug interactions can ↑ the concentration of QT interval-prolonging drugs. Coadministration of QT interval-prolonging drugs can have additive effects. Avoid these (and other) drugs in congenital prolonged QT syndrome (www.qtdrugs.org). *Torsades reported in product labeling/case reports. †↑Risk in women. ‡QT prolongation: thioridazine>ziprasidone>risperidone, quetiapine, haloperidol. §May be due to electrolyte imbalance. ¶QT prolongation documented for chlorpromazine*, mesoridazine*, thioridazine*.

Antirheumatic Agents - Immunomodulators

anakinra (Kineret): RA: 100 mg SC daily. [Trade: 100 mg pre-filled glass syringes with needles, 7 or 28 per box.] ▶K ♀B ▷? $$$$$

etanercept (Enbrel): RA, psoriatic arthritis, ankylosing spondylitis: 50 mg SC q week. Plaque psoriasis: 50 mg SC twice weekly x 3 months, then 50 mg SC q week. JRA 4-17 yo: 0.8 mg/kg SC q week, to max single dose of 50 mg. Max dose per injection site is 25 mg. [Supplied in a carton containing four dose trays. Each dose tray contains one 25 mg single-use vial of etanercept, one syringe (1 mL sterile bacteriostatic water for injection, containing 0.9% benzyl alcohol), one plunger, and two alcohol swabs.] ▶Serum ♀B ▷- $$$$$

infliximab (Remicade): RA: 3 mg/kg IV in combo with methotrexate at 0, 2, and 6 wks. Ankylosing spondylitis: 5 mg/kg IV at 0, 2, and 6 wks. Psoriatic arthritis: 5 mg/kg IV at 0, 2, and 6 wks with or without methotrexate. ▶Serum ♀B ▷? $$$$$

leflunomide (Arava): RA: 100 mg PO qd x 3 days. Maintenance: 10-20 mg PO qd. [Trade: Tabs 10, 20, & 100 mg.] ▶LK ♀X ▷- $$$$$

Antirheumatic Agents - Other

azathioprine (Azasan, Imuran, ✚Immunoprin, Oprisine): RA: Initial dose 1 mg/kg (50-100 mg) PO daily or divided bid. Increase after 6-8 weeks. [Generic/Trade: Tabs 50 mg, scored. Trade (Azasan): 25, 75 & 100 mg, scored.] ▶LK ♀D ▷- $$$

hydroxychloroquine (Plaquenil): RA: start 400-600 mg PO daily, then taper to 200-400 mg daily. SLE: 400 PO daily-bid to start, then taper to 200-400 mg daily. [Generic/Trade: Tabs 200 mg, scored.] ▶K ♀C ▷+ $$

methotrexate (Rheumatrex, Trexall): RA, psoriasis: Start with 7.5 mg/week PO single dose or 2.5 mg PO q12h x 3 doses given as a course once weekly. Max dose 20 mg/week. Supplement with 1 mg/day of folic acid. [Trade: Tabs 5, 7.5, 10 & 15 mg. Generic/Trade: Tabs 2.5 mg, scored.] ▶LK ♀X ▷- $$

sulfasalazine (Azulfidine, Azulfidine EN-tabs, ✚Salazopyrin, Salazopyrin EN-Tabs, S.A.S.): RA: 500 mg PO daily-bid after meals up to 1g PO bid. May turn body fluids, contact lenses or skin orange-yellow. [Generic/Trade: Tabs 500 mg, scored. Enteric coated, Delayed-release (EN-Tabs) 500 mg.] ▶L ♀B ▷- $

Muscle Relaxants

baclofen (Lioresal): Spasticity related to MS or spinal cord disease/injury: Start 5 mg PO tid, then increase by 5 mg/dose q 3 days until 20 mg PO tid. Max dose 20 mg qid. [Generic/Trade: Tabs 10 & 20 mg, trade scored.] ▶K ♀C ▷+ $$

carisoprodol (Soma): Musculoskeletal pain: 350 mg PO tid-qid. Abuse potential. [Generic/Trade: Tabs 350 mg.] ▶LK ♀? ▷- $

chlorzoxazone (Parafon Forte DSC): Musculoskeletal pain: 500-750 mg PO tid-qid to start. Decrease to 250 mg tid-qid. [Generic/Trade: Tabs & caplets 250 & 500 mg (Parafon Forte DSC 500 mg tablets scored).] ▶LK ♀C ▷? $$

cyclobenzaprine (Flexeril): Musculoskeletal pain: Start 5-10 mg PO tid, max 60 mg/day. Not recommended in elderly. [Generic/Trade: Tab 10 mg. Trade: Tab 5 mg.] ▶LK ♀B ▷? $

dantrolene (Dantrium): Chronic spasticity related to spinal cord injury, stroke, cerebral palsy, MS: 25 mg PO daily to start, up to max of 100 mg bid-qid if necessary. Malignant hyperthermia: 2.5 mg/kg rapid IV push q 5-10 minutes continuing until symptoms subside or to a maximum 10 mg/kg. [Generic/Trade: Caps 25, 50, 100 mg.] ▶LK ♀C ▷- $$$$

diazepam (Valium, Diastat, ✚Vivol, E Pam): Skeletal muscle spasm, spasticity related to cerebral palsy, paraplegia, athetosis, stiff man syndrome: 2-10 mg PO/

PR tid-qid. [Generic/Trade: Tabs 2, 5 & 10 mg, trade scored. Generic: Oral drops 2 mg/ml, oral soln 1mg/ml, 5 mg/5 ml & concentrated soln 5 mg/ml, 10 mg/ml. Trade only: Rectal gel: 2.5 mg & 5 mg, 10 mg, 15 mg & 20 mg, in twin packs.] ▶LK ♀D ▶– ⊚IV $

metaxalone (***Skelaxin***): Musculoskeletal pain: 800 mg PO tid-qid. [Trade: Tabs 400 & 800 mg, scored.] ▶LK ♀? ▶? $$$

methocarbamol (***Robaxin, Robaxin-750***): Acute musculoskeletal pain: 1500 mg PO qid or 1000 mg IM/IV tid x 48-72h. Maintenance: 1000 mg PO qid, 750 mg PO q4h, or 1500 mg PO tid. Tetanus: specialized dosing. [Generic/Trade: Tabs 500 & 750 mg. OTC in Canada.] ▶LK ♀C ▶? $

orphenadrine (***Norflex***): Musculoskeletal pain: 100 mg PO bid. 60 mg IV/IM bid. [Generic: 100 mg extended release. OTC in Canada.] ▶LK ♀C ▶? $$

quinine sulfate: Commonly prescribed for nocturnal leg cramps, but not FDA approved for this indication: 260-325 mg PO qhs. Cinchonism with overdose. Hemolysis with G6PD deficiency, hypersensitivity. [Rx: Generic: Caps 130, 200, 260, 300, 324, 325, 650 mg. Tabs 250, 260, 325 mg.] ▶L ♀X ▶+ $

tizanidine (***Zanaflex***): Muscle spasticity due to MS or spinal cord injury: 4-8 mg PO q6-8h prn, max 36 mg/d. [Generic/Trade: Tabs 2 & 4 mg, scored. Trade 6 mg.] ▶LK ♀C ▶? $$$$

Non-Opioid Analgesic Combinations

Ascriptin (aspirin + aluminum hydroxide + magnesium hydroxide + calcium carbonate): Multiple strengths. 1-2 tabs PO q4h. [OTC: Trade: Tabs 325 mg ASA/50 mg magnesium hydroxide/50 mg aluminum hydroxide/calcium carbonate (Ascriptin). 325 mg ASA/75 mg magnesium hydroxide/75 mg aluminum hydroxide/calcium carbonate (Ascriptin A/D). 500 mg ASA/80 mg magnesium hydroxide/80 mg aluminum hydroxide/calcium carb (Ascriptin Extra Strength).] ▶K ♀D ▶? $

Bufferin (aspirin + calcium carbonate + magnesium oxide + magnesium carbonate): 1-2 tabs/caplets PO q4h. [OTC: Trade: Tabs/caplets 325 mg ASA/158 mg Ca carbonate/63 mg of Mg oxide/34 mg of Mg carbonate. Bufferin ES: 500 mg ASA/222.3 mg Ca carb/88.9 mg of Mg oxide/55.6 mg of Mg carb] ▶K ♀D ▶? $

Esgic (acetaminophen + butalbital + caffeine): 1-2 tabs or caps PO q4h. Max 6 in 24 hours. [Generic/Trade: Tabs/caps Esgic = 325/50/40 mg of acetaminophen/butalbital/caffeine. Esgic Plus = 500/50/40 mg.] ▶LK ♀C ▶? $$

Excedrin Migraine (acetaminophen + aspirin + caffeine): 2 tabs/caps/geltabs PO q6h while symptoms persist. Max 8 in 24 hours. [OTC/Generic/Trade: Tabs/caplets/geltabs acetaminophen 250 mg/ASA 250 mg/caffeine 65 mg.] ▶LK ♀C ▶? $

Fioricet (acetaminophen + butalbital + caffeine): 1-2 tabs PO q4h. Max 6 in 24 hours. [Generic/Trade: Tab 325 mg acetaminophen//50 mg butalbital/40 mg caffeine.] ▶LK ♀C ▶? $$

Fiorinal (aspirin + butalbital + caffeine, ✚***Tecnal, Trianal***): 1-2 tabs PO q4h. Max 6 tabs in 24 hours. [Generic/Trade: Cap 325 mg aspirin/50 mg butalbital/40 mg caffeine.] ▶KL ♀D ▶– ⊚III $$

Goody's Extra Strength Headache Powder (acetaminophen + aspirin + caffeine): One powder PO followed with liquid, or stir powder into a glass of water or other liquid. Repeat in 4-6 hours prn. Max 4 powders in 24 hours. [Trade: 260 mg acetaminophen/520 mg ASA/32.5 mg caffeine per powder paper.] ▶LK ♀D ▶? $

Norgesic (orphenadrine + aspirin + caffeine): Multiple strengths; write specific product on Rx. Norgesic: 1-2 tabs PO tid-qid. Norgesic Forte, 1 tab PO tid-qid. [Trade: Tabs Norgesic 25 mg orphenadrine/385 mg aspirin/30 mg caffeine. Norgesic Forte 50 mg orphenadrine/770 mg aspirin/60 mg caffeine.] ▶KL ♀D ▶? $$$

Phrenilin (acetaminophen + butalbital): Tension or muscle contraction headache: 1-2 tabs PO q4h. Max 6 in 24 hours. [Trade: Tabs Phrenilin 325/50 mg acetaminophen/butalbital. Phrenilin Forte 650/50 mg.] ▶LK ♀C ▶? $

Sedapap (acetaminophen + butalbital): 1-2 tabs PO q4h. Max 6 tabs in 24 hours. [Generic/Trade: Tab 650 mg acetaminophen//50 mg butalbital.] ▶LK ♀C ▶? $

Soma Compound (carisoprodol + aspirin): 1-2 tabs PO qid. Abuse potential. [Generic/Trade: Tab 200 mg carisoprodol/325 mg ASA.] ▶LK ♀D ▶- $

Ultracet (tramadol + acetaminophen): Acute pain: 2 tabs PO q4-6h prn, max 8 tabs/day for ≤5 days. Adjust dose in elderly & renal dysfunction. Avoid in opioid-dependent patients. Seizures may occur if concurrent antidepressants or seizure disorder. [Generic/trade: Tab 37.5 mg tramadol/325 mg acet.] ▶KL ♀C ▶- $$

Nonsteroidal Anti-Inflammatories - COX-2 Inhibitors

celecoxib (*Celebrex*): OA, ankylosing spondylitis: 200 mg PO daily or 100 mg PO bid. RA: 100-200 mg PO bid. Familial adenomatous polyposis: 400 mg PO bid with food. Acute pain, dysmenorrhea: 400 mg x 1, then 200 bid prn. An additional 200 mg dose may be given on day 1 if needed. Contraindicated in sulfonamide allergy. [Trade: Caps 100, 200, & 400 mg.] ▶L ♀C (D in 3rd trimester) ▶? $$$

Nonsteroidal Anti-Inflammatories - Salicylic Acid Derivatives

aspirin (*Ecotrin, Bayer, Anacin, ASA, ♣Asaphen, Entrophen, Novasen*): 325-650 mg PO/PR q4-6h. [OTC: Tabs 65, 81, 162.5, 300, 320, 324, 325, 486, 500, 640, 650, controlled-release tabs 650 (scored). Rx only: 800 mg controlled-release tabs & 975 mg enteric coated. OTC: suppositories 120, 125, 300, & 600 mg.] ▶K ♀D ▶? $

choline magnesium trisalicylate (*Trilisate*): 1500 mg PO bid. [Generic/Trade: Tabs 500, 750, & 1000 mg, scored.] ▶K ♀C (D in 3rd trimester) ▶? $$

diflunisal (*Dolobid*): Pain: 500-1000 mg initially, then 250-500 mg PO q8-12h. RA/OA: 500 mg-1g PO divided bid. [Generic/Trade: Tabs 250 & 500 mg.] ▶K ♀C (D in 3rd trimester) ▶- $$

salsalate (*Salflex, Disalcid, Amigesic*): 3000 mg/day PO divided q8-12h. [Generic/Trade: Tabs 500 & 750 mg, scored.] ▶K ♀C (D in 3rd trimester) ▶? $

Nonsteroidal Anti-Inflammatories - Other

Arthrotec (diclofenac + misoprostol): OA: one 50/200 tab PO tid. RA: one 50/200 tab PO tid-qid. If intolerant, may use 50/200 or 75/200 PO bid. Misoprostol is an abortifacient. [Trade: Tab 50/200 mcg & 75 mg/200 mcg diclofenac/misoprostol.] ▶LK ♀X ▶- $$$$

diclofenac (*Voltaren, Voltaren XR, Cataflam, ♣Voltaren Rapide*): Multiple strengths; write specific product on Rx. Immediate or delayed release 50 mg PO bid-tid or 75 mg PO tid. Extended release (Voltaren XR): 100-200 mg PO daily. [Generic/Trade: Tabs, immediate-release (Cataflam) 25, 50 mg. Tabs, delayed-release (Voltaren) 25, 50, & 75 mg. Tabs, extended-release (Voltaren XR) 100 mg.] ▶L ♀B (D in 3rd trimester) ▶- $$$

etodolac (*Lodine, Lodine XL, ♣Ultradol*): Multiple strengths; write specific product on Rx. Immediate release 200-400 mg PO bid-tid. Extended release (Lodine XL): 400-1200 mg PO daily. [Generic/Trade: Tabs, immediate-release (Lodine) 400,500 mg. Caps, immediate-release (Lodine) 200,300 mg. Generic/Trade: tabs, extended-release (Lodine XL) 400,500,600 mg.] ▶L ♀C (D in 3rd trimester) ▶- $$

flurbiprofen (*Ansaid, ♣Froben, Froben SR*): 200-300 mg/day PO divided bid-qid. [Generic/Trade: Tabs immed. release 50,100 mg.] ▶L ♀B (D in 3rd trimester) ▶+ $

NSAIDs – If one class fails, consider another. *Salicylic acid derivatives:* aspirin, diflunisal, salsalate, Trilisate. *Propionic acids:* flurbiprofen, ibuprofen, ketoprofen, naproxen, oxaprozin. *Acetic acids:* diclofenac, etodolac, indomethacin, ketorolac, nabumetone, sulindac, tolmetin. *Fenamates:* meclofenamate. *Oxicams:* meloxicam, piroxicam. *COX-2 inhibitors:* celecoxib.

ibuprofen (*Motrin, Advil, Nuprin, Rufen*): 200-800 mg PO tid-qid. Peds >6 mo: 5-10 mg/kg PO q6-8h. [OTC: Cap 200 mg. Tabs 100, 200 mg. Chewable tabs 50 mg. Liquid & suspension 50 mg/1.25ml, 100 mg/5 ml, suspension 100 mg/2.5 ml. Infant drops, 50 mg/1.25 ml (calibrated dropper). Rx only: Tabs 400, 600 & 800 mg.] ▶L ♀B (D in 3rd trimester) ▶+ $

indomethacin (*Indocin, Indocin SR, ✦Rhodacine*): Multiple strengths; write specific product on Rx. Immediate release preparations 25-50 mg cap or supp PO/PR tid. Sustained release: 75 mg cap PO daily-bid. [Generic/Trade: Caps, immediate-release 25 & 50 mg. Oral suspension 25 mg/5 ml. Suppositories 50 mg. Cap, sustained-release 75 mg.] ▶L ♀B (D in 3rd trimester) ▶+ $

ketoprofen (*Orudis, Orudis KT, Actron, Oruvail, ✦Rhodis, Rhodis EC, Rhodis SR, Rhovail, Orudis SR*): Immediate release: 25-75 mg PO tid-qid. Extended release: 100-200 mg cap PO daily. [OTC: Tab, immediate-release 12.5 mg. Rx: Generic/Trade: Caps, immediate-release 25, 50 & 75 mg. Caps, extended-release 100, 150 & 200 mg.] ▶L ♀B (D in 3rd trimester) ▶? $

ketorolac (*Toradol*): Moderately severe acute pain: 15-30 mg IV/IM q6h or 10 mg PO q4-6h prn. Combined duration IV/IM and PO is not to exceed 5 days. [Generic/Trade: Tab 10 mg.] ▶L ♀C (D in 3rd trimester) ▶+ $

mefenamic acid (*Ponstel, ✦Ponstan*): Mild to moderate pain, primary dysmenorrhea: 500 mg PO initially, then 250 mg PO q6h prn for ≤1 week. [Trade: Cap 250 mg.] ▶L ♀D ▶- $

meloxicam (*Mobic, ✦Mobicox*): RA/OA: 7.5 mg PO daily. JRA, ≥2 yo: 0.125 mg/kg PO daily. [Trade: Tabs 7.5, 15 mg. Suspension 7.5 mg/5 ml (1.5 mg/ml).] ▶L ♀C (D in 3rd trimester) ▶? $$$

nabumetone (*Relafen*): RA/OA: Initial: two 500 mg tabs (1000 mg) PO daily. May increase to 1500-2000 mg PO daily or divided bid. [Generic/Trade: Tabs 500 & 750 mg.] ▶L ♀C (D in 3rd trimester) ▶- $$$

naproxen (*Naprosyn, Aleve, Anaprox, EC-Naprosyn, Naprelan*): Immediate release: 250-500 mg PO bid. Delayed release: 375-500 mg PO bid (do not crush or chew). Controlled release: 750-1000 mg PO daily. JRA ≤13 kg: 2.5 mg PO bid. 14-25 kg: 5 ml PO bid. 26-38 kg: 7.5 ml PO bid. 500 mg naproxen = 550 mg naproxen sodium. [OTC: Generic/Trade: Tab immediate-release 200 mg. OTC Trade: Capsules & Gelcaps immediate-release 200 mg. Rx: Generic/Trade: Tabs immediate-release 250, 375 & 500 mg. Delayed-release 375 & 500 mg. Rx: Trade: Tabs delayed-release enteric coated (EC-Naprosyn), 375 & 500 mg. Tabs, controlled-release (Naprelan), 375 & 500 mg. Generic/Trade: Suspension 125 mg/5 ml.] ▶L ♀B (D in 3rd trimester) ▶+ $$$

oxaprozin (*Daypro, Daypro Alta*): 1200 mg PO daily. [Generic/Trade (Daypro): Caplets, tabs 600 mg, trade scored. Trade (Daypro Alta): Tabs 600 mg.] ▶L ♀C (D in 3rd trimester) ▶- $$

piroxicam (*Feldene, Fexicam*): 20 mg PO daily. [Generic/Trade: Caps 10 & 20 mg.] ▶L ♀B (D in 3rd trimester) ▶+ $

sulindac (*Clinoril*): 150-200 mg PO bid. [Generic/Trade: Tabs 150 & 200 mg.] ▶L ♀B (D in 3rd trimester) ▶- $

tiaprofenic acid (✸**Surgam, Surgam SR**): Canada only. 600 mg PO daily of sustained release, or 300 mg PO bid of regular release. [Trade: Cap, sustained-release 300 mg. Generic/Trade: Tab 300 mg] ▶K ♀C (D in 3rd trimester) ▶- $$

tolmetin (**Tolectin**): 200-600 mg PO tid. [Generic/Trade: Tabs 200 (trade scored) & 600 mg. Cap 400 mg.] ▶L ♀C (D in 3rd trimester) ▶+ $$$

Opioid Agonist-Antagonists

buprenorphine (**Buprenex**): 0.3-0.6 mg IV/IM q6h prn. ▶L ♀C ▶- ©III $

butorphanol (**Stadol, Stadol NS**): 0.5-2 mg IV or 1-4 mg IM q3-4h prn. Nasal spray (Stadol NS): 1 spray (1 mg) in 1 nostril q3-4h. Abuse potential. [Generic/Trade: Nasal spray 1 mg/spray, 2.5 ml bottle (14-15 doses/bottle).] ▶LK ♀C ▶+ ©IV $$$

nalbuphine (**Nubain**): 10-20 mg IV/IM/SC q3-6h prn. ▶LK ♀? ▶? $

pentazocine (**Talwin, Talwin NX**): 30 mg IV/IM q3-4h prn (Talwin). 1 tab PO q3-4h. (Talwin NX = 50 mg pentazocine/0.5 mg naloxone). [Generic/Trade: Tab 50 mg with 0.5 mg naloxone, trade scored.] ▶LK ♀C ▶? ©IV $$$

FENTANYL TRANSDERMAL DOSE (based on ongoing morphine requirement)*

morphine (IV/IM)	morphine (PO)	Transdermal fentanyl
8-22 mg/day	45-134 mg/day	25 mcg/hr
23-37 mg/day	135-224 mg/day	50 mcg/hr
38-52 mg/day	225-314 mg/day	75 mcg/hr
53-67 mg/day	315-404 mg/day	100 mcg/hr

For higher morphine doses see product insert for transdermal fentanyl equivalencies.

Opioid Agonists

NOTE: May cause drowsiness and/or sedation, which may be enhanced by alcohol & other CNS depressants. Patients with chronic pain may require more frequent & higher dosing. All opioids are pregnancy class D if used for prolonged periods or in high doses at term.

codeine: 0.5-1 mg/kg up to 15-60 mg PO/IM/IV/SC q4-6h. Do not use IV in children. [Generic: Tabs 15, 30, & 60 mg. Oral soln: 15 mg/5 ml.] ▶LK ♀C ▶+ ©II $

fentanyl (**Duragesic, Actiq, Sublimaze**): Transdermal (Duragesic): 1 patch q72 hrs (some chronic pain pts may req q48 h dosing). May wear more than one patch to achieve the correct analgesic effect. Transmucosal lozenge (Actiq) for break-through cancer pain: 200-1600 mcg, goal is 4 lozenges on a stick/day in conjunction with long-acting opioid. Adult analgesia/procedural sedation: 50-100 mcg slow IV over 1-2 minutes; carefully titrate to effect. Analgesia: 50-100 mcg IM q1-2h prn. [Generic/Trade: Transdermal patches (Duragesic) 12, 25, 50, 75, 100 mcg/h. Transmucosal forms: Actiq lozenges on a stick, raspberry flavored 200, 400, 600, 800, 1,200, 1,600 mcg.] ▶L ♀C ▶? ©II $$$$

hydromorphone (**Dilaudid, Dilaudid-5**, ✸**Hydromorph Contin**): Adults: 2-4 mg PO q4-6h. Titrate dose as high as necessary to relieve cancer pain or other types of non-malignant pain where chronic opioids are necessary. 0.5-2 mg IM/SC or slow IV q4-6h. 3 mg PR q6-8h. Peds ≤12 yo: 0.03-0.08 mg/kg PO q4-6h prn. 0.015 mg/kg/dose IV q4-6h prn. [Generic/Trade: Tabs 2, 4, & 8 mg (8 mg trade scored). Liquid 5 mg/5 ml. Suppositories 3 mg. Trade only: Tabs 1 & 3 mg.] ▶L ♀C ▶? ©II $$$

levorphanol: 2 mg PO q6-8h prn. [Generic: Tabs 2 mg, scored.] ▶L ♀C ▶? ©II $$$

meperidine (**Demerol, pethidine**): 1-1.8 mg/kg up to 150 mg IM/SC/PO or slow IV q3-4h. 75 mg meperidine IV,IM,SC = 300 mg meperidine PO. [Generic/Trade: Tabs 50 (trade scored) & 100 mg. Syrup 50 mg/5 ml (trade banana flavored).] ▶LK ♀C but + ▶+ ©II $$$

OPIOIDS*

	Approximate equianalgesic		Recommended starting dose			
			Adults >50kg		Children/Adults 8 to 50 kg	
	IV / SC / IM	PO	IV / SC / IM	PO	IV / SC / IM	PO
Opioid Agonists						
morphine	10 mg q3-4h	†30 mg q3-4h / †60 mg q3-4h	10 mg q3-4h	30 mg q3-4h	0.1 mg/kg q3-4h	0.3 mg/kg q3-4h
codeine	75 mg q3-4h	130 mg q3-4h	60 mg q2h	60 mg q3-4h	n/r	1 mg/kg q3-4h
fentanyl	0.1 mg q1h	n/a	0.1 mg q1h	n/a	n/r	n/a
hydromorphone	1.5 mg q3-4h	7.5 mg q3-4h	1.5 mg q3-4h	6 mg q3-4h	0.015 mg/kg q3-4h	0.06 mg/kg q3-4h
hydrocodone	n/a	30 mg q3-4h	n/a	10 mg q3-4h	n/a	0.2 mg/kg q3-4h
levorphanol	2 mg q6-8h	4 mg q6-8h	2 mg q6-8h	4 mg q6-8h	0.02 mg/kg q6-8h	0.04 mg/kg q6-8h
meperidine§	100 mg q3h	300 mg q2-3h	100 mg q3h	n/r	0.75 mg/kg q2-3h	n/r
oxycodone	n/a	30 mg q3-4h	n/a	10 mg q3-4h	n/a	0.2 mg/kg q3-4h
oxymorphone	1 mg q3-4h	n/a	1 mg q3-4h	n/a	n/r	n/r
Opioid Agonist-Antagonist and Partial Agonist						
buprenorphine	0.3-0.4 mg q6-8h	n/a	0.4 mg q6-8h	n/a	0.004 mg/kg q6-8h	n/a
butorphanol	2 mg q3-4h	n/a	2 mg q3-4h	n/a	n/r	n/a
nalbuphine	10 mg q3-4h	n/a	10 mg q3-4h	n/a	0.1 mg/kg q3-4h	n/a
pentazocine	60 mg q3-4h	150 mg q3-4h	n/r	50 mg q4-6h	n/r	n/r

*Approximate dosing, adapted from 1992 AHCPR guidelines, www.ahcpr.gov. IV doses should be titrated slowly with appropriate monitoring. All PO dosing is with immediate-release preparations. Use lower doses initially in those not currently taking opioids. Individualize all dosing, especially in the elderly, children, and patients with chronic pain, opioid tolerance, or hepatic/renal insufficiency. Many recommend initially using lower than equivalent doses when switching between different opioids. Not available = "n/a". Not recommended = "n/r". Methadone is excluded due to poor consensus on equivalence.
†30 mg with around the clock dosing, and 60 mg with a single dose or short-term dosing (ie, the opioid-naive).
§Doses should be limited to <600 mg/24 hrs and total duration of use <48 hrs; not for chronic pain.

methadone (***Dolophine, Methadose, ♣Metadol***): Severe pain in opioid-tolerant patients: 2.5-10 mg IM/SC/PO q3-4h prn. Titrate dose as high as necessary to relieve cancer pain or other types of non-malignant pain where chronic opioids are necessary. Opioid dependence: 20-100 mg PO daily. Treatment >3 wks is maintenance and only permitted in approved treatment programs. [Generic/Trade: Tabs 5, 10, various scored. Dispersible tabs 40 mg. Oral concentrate: 10 mg/ml. Generic only: Oral soln 5 & 10 mg/5 ml.] ▶L ♀C ▶+ ©II $

morphine (***MS Contin, Kadian, Avinza, Roxanol, Oramorph SR, MSIR, DepoDur, ♣Statex, M-Eslon, M.O.S., Doloral***): Controlled-release tabs (MS Contin, Oramorph SR): Start at 30 mg PO q8-12h. Controlled-release caps (Kadian): 20 mg PO q12-24h. Extended-release caps (Avinza): Start at 30 mg PO daily. Do not break, chew, or crush MS Contin or Oramorph SR. Kadian & Avinza caps may be opened & sprinkled in applesauce for easier administration, however the pellets should not be crushed or chewed. 0.1-0.2 mg/kg up to 15 mg IM/SC or slow IV q4h. Titrate dose as high as necessary to relieve cancer pain or other types of non-malignant pain where chronic opioids are necessary. [Generic/Trade: Tabs, immediate-release: 15 & 30 mg. Trade: Caps 15 & 30 mg. Generic/Trade: Oral soln: 10 mg/5 ml, 10 mg/2.5 ml, 20 mg/5 ml, 20 mg/ml (concentrate) & 100 mg/5 ml (concentrate). Rectal suppositories 5, 10, 20 & 30 mg. Controlled-release tabs (MS Contin, Oramorph SR) 15, 30, 60, 100; 200 mg MS Contin only. Controlled-release caps (Kadian) 20, 30, 50, 60 & 100 mg. Extended release caps (Avinza) 30, 60, 90 & 120 mg.] ▶LK ♀C ▶+ ©II $$$$$

oxycodone (***Roxicodone, OxyContin, Percolone, OxyIR, OxyFAST, ♣Endocodone, Supeudol***): Immediate-release preparations: 5 mg PO q4-6h prn. Controlled-release (OxyContin) 10-40 mg PO q12h (no supporting data for shorter dosing intervals for controlled-release tabs.) Titrate dose as high as necessary to relieve cancer pain or other types of non-malignant pain where chronic opioids are necessary. Do not break, chew, or crush controlled release preparations. [Generic /Trade: Immediate-release: Tabs (scored) & caps 5 mg. Tabs 15,30 mg. Oral soln 5 mg/5 ml. Oral concentrate 20 mg/ml. Trade: Controlled-release tabs (OxyContin): 10, 20, 40. Generic/Trade: Controlled-release tabs: 80 mg.] ▶L ♀C ©II $$$

oxymorphone (***Numorphan***): 1-1.5 mg IM/SC q4-6h prn. 0.5 mg IV q4-6h prn, increase dose until pain adequately controlled. 5 mg PR q4-6h prn. [Trade: Suppositories 5 mg.] ▶L ♀C ▶? ©II $

propoxyphene (***Darvon-N, Darvon Pulvules***): 65-100 mg PO q4h prn. [Generic/Trade: Caps 65 mg. Trade: 100 mg (Darvon-N).] ▶L ♀C ▶+ ©IV $

Opioid Analgesic Combinations

NOTE: Refer to individual components for further information. May cause drowsiness and/or sedation, which may be enhanced by alcohol & other CNS depressants. Opioids, carisoprodol, and butalbital may be habit-forming. Avoid exceeding 4 g/day of acetaminophen in combination products. Caution people who drink ≥3 alcoholic drinks/day to limit acetaminophen use to 2.5 g/day due to additive liver toxicity. Opioids commonly cause constipation − concurrent laxatives are recommended. All opioids are pregnancy class D if used for prolonged periods or in high doses at term.

Anexsia (hydrocodone + acetaminophen): Multiple strengths; write specific product on Rx. 1 tab PO q4-6h prn. [Generic/Trade: Tabs 5/500, 7.5/325, 7.5/650, 10/660 mg hydrocodone/mg acetaminophen, scored.] ▶LK ♀C ▶- ©III $

Capital with Codeine suspension (acetaminophen + codeine): 15 ml PO q4h prn. >12yo use adult dose. 7-12 yo 10 ml/dose q4-6h prn. 3-6 yo 5 ml/dose q4-6h prn. [Generic = oral soln. Trade = suspension. Both codeine 12 mg/acetaminophen 120 mg/5 ml (trade, fruit punch flavor).] ▶LK ♀C ▶? ©V $

Combunox (oxycodone + ibuprofen): 1 tab PO q6h prn for ≤7 days. Max 4 tabs/24h. [Generic/Trade: Tab 5 mg oxycodone/400 mg ibuprofen.] ▶L ♀C (D in 3rd trimester) ▶? ©II ?

Darvocet (propoxyphene + acetaminophen): Multiple strengths; write specific product on Rx. 50/325, 2 tabs PO q4h prn. 100/500 or 100/650, 1 tab PO q4h prn. [Generic/Trade: Tabs 50/325 (Darvocet N-50), 100/650 (Darvocet N-100), & 100/500 (Darvocet A500), mg propoxyphene/mg acetaminophen.] ▶L ♀C ▶+ ©IV $

Darvon Compound Pulvules (propoxyphene + aspirin + caffeine, ✦*692 tablet*): 1 cap PO q4h prn. [Generic/Trade: Cap 65 mg propox/389 mg ASA/32.4 mg caffeine. Trade: 32 mg propox/389 mg ASA/32.4 mg caffeine.] ▶LK ♀D ▶- ©IV $$

Empirin with Codeine (aspirin + codeine, ✦*292 tablet*): Multiple strengths; write specific product on Rx. 1-2 tabs PO q4h prn. [Generic/Trade: Tab 325/30 & 325/60 mg ASA/mg codeine. Empirin brand no longer made.] ▶LK ♀D ▶- ©III $

Fioricet with Codeine (acetaminophen + butalbital + caffeine + codeine): 1-2 caps PO q4h prn. [Generic/Trade: Cap 325 mg acetaminophen/50 mg butalbital/40 mg caffeine/30 mg codeine.] ▶LK ♀C ▶- ©III $$$

Fiorinal with Codeine (aspirin + butalbital + caffeine + codeine, ✦*Fiorinal C-1/4, Fiorinal C-1/2, Tecnal C-1/4, Tecnal C-1/2*): 1-2 caps PO q4h prn. [Trade: Cap 325/50/40/30 mg of ASA/butalbital/caffeine/codeine.] ▶LK ♀D ▶- ©III $$$$

Lorcet (hydrocodone + acetaminophen): Multiple strengths; write specific product on Rx. 5/500: 1-2 tabs PO q4-6h prn. 7.5/650 & 10/650: 1 tab PO q4-6h prn. [Generic/Trade: Caps, 2.5/500, 5/500, 7.5/500, 7.5/750, 10/325, 10/500. (Lorcet HD) Tabs, 7.5/650 (Lorcet Plus). Trade: Lorcet -10/650, mg hydrocodone/mg acetaminophen, scored. Elixir: 7.5/500 (15 ml)] ▶LK ♀C ▶- ©III $$

Lortab (hydrocodone + acetaminophen): Multiple strengths; write specific product on Rx. 1-2 tabs PO q4-6h prn (2.5/500 & 5/500). 1 tab PO q4-6h prn (7.5/500 & 10/500). Elixir: 15 ml PO q4-6h prn. [Trade: Tabs Lortab 2.5/500. Generic/Trade: Lortab 5/500 (scored), Lortab 7.5/500 (trade scored) & Lortab 10/500 mg hydroco/ acet. Elixir: 7.5/500 mg hydrocodone/mg acetaminophen/15 ml.] ▶LK ♀C ▶- ©III $$

Maxidone (hydrocodone + acetaminophen): 1 tab PO q4-6h prn, max dose 5 tabs/ day. [Trade: Tab 10/750 mg hydrocodone/mg acet.] ▶LK ♀C ▶- ©III $$$

Mersyndol with Codeine (acetaminophen + codeine + doxylamine): Canada only. 1-2 tabs PO q4-6h prn. Max 12 tabs/24 hours. [Trade OTC Tab acetaminophen 325 mg + codeine phosphate 8 mg + doxylamine 5 mg.] ▶LK ♀C ▶? $

Norco (hydrocodone + acetaminophen): 1 tab PO q4-6h prn. [Trade: Tabs 5/325, 7.5/325 & 10/325 mg hydrocodone mg acetaminophen, scored.] ▶L ♀C ▶? ©III $$

Percocet (oxycodone + acetaminophen, ✦*Percocet-demi, Oxycocet, Endocet*): Multiple strengths; write specific product on Rx. 1-2 tabs PO q4-6h prn (2.5/325 & 5/325). 1 tab PO q4-6 prn (7.5/500 & 10/650). [Trade: Tabs 2.5/325, 7.5/500, 10/ 650 oxycodone/acet. Generic/Trade: tabs 5/325, 7.5/325, 10/325.] ▶L ♀C ▶- ©II $

Percodan (oxycodone + aspirin, ✦*Oxycodan, Endodan*): Percodan: 1 tab PO q6h prn. Percodan Demi: 1-2 tabs PO q6h prn. [Generic/Trade: Tab Percodan 4.88/ 325 mg oxycodone/ASA (trade scored). Trade only: Percodan Demi 2.44/325 mg scored.] ▶LK ♀D ▶- ©II $

Propacet (propoxyphene + acetaminophen): Moderate pain: 1 tab (100/650) PO q4h prn. [Generic/Trade: Tab 100/650 mg propoxy/mg acet.] ▶L ♀C ▶+ ©IV $$

Roxicet (oxycodone + acetaminophen): Multiple strengths; write specific product on Rx. 1 tab PO q6h prn. Soln: 5 ml PO q6h prn. [Generic/Trade: tab Roxicet 5/325, scored. Caplet Roxicet 5/500, scored. Generic: Cap 5/500. Trade only: Roxicet oral soln 5/325 per 5 ml, mg oxycodone/mg acetaminophen.] ▶L ♀C ▶- ©II $$

Soma Compound with Codeine (carisoprodol + aspirin + codeine): Moderate to severe musculoskeletal pain: 1-2 tabs PO qid prn. [Trade: Tab 200 mg carisoprodol/325 mg ASA/16 mg codeine.] ▶L ♀D ▶– ©III $$$

Synalgos-DC (dihydrocodeine + aspirin + caffeine): 2 caps PO q4h prn. [Trade: Cap 16/356.4/30 mg dihydrocodeine/ASA/caffeine.] ▶L ♀C ▶– ©III $

Talacen (pentazocine + acetaminophen): 1 tab PO q4h prn. [Trade: Tab 25 mg pentazocine/650 mg acetaminophen, scored.] ▶L ♀C ▶? ©IV $$$

Tylenol with Codeine (codeine + acetaminophen; ♣**Lenoltec, Emtec, Triatec**): Multiple strengths; write specific product on Rx. 1-2 tabs PO q4h prn. Elixir 3-6 yo 5 ml/dose. 7-12 yo 10 ml/dose q4-6h prn. [Generic/Trade: Tabs Tylenol #2 (15/300), Tylenol #3 (30/300), Tylenol #4 (60/300). Tylenol with Codeine Elixir 12/120 per 5 ml, mg codeine/mg acetaminophen. Canadian forms come with (Lenoltec, Tylenol) or without (Empracet, Emtec) caffeine.] ▶LK ♀C ▶? ©III (Tabs), V(elixir) $

Tylox (oxycodone + acetaminophen): 1 cap PO q6h prn. [Generic/Trade: Cap 5 mg oxycodone/500 mg acetaminophen.] ▶L ♀C ▶– ©II $

Vicodin (hydrocodone + acetaminophen): Multiple strengths; write specific product on Rx. 5/500 & 7.5/750: 1-2 tabs PO q4-6h prn. 10/660: 1 tab PO q4-6h prn. [Generic/Trade: Tabs Vicodin (5/500), Vicodin ES (7.5/750), Vicodin HP (10/660), scored, mg hydrocodone/mg acetaminophen.] ▶LK ♀C ▶? ©III $

Vicoprofen (hydrocodone + ibuprofen): 1 tab PO q4-6h prn. [Generic/Trade: Tab 7.5 mg hydrocodone/200 mg ibuprofen.] ▶LK ♀– ▶? ©III $$$

Wygesic (propoxyphene + acetaminophen): 1 tab PO q4h prn. [Generic/Trade: Tab 65 mg propoxyphene/650 mg acetaminophen.] ▶L ♀C ▶? ©IV $

Zydone (hydrocodone + acetaminophen): Multiple strengths; write specific product on Rx: 1-2 tabs PO q4-6h prn (5/400). 1 tab q4-6h prn (7.5/400,10/400). [Trade: Tabs 5/400, 7.5/400, & 10/400 mg hydrocodone/mg acet.] ▶LK ♀C ▶? ©III $$

Opioid Antagonists

nalmefene (***Revex***): Opioid overdose: 0.5 mg/70 kg IV. If needed, this may be followed by a second dose of 1 mg/70 kg, 2-5 minutes later. Max cumulative dose 1.5 mg/70 kg. If suspicion of opioid dependency, initially administer a challenge dose of 0.1 mg/70 kg. Post-operative opioid reversal: 0.25 mcg/kg IV followed by 0.25 mcg/kg incremental doses at 2-5 minute intervals, stopping as soon as the desired degree of opioid reversal is obtained. Max cumulative dose 1 mcg/kg. [Trade: Injection 100 mcg/ml nalmefene for postoperative reversal (blue label). 1 mg/ml nalmefene for opioid overdose (green label).] ▶L ♀B ▶? $$$

naloxone (***Narcan***): Opioid overdose: 0.4-2.0 mg q2-3 min prn. Adult post-op reversal 0.1-0.2 mg. Ped post-op reversal: 0.005-0.01 mg. IV/IM/SC/ET. ▶LK ♀B ▶? $

Other Analgesics

acetaminophen (***Tylenol, Panadol, Tempra, paracetamol***, ♣**Abenol, Atasol, Pediatrix***): 325-650 mg PO/PR q4-6h prn. Max dose 4 g/day, 2.5 g/day if ≥3 alcoholic drinks/day. OA: 2 extended release caplets (ie, 1300 mg) PO q8h around the clock. Peds: 10-15 mg/kg/dose PO/PR q4-6h prn. [OTC tabs 160,325,500,650 mg. Chewable Tabs 80 mg. Gelcaps 500 mg. Caps 325 & 500 mg. Sprinkle Caps 80,160 mg. Extended-release caplets 650 mg. Liquid 160 mg/5 ml, 500 mg/15 ml. Drops 80 mg/0.8 ml. Suppositories 80,120,125,300,325,650 mg.] ▶LK ♀B ▶+ $

tramadol (***Ultram***): Moderate to moderately severe pain: 50-100 mg PO q4-6h prn, max 400 mg/day. Adjust dose in elderly, renal & hepatic dysfunction. Avoid in opioid-dependent. Seizures may occur with concurrent antidepressants or seizure disorder. [Generic/Trade: Tab, immediate-release 50 mg.] ▶LK ♀C ▶– $$$

Women's Tylenol Menstrual Relief (acetaminophen + pamabrom): 2 caplets PO q4-6h. [OTC: Caplet 500 mg acet. /25 mg pamabrom (diuretic).] ▶LK ♀B ▶+ $
ziconotide (**Prialt**): Severe intractable chronic pain: Specialized intrathecal dosing. ▶Plasma ♀C ▶? $$$$

ANESTHESIA

Anesthetics & Sedatives

dexmedetomidine (**Precedex**): ICU sedation <24h: Load 1 mcg/kg over 10 min followed by infusion 0.2-0.7 mcg/kg/h titrated to desired sedation endpoint. Beware of bradycardia and hypotension. ▶LK ♀C ▶? $$
etomidate (**Amidate**): Induction 0.3 mg/kg IV. ▶L ♀C ▶? $
ketamine (**Ketalar**): 1-2 mg/kg IV over 1-2 min or 4 mg/kg IM induces 10-20 min dissociative state. Concurrent atropine minimizes hypersalivation. ▶L ♀? ▶? ©III $
methohexital (**Brevital**): Induction 1-1.5 mg/kg IV, duration 5 min. ▶L ♀B ▶? ©IV $
midazolam (**Versed**): Adult sedation/anxiolysis: 5 mg or 0.07 mg/kg IM; or 1 mg IV slowly q2-3 min up to 5 mg. Peds: 0.25-1.0 mg/kg to max of 20 mg PO, or 0.1-0.15 mg/kg IM. IV route (6 mo to 5 yo): Initial dose 0.05-0.1 mg/kg IV, then titrated to max 0.6 mg/kg. IV route (6-12 yo): Initial dose 0.025-0.05 mg/kg IV, then titrated to max 0.4 mg/kg. Monitor for respiratory depression. [Oral liquid 2 mg/ml] ▶LK ♀D ▶- ©IV $
pentobarbital (**Nembutal**): Pediatric sedation: 1-6 mg/kg IV, adjusted in increments of 1-2 mg/kg to desired effect, or 2-6 mg/kg IM, max 100 mg. ▶LK ♀D ▶? ©II $$
propofol (**Diprivan**): Induction 2-2.5 mg/kg IV. ICU ventilator sedation: infusion 5-50 mcg/kg/min. ▶L ♀B ▶- $$$
thiopental (**Pentothal**): Induction 3-5 mg/kg IV, duration 5 min. ▶L ♀C ▶? ©III $

Local Anesthetics

articaine (**Septocaine, Zorcaine**): 4% injection (includes epinephrine). [4% (includes epinephrine 1:100,000)/] ▶LK ♀C ▶? ?
bupivacaine (**Marcaine, Sensorcaine**): 0.25% injection. [0.25%, 0.5%, 0.75%, all with or without epinephrine.] ▶LK ♀C ▶? ?
Duocaine (bupivacaine + lidocaine): Local anesthesia, nerve block for eye surgery. [Vials contain bupivacaine 0.375% + lidocaine 1%.] ▶LK ♀C ▶? ?
levobupivacaine (**Chirocaine**): Local & epidural anesthesia, nerve block. [2.5, 5, 7.5 mg/ml injection.] ▶LK ♀B ▶? ?
lidocaine (**Xylocaine**): 0.5-1% injection with and without epinephrine. [0.5,1,1.5,2%. With epi: 0.5,1,1.5,2%.] ▶LK ♀B ▶? $
mepivacaine (**Carbocaine, Polocaine**): 1-2% injection. [1,1.5,2,3%.] ▶LK ♀C ▶? $

Neuromuscular Blockers

Should be administered only by those skilled in airway management and respiratory support.

atracurium (**Tracrium**): 0.4-0.5 mg/kg IV. Duration 15-30 min. ▶Plasma ♀C ▶? $
cisatracurium (**Nimbex**): 0.1-0.2 mg/kg IV. Duration 30-60 min. ▶Plasma ♀B ▶? $$
doxacurium (**Nuromax**): 0.05 mg/kg IV. Duration ~100 minutes. ▶KL ♀C ▶? $$
mivacurium (**Mivacron**): 0.15 mg/kg IV. Duration 20 minutes. ▶Plasma ♀C ▶? $$
pancuronium (**Pavulon**): 0.04 to 0.1 mg/kg IV. Duration 45 min. ▶Plasma ♀C ▶? $
rocuronium (**Zemuron**): 0.6 mg/kg IV. Duration 30 min. ▶L ♀B ▶? $$
succinylcholine (**Anectine, Quelicin**): 0.6-1.1 mg/kg IV. Peds: 2 mg/kg IV, consider pretreatment with atropine 0.02 mg/kg if <5 yo. ▶Plasma ♀C ▶? $
vecuronium (**Norcuron**): 0.08-0.1 mg/kg IV. Duration 15-30 min. ▶LK ♀C ▶? $

ANTIMICROBIALS

Aminoglycosides

NOTE: See also Dermatology and ophthalmology

amikacin (*Amikin*): 15 mg/kg up to 1500 mg/day IM/IV divided q8-12h. Peak 20-35 mcg/ml, trough <5 mcg/ml. Alternative 15 mg/kg IV q24h. ▶K ♀D ▶? $$$

gentamicin (*Garamycin*): Adults: 3-5 mg/kg/day IM/IV divided q8h. Peak 5-10 mcg/ml, trough <2 mcg/ml. Alternative 5-7 mg/kg IV q24h. Peds: 2-2.5 mg/kg q8h. ▶K ♀D ▶+ $$

streptomycin: Combo therapy for TB: 15 mg/kg up to 1 g IM daily. 10 mg/kg up to 750 mg if >59 yo. Peds: 20-40 mg/kg up to 1 g IM daily. Nephrotoxicity, ototoxicity. [Generic: 1 g vials for parenteral use.] ▶K ♀C ▶+ $$$$$

tobramycin (*Nebcin, TOBI*): Adults: 3-5 mg/kg/day IM/IV divided q8h. Peak 5-10 mcg/ml, trough <2 mcg/ml. Alternative 5-7 mg/kg IV q24h. Peds: 2-2.5 mg/kg q8h. Cystic fibrosis (TOBI): 300 mg neb bid 28 days on, then 28 days off. [Trade: TOBI 300 mg ampules for nebulizer.] ▶K ♀D ▶? $$$$

Antifungal Agents

amphotericin B deoxycholate (*Fungizone*): Test dose 0.1 mg/kg up to 1 mg slow IV. Wait 2-4 h, and if tolerated then begin 0.25 mg/kg IV daily and advance to 0.5-1.5 mg/kg/day depending on fungal type. Maximum dose 1.5 mg/kg/day. ▶Tissues ♀B ▶? $$$$

amphotericin B lipid formulations (*Amphotec, Abelcet, AmBisome*): Abelcet: 5 mg/kg/day IV at 2.5 mg/kg/hr. AmBisome: 3-5 mg/kg/day IV over 2 h. Amphotec: Test dose of 10 ml over 15-30 minutes, observe for 30 minutes, then 3-4 mg/kg/day IV at 1 mg/kg/h. ▶? ♀B ▶? $$$$$

caspofungin (*Cancidas*): 70 mg IV loading dose on day 1, then 50 mg IV daily. Infuse over 1 h. ▶KL ♀C ▶? $$$$$

clotrimazole (*Mycelex, ✚Canesten, Clotrimaderm*): Oral troches 5 x/day x 14 days. [Generic/Trade: Oral troches 10 mg.] ▶L ♀C ▶? $$$

fluconazole (*Diflucan*): Vaginal candidiasis: 150 mg PO single dose ($). All other dosing regimens IV/PO. Oropharyngeal/ esophageal candidiasis: 200 mg first day, then 100 mg daily. Systemic candidiasis, cryptococcal meningitis: 400 mg daily. Peds: Oropharyngeal/esophageal candidiasis: 6 mg/kg first day, then 3 mg/kg daily. Systemic candidiasis: 6-12 mg/kg daily. Cryptococcal meningitis: 12 mg/kg on first day, then 6 mg/kg daily. [Generic/Trade: Tabs 50,100,200 mg; 150 mg tab in single-dose blister pack; susp 10 & 40 mg/mL (35 mL).] ▶K ♀C ▶? $$$

flucytosine (*Ancobon*): 50-150 mg/kg/day PO divided qid. Myelosuppression. [Trade: Caps 250, 500 mg.] ▶K ♀C ▶? $$$$$

griseofulvin (*Grisactin 500, Grifulvin V, ✚Fulvicin*): Tinea capitis: 500 mg PO daily in adults; 15-20 mg/kg up to 1 g PO daily in peds. Treat x 4-6 weeks, continuing for 2 weeks past symptom resolution. [Generic/Trade: Susp 125 mg/5 ml (120 ml), Trade only: tabs 500 mg.] ▶Skin ♀C ▶? $$$

itraconazole (*Sporanox*): Oral caps for onychomycosis "pulse dosing": 200 mg PO bid for 1st wk of month x 2 months (fingernails) or 3-4 months (toenails). Oral soln for oropharyngeal or esophageal candidiasis: 100-200 mg PO daily or 100 mg bid swish & swallow in 10 ml increments on empty stomach. For life-threatening infections, load with 200 mg IV bid x 4 doses or 200 mg PO tid x 3 days. Empiric therapy of suspected fungal infection in febrile neutropenia: 200 mg IV bid x 4 doses, then 200 mg IV daily for ≤14 days. Continue with oral soln 200 mg (20 ml)

PO bid until significant neutropenia resolved. Contraindicated with cisapride, dofetilide, lovastatin, PO midazolam, pimozide, quinidine, simvastatin, triazolam. Negative inotrope; do not use for onychomycosis if ventricular dysfunction. [Generic/Trade: Cap 100 mg. Trade: Oral soln 10 mg/ml (150 mL).] ▶L ♀C ▶- $$$$$

ketoconazole (*Nizoral*): 200-400 mg PO daily. Hepatotoxicity. Contraindicated with cisapride, midazolam, pimozide, triazolam. H2 blockers, proton pump inhibitors, antacids impair absorption. [Generic/Trade: Tabs 200 mg.] ▶L ♀C ▶?+ $$$

micafungin (*Mycamine*): Infuse IV over 1 h. Esophageal candidiasis: 150 mg once daily. Prevention of candidal infections in bone marrow transplant patients: 50 mg once daily. ▶L, feces ♀C ▶? $$$$$

nystatin (*Mycostatin*, ✚*Nilstat, Nyaderm, Candistatin*): Thrush: 4-6 ml PO swish & swallow qid. Infants: 2 ml/dose with 1 ml in each cheek qid. [Generic/Trade: Susp 100,000 units/ml. Trade: Troches 200,000 units.] ▶Not absorbed ♀B ▶? $$$

terbinafine (*Lamisil*): Onychomycosis: 250 mg PO daily x 6 weeks for fingernails, x 12 weeks for toenails. "Pulse dosing": 500 mg PO daily for first week of month x 2 months (fingernails) or 4 months (toenails). [Trade: Tabs 250 mg.] ▶LK ♀B ▶- $$$$$

voriconazole (*Vfend*): IV: 6 mg/kg q12h x 2, then 3-4 mg/kg IV q12h (use 4 mg/kg for non-candidal infections). Infuse over 2 h. PO: 200 mg q12h if >40 kg, 100 mg PO q12 h if <40 kg. Take 1 h before/after meals. Treat esophageal candidiasis with oral regimen for ≥2 weeks & continuing for >1 week past symptom resolution. Treat systemic candidal infections for ≥2 weeks past symptom resolution or last positive culture, whichever is longer. Many drug interactions. [Trade: Tabs 50,200 mg (contains lactose), susp 40 mg/mL (75mL).] ▶L ♀D ▶? $$$$$

Antimalarials

> **NOTE:** For help treating malaria or getting antimalarials, call the CDC "malaria hotline" (770) 488-7788 Monday-Friday 8 am to 4:30 pm EST. After hours / weekend (404) 639-2888. Information is also available at: http://www.cdc.gov.

chloroquine (*Aralen*): Malaria prophylaxis, chloroquine-sensitive areas: 8 mg/kg up to 500 mg PO q wk from 1-2 weeks before exposure to 4 weeks after. Chloroquine resistance widespread. [Generic: Tabs 250 mg. Generic/Trade: Tabs 500 mg (500 mg phosphate equivalent to 300 mg base).] ▶KL ♀C but ✓ ▶+ $$

doxycycline (*Adoxa, Vibramycin, Vibra-Tabs, Doryx, Monodox*, ✚*Doxycin*): Malaria prophylaxis: 2 mg/kg/day up to 100 mg PO daily starting 1-2 days before exposure until 4 weeks after. 100 mg IV/PO bid for severe bacterial infections. Avoid in children <8 yo due to teeth staining. [Generic/Trade: Tabs 75,100 mg, caps 50,100 mg. Trade: Vibramycin Susp 25 mg/5 ml (60 mL), Syrup 50 mg/5 ml (480 mL). Periostat caps 20 mg.] ▶LK ♀D ▶? $

Fansidar (sulfadoxine + pyrimethamine): Chloroquine-resistant P falciparum malaria: 2-3 tabs PO single dose. Peds: 5-10 kg: ½ tab. 11-20 kg: 1 tab. 21-30 kg: 1½ tab. 31-45 kg: 2 tabs. >45 kg: 3 tabs. Do not use in infants <2 mo; may cause kernicterus. Stevens-Johnson syndrome, toxic epidermal necrolysis. Fansidar resistance common in many malarious areas. [Trade: Tabs sulfadoxine 500 mg + pyrimethamine 25 mg.] ▶KL ♀C ▶- $

Malarone (atovaquone+proguanil): Prevention of malaria: 1 adult tab PO daily from 1-2 days before exposure until 7 days after. Treatment of malaria: 4 adult tabs PO daily x 3 days. Take with food or milky drink. [Trade: Adult tabs 250/100 mg atovaquone/proguanil; peds tabs 62.5/25 mg.] ▶Fecal excretion; LK ♀C ▶? $$$$

mefloquine (*Lariam*): Malaria prophylaxis for chloroquine-resistant areas: 250 mg PO q week from 1 week before exposure to 4 weeks after. Treatment: 1250 mg

PO single dose. Peds. Malaria prophylaxis: Give PO once weekly starting 1 week before exposure to 4 weeks after: <15 kg, 5 mg/kg (prepared by pharmacist); 15-19 kg, ¼ tab; 20-30 kg, ½ tab; 31-45 kg, ¾ tab; >45 kg, 1 tab. Treatment: 20-25 mg/kg PO; can divide into 2 doses given 6-8 h apart. Take on full stomach. [Generic/Trade: Tabs 250 mg.] ▶L ♀C ▶? $$

primaquine: 30 mg base PO daily x 14 days. [Generic: Tabs 26.3 mg (equiv to 15 mg base).] ▶L ♀- ▶- $

quinidine: Life-threatening malaria: Load with 10 mg/kg (max 600 mg) IV over 1-2 h, then 0.02 mg/kg/min. Treat x 72 h, until parasitemia <1%, or PO meds tolerated. Dose given as quinidine gluconate. ▶LK ♀C ▶+ $$$$

quinine: Malaria: 600-650 mg PO tid. Peds: 25-30 mg/kg/day up to 2 g/day PO divided q8h. Treat for 3-7 days. Also give doxycycline or Fansidar. [Generic: Tabs 260 mg, caps 200,325 mg.] ▶L ♀X ▶+? $

Antimycobacterial Agents

> **NOTE:** Two or more drugs are needed for the treatment of active mycobacterial infections. See guidelines at http://www.thoracic.org/statements/.

dapsone: Pneumocystis prophylaxis, leprosy: 100 mg PO daily. Pneumocystis treatment: 100 mg PO daily with trimethoprim 5 mg/kg PO tid x 21 days. [Generic: Tabs 25,100 mg.] ▶LK ♀C ▶+? $

ethambutol (Myambutol, ✚Etibi): 15-20 mg/kg PO daily. Dose with whole tabs: Give PO daily 800 mg if 40-55 kg, 1200 mg if 56-75 kg, 1600 mg if 76-90 kg. Base dose on estimated lean body weight. Peds: 15-20 mg/kg up to 1 g PO daily. [Generic/Trade: Tabs 100,400 mg.] ▶LK ♀C but + ▶? $$$

isoniazid (INH, ✚Isotamine): Adults: 5 mg/kg up to 300 mg PO daily. Peds: 10-15 mg/kg up to 300 mg PO daily. Hepatotoxicity. Consider supplemental pyridoxine 10-50 mg PO daily. [Generic: Tabs 100,300 mg, syrup 50 mg/5 ml.] ▶LK ♀C but + ▶+ $

pyrazinamide (PZA, ✚Tebrazid): 20-25 mg/kg up to 2000 mg PO daily. Dose with whole tabs: Give PO daily 1000 mg if 40-55 kg, 1500 mg if 56-75 kg, 2000 mg if 76-90 kg. Base dose on estimated lean body weight. Peds: 15-30 mg/kg up to 2000 mg PO daily. Hepatotoxicity. [Generic: Tabs 500 mg.] ▶LK ♀C ▶? $$$

rifabutin (Mycobutin): 300 mg PO daily or 150 mg PO bid. [Trade: Caps 150 mg.] ▶L ♀B ▶? $$$$$

Rifamate (isoniazid + rifampin): 2 caps PO daily. [Trade: Caps isoniazid 150 mg + rifampin 300 mg.] ▶LK ♀C but + ▶+ $$$$

rifampin (Rimactane, Rifadin, ✚Rofact): TB: 10 mg/kg up to 600 mg PO/IV daily. Peds: 10-20 mg/kg up to 600 mg PO/IV daily. IV and PO doses are the same. [Generic/Trade: Caps 150,300 mg. Pharmacists can make oral suspension.] ▶L ♀C but + ▶+ $$$

rifapentine (Priftin): 600 mg PO twice weekly x 2 months, then once weekly x 4 months. Use for continuation therapy only in selected HIV-negative patients. [Trade: Tabs 150 mg.] ▶ Esterases, fecal ♀C ▶? $$$$

Rifater (isoniazid + rifampin + pyrazinamide): 6 tabs PO daily if ≥55 kg, 5 daily if 45-54 kg, 4 daily if ≤44 kg. [Trade: Tab Isoniazid 50 mg + rifampin 120 mg + pyrazinamide 300 mg.] ▶LK ♀C ▶? $$$$$

Antiparasitics

albendazole (Albenza): Hydatid disease, neurocysticercosis: 400 mg PO bid. 15 mg/kg/day up to 800 mg/day if <60 kg. [Trade: Tabs 200 mg.] ▶L ♀C ▶? $$$

atovaquone (**Mepron**): Pneumocystis treatment: 750 mg PO bid x 21 days. Pneumocystis prevention: 1500 mg PO daily. Take with meals. [Trade: Susp 750 mg/5 ml, foil pouch 750 mg/5 ml.] ▶Fecal ♀C ▶? $$$$$

ivermectin (**Stromectol**): Single PO dose of 200 mcg/kg for strongyloidiasis, scabies (not for children <15 kg), 150 mcg/kg for onchocerciasis. Take on empty stomach with water. [Trade: Tab 3, 6 mg.] ▶L ♀C ▶+ $

mebendazole (**Vermox**): Pinworm: 100 mg PO x 1; repeat in 2 wks. Roundworm, whipworm, hookworm: 100 mg PO bid x 3d. [Generic/Trade: Chew tab 100 mg.] ▶L ♀C ▶? $$

metronidazole (**Flagyl**, ✦**Trikacide, Florazole ER, Nidazol**): Trichomoniasis: 2g PO single dose for patient & sex partners. Giardia: 250 mg (5 mg/kg/dose for peds) PO tid x 5-7 days. [Generic/Trade: Tabs 250,500 mg, ER tabs 750 mg, Caps 375 mg.] ▶KL ♀B ▶- $

nitazoxanide (**Alinia**): Cryptosporidial or Giardial diarrhea: 100 mg bid for 1-3 yo, 200 mg bid for 4-11 yo, 500 mg bid for adults and children ≥12 yo. Give PO with food x 3 days. Use susp for <12 yo. [Trade: Oral susp 100 mg/5 ml 60 ml bottle, tab 500 mg.] ▶L ♀B ▶? $$$

paromomycin (**Humatin**): 25-35 mg/kg/day PO divided tid with or after meals. [Generic/Trade: Caps 250 mg.] ▶Not absorbed ♀C ▶? $$

pentamidine (**Pentam, NebuPent**, ✦**Pentacarinat**): Pneumocystis treatment: 4 mg/kg IM/IV daily x 21 days. Pneumocystis prevention: 300 mg nebulized q 4 weeks. [Trade: Aerosol 300 mg.] ▶K ♀C ▶- $$$

praziquantel (**Biltricide**): Schistosomiasis: 20 mg/kg PO q4-6h x 3 doses. Neurocysticercosis: 50 mg/kg/day PO divided tid x 15 days (up to 100 mg/kg/day for peds). [Trade: Tabs 600 mg.] ▶LK ♀B ▶- $$$

pyrantel (**Antiminth, Pin-X, Pinworm**, ✦**Combantrin**): Pinworm and roundworm: 11 mg/kg up to 1 g PO single dose. [OTC: Caps 62.5 mg, liquid 50 mg/ml.] ▶Not absorbed ♀- ▶? $

pyrimethamine (**Daraprim**): CNS toxoplasmosis in AIDS. Acute therapy: 200 mg PO x 1, then 50 mg (<60 kg) to 75 mg (≥60 kg) PO once daily + sulfadiazine + leucovorin 10-20 mg PO once daily (can increase to ≥50 mg/day) for ≥6 weeks. Secondary prevention: Pyrimethamine 25-50 mg PO once daily + sulfadiazine + leucovorin 10-25 mg PO once daily. [Trade: Tabs 25 mg.] ▶L ♀C ▶+ $$$

thiabendazole (**Mintezol**): Helminths: 22 mg/kg/dose up to 1500 mg PO bid after meals. Treat x 2 days for strongyloidiasis, cutaneous larva migrans. [Trade: Chew tab 500 mg, susp 500 mg/5 ml (120 mL).] ▶LK ♀C ▶? $$

tinidazole (**Tindamax**): Adults: 2 g PO daily x 1 day for trichomoniasis or giardiasis, x 3 days for amebiasis. Peds, >3 yo: 50 mg/kg (up to 2 g) PO daily x 1 day for giardiasis, x 3 days for amebiasis. Take with food. [Trade: Tabs 250,500 mg. Pharmacists can compound oral suspension.] ▶KL ♀C ▶? $

trimetrexate (**Neutrexin**): 45 mg/m² IV infused over 1h daily x 21 days. Give leucovorin 20 mg/m² IV/PO q6h x 24 days (until 72 h after last trimetrexate dose). ▶LK ♀D ▶- $$$$$

Antiviral Agents - Anti-CMV

cidofovir (**Vistide**): CMV retinitis in AIDS: 5 mg/kg IV q wk x 2, then 5 mg/kg q2 wks. Nephrotoxicity. ▶K ♀C ▶- $$$$$

foscarnet (**Foscavir**): CMV retinitis: 60 mg/kg IV (over 1 h) q8h or 90 mg/kg IV (over 1.5-2 h) q12h x 2-3 weeks, then 90-120 mg/kg/day IV over 2h. HSV infection: 40 mg/kg (over 1 h) q8-12h. Nephrotoxicity, seizures. ▶K ♀C ▶? $$$$$

ganciclovir (**DHPG, Cytovene**): CMV retinitis: Induction 5 mg/kg IV q12h for 14-21 days. Maintenance 6 mg/kg IV daily for 5 days per week. Oral: 1000 mg PO tid or 500 mg 6 times daily. Myelosuppression. Potential carcinogen, teratogen. May impair fertility. [Generic/Trade: Caps 250, 500 mg.] ▶K ♀C ▶- $$$$$

valganciclovir (**Valcyte**): CMV retinitis: 900 mg PO bid x 21 days, then 900 mg PO daily. Prevention of CMV disease in high-risk kidney, kidney-pancreas, heart transplant patients: 900 mg PO daily from within 10 days after transplant until 100 days post-transplant. Give with food. Impaired fertility, myelosuppression, potential carcinogen & teratogen. [Trade: Tabs 450 mg.] ▶K ♀C ▶- $$$$$

Antiviral Agents - Anti-Herpetic

acyclovir (**Zovirax**): Genital herpes: 400 mg PO tid x 7-10 days for first episode, x 5 days for recurrent episodes. Chronic suppression of genital herpes: 400 mg PO bid, 400-800 mg PO bid-tid in HIV infection. Zoster: 800 mg PO 5 times/day x 7-10 days. Chickenpox: 20 mg/kg up to 800 mg PO qid x 5 days. Adult IV: 5-10 mg/kg IV q8h, each dose over 1h. Peds, herpes encephalitis: 20 mg/kg IV q8h x 10 days for 3 mo-12 yo, adult dose for ≥12 yo. [Generic/Trade: Caps 200 mg, tabs 400,800 mg. Susp 200 mg/5 ml.] ▶K ♀B ▶+ $

famciclovir (**Famvir**): First-episode genital herpes: 250 mg PO tid x 7-10 days. Recurrent genital herpes: 125 mg PO bid x 5 days. Chronic suppression of genital herpes: 250 mg PO bid, 500 mg PO bid if HIV infection. Recurrent oral/genital herpes in HIV patients: 500 bid x 7 days. Zoster: 500 mg PO tid for 7 days. [Trade: Tabs 125,250,500 mg.] ▶K ♀B ▶- $$

valacyclovir (**Valtrex**): First-episode genital herpes: 1000 mg PO bid x 10 days. Recurrent genital herpes: 500 mg PO bid x 3 days, 1 g PO bid x 5-10 days in HIV infection. Chronic suppression of genital herpes: 500-1000 mg PO daily; 500 mg PO bid if HIV infection. Reduction of genital herpes transmission in immunocompetent patients with ≤9 recurrences/year: 500 mg PO daily by source partner, in conjunction with safer sex practices. Herpes labialis: 2 g PO q12h x 2 doses. Zoster: 1000 mg PO tid x 7 days. [Trade: Tabs 500,1000 mg.] ▶K ♀B ▶+ $$$$

Antiviral Agents - Anti-HIV - Fusion Inhibitors

enfuvirtide (**Fuzeon, T-20**): 90 mg SC bid. Peds, ≥6 yo: 2 mg/kg up to 90 mg SC bid. [30-day kit with vials, diluent, syringes, alcohol wipes. Single-dose vials contain 108 mg to provide 90 mg enfuvirtide.] ▶Serum ♀B ▶- $$$$$

Antiviral Agents - Anti-HIV - Non-Nucleoside Reverse Transcript. Inhibitors

> NOTE: AIDS treatment guidelines available online at www.aidsinfo.nih.gov. Many serious drug interactions - always check before prescribing!

efavirenz (**Sustiva, EFV**): Adults & children >40 kg: 600 mg PO qhs. Peds: ≥3 yo: 10-15 kg: 200 mg PO qhs. 15-20 kg: 250 mg qhs. 20 to <25 kg: 300 mg qhs. 25 to <32.5 kg: 350 mg qhs. 32.5 to <40 kg: 400 mg qhs. Do not give with high-fat meal. [Caps 50,100,200 mg, tabs 600 mg.] ▶L ♀D ▶- $$$$$

nevirapine (**Viramune, NVP**): 200 mg PO daily x 14 days initially. If tolerated, ↑ to 200 mg PO bid. Peds <8 yo: 4 mg/kg PO daily x 14 days, then 7 mg/kg PO bid. ≥8 yo: 4 mg/kg PO daily x 14 days, then 4 mg/kg PO bid. Severe skin reactions, hepatotoxicity. [Trade: Tabs 200 mg, susp 50 mg/5 ml] ▶LK ♀C ▶- $$$$$

Antiviral Agents - Anti-HIV - Nucleoside/Nucleotide Reverse Transcrip Inhib

> NOTE: AIDS treatment guidelines available online at www.aidsinfo.nih.gov. Consider monitoring LFTs in patients receiving highly active anti-retroviral therapy (HAART).

abacavir (*Ziagen, ABC*): Adult: 300 mg PO bid or 600 mg PO daily. Children >3 mo: 8 mg/kg up to 300 mg PO bid. Potentially fatal hypersensitivity; never rechallenge if this occurs. Severe hypersensitivity may be more common with once-daily regimen. [Trade: Tabs 300 mg, oral soln 20 mg/ml (240 mL).] ▶L ♀C ▶- $$$$$

Combivir (lamivudine + zidovudine): 1 tab PO bid. [Trade: Tabs lamivudine 150 mg + zidovudine 300 mg.] ▶LK ♀C ▶- $$$$$

didanosine (*Videx, Videx EC, ddI*): Adult, buffered tabs: 200 mg PO bid if ≥60 kg, 125 mg PO bid if <60 kg. Peds: 120 mg/m² PO bid. Videx EC, adults: 400 mg PO daily if ≥60 kg, 250 mg PO daily if <60 kg. Dosage reduction of Videx EC with tenofovir: 250 mg if ≥60 kg, 200 mg if <60 kg. Dosage reduction unclear with tenofovir if CrCl <60 mL/min. All formulations usually taken on empty stomach. [Trade: Chew/dispersible buffered tabs 25,50,100,150, 200 mg. Packets of buffered powder for oral soln 100,167,250 mg. Pediatric powder for oral soln 10 mg/ml (buffered with antacid). Generic/Trade: Delayed-release caps 200,250,400 mg. Trade only: (Videx EC) delayed-release caps 125 mg. All forms except delayed release caps ▶LK ♀B ▶- $$$$$

emtricitabine (*Emtriva, FTC*): 200 mg PO daily. [Trade: Caps 200 mg.] ▶K ♀B ▶- $$$$$

Epzicom (abacavir + lamivudine): 1 tab PO daily. [Trade: Tabs abacavir 600 mg + lamivudine 300 mg.] ▶LK ♀C ▶- $$$$$

lamivudine (*Epivir, Epivir-HBV, 3TC, ♥Heptovir*): Epivir for HIV infection. Adults: 150 mg PO bid or 300 mg PO daily. Peds: 4 mg/kg up to 150 mg PO bid. Epivir-HBV for hepatitis B: Adults: 100 mg PO daily. Peds: 3 mg/kg up to 100 mg PO daily. [Trade: Epivir, 3TC: Tabs 150, 300 mg, oral soln 10 mg/ml. Epivir-HBV, Heptovir: Tabs 100 mg, oral soln 5 mg/ml.] ▶K ♀C ▶- $$$$$

stavudine (*Zerit, d4T*): 40 mg PO q12h, or 30 mg q12h if <60 kg. Peds (<30 kg): 1 mg/ kg PO bid. [Trade: Caps 15,20,30,40 mg; oral soln 1 mg/ml (200 mL).] ▶LK ♀C ▶- $$$$$

tenofovir (*Viread, TDF*): 300 mg PO daily with a meal. [Trade: Tab 300 mg.] ▶K ♀B ▶- $$$$$

Trizivir (abacavir + lamivudine + zidovudine): 1 tab PO bid. [Trade: Tabs abacavir 300 mg + lamivudine 150 mg + zidovudine 300 mg.] ▶LK ♀C ▶- $$$$$

Truvada (emtricitabine + tenofovir): 1 tab PO daily. [Trade: Tabs emtricitabine 200 mg + tenofovir 300 mg.] ▶K ♀B ▶- $$$$$

zalcitabine (*Hivid, ddC*): 0.75 mg PO q8h on an empty stomach. [Trade: Tabs 0.375, 0.75 mg.] ▶K ♀C ▶- $$$$$

zidovudine (*Retrovir, AZT, ZDV*): 200 mg PO tid or 300 bid. Peds: 160 mg/m² up to 200 mg PO q8h. [Trade: Cap 100 mg, tab 300 mg, syrup 50 mg/5 ml (240 mL).] ▶LK ♀C ▶- $$$$$

Antiviral Agents - Anti-HIV - Protease Inhibitors

NOTE: Many serious drug interactions - always check before prescribing! Contraindicated with most antiarrhythmics, cisapride, ergot alkaloids, lovastatin, pimozide, simvastatin, St. John's wort, triazolam. See http://www.cdc.gov/nchstp/tb/TB_HIV_Drugs/TOC.htm or www.aidsinfo.nih.gov for use of rifamycins with protease inhibitors.

atazanavir (*Reyataz, ATV*): Therapy-naive patients: 400 mg PO daily. Efavirenz regimen, therapy-naive patients: atazanavir 300 mg + ritonavir 100 mg + efavirenz 600 mg all PO daily. Therapy-experienced patients: atazanavir 300 mg PO daily + ritonavir 100 mg PO daily. Tenofovir regimen (must include ritonavir): atazanavir 300 mg + ritonavir 100 mg + tenofovir 300 mg all PO daily with food. Give atazanavir with food; give 2 h before or 1 h after buffered didanosine. [Trade: Caps 100,150,200 mg.] ▶L ♀B ▶- $$$$$

fosamprenavir (*Lexiva, 908*): Therapy-naïve patients: 1400 mg PO bid (without ritonavir). OR fosamprenavir 1400 mg + ritonavir 200 mg both PO daily. OR 700 mg fosamprenavir + 100 mg ritonavir both PO bid. Protease inhibitor-experienced patients: 700 mg fosamprenavir + 100 mg ritonavir both PO bid. Do not use once-daily regimen. If once-daily ritonavir-boosted regimen given with efavirenz, increase ritonavir to 300 mg/day; no increase of ritonavir dose needed for bid regimen with efavirenz. No meal restrictions. [Trade: Tabs 700 mg (equivalent to amprenavir 600 mg).] ▶L ♀C ▶- $$$$$

indinavir (*Crixivan, IDV*): 800 mg PO q8h between meals with water (at least 48 ounces/day to prevent kidney stones). [Trade: Caps 100,200,333,400 mg.] ▶LK ♀C ▶- $$$$$

lopinavir-ritonavir (*Kaletra, LPV/r*): 3 caps or 5 ml PO bid. Increase to 4 caps or 6.5 ml PO bid with efavirenz/nevirapine. Can give once-daily therapy of 6 caps or 10 ml to therapy-naïve patients only (do not use once daily with efavirenz, nevirapine, amprenavir, or nelfinavir). Peds 6 mo-12 yo: lopinavir 12 mg/kg PO bid for 7 to <15 kg, 10 mg/kg PO bid for 15-40 kg, adult dose for >40 kg. With efavirenz/nevirapine, increase to 13 mg/kg PO bid for 7 to <15 kg, 11 mg/kg PO bid for 15-45 kg, adult dose for >45 kg. Take with food. [Trade: Caps 133.3/33.3 mg of lopinavir/ritonavir. Oral soln 80/20 mg/ml (160 mL).] ▶L ♀C ▶- $$$$$

nelfinavir (*Viracept, NFV*): 750 mg PO tid or 1250 mg PO bid. Peds: 20-45 mg/kg PO tid. Take with meals. [Trade: Tab 250,625 mg, powder 50 mg/g (114 g).] ▶L ♀B ▶- $$$$$

ritonavir (*Norvir, RTV*): Full-dose regimen (600 mg PO bid) poorly tolerated. Adult doses of 100 mg PO daily to 400 mg PO bid used to boost levels of other protease inhibitors. [Trade: Cap 100 mg, oral soln 80 mg/ml.] ▶L ♀B ▶- $$$$$

saquinavir (*Fortovase, Invirase, SQV, FTV*): Do not use Invirase as sole protease inhibitor; low dose in combo with ritonavir preferred (such as Invirase 400 mg PO bid with ritonavir 400 mg PO bid with no regard to meals). Fortovase: 1200 mg PO tid. Peds: 33 mg/kg Fortovase PO tid. Take with/after meals. [Trade: Fortovase (soft gel), Invirase (hard gel) caps 200 mg, tabs 500 mg. Fortovase will be discontinued by Feb 15, 2006.] ▶L ♀B ▶? $$$$$

tipranavir (*Aptivus*): 500 mg boosted by ritonavir 200 mg PO bid with food. Hepatotoxicity. [Trade: Caps 250 mg.] ▶Feces ♀C ▶- $$$$$

Antiviral Agents - Anti-Influenza

amantadine (*Symmetrel*, ✦*Endantadine*): Influenza A: 100 mg PO bid. Elderly: 100 mg daily. Peds: 5 mg/kg up to 150 mg/day. [Generic: Cap 100 mg. Generic/Trade: Tab 100 mg, syrup 50 mg/5 ml (120 mL).] ▶K ♀C ▶? $

oseltamivir (*Tamiflu*): 75 mg PO bid x 5 days starting within 2 days of symptom onset. 75 mg PO daily for prophylaxis. Peds treatment: 2 mg/kg PO bid x 5 days. Take with food to improve tolerability. [Trade: Caps 75 mg, susp 12 mg/ml (25 mL).] ▶LK ♀C ▶? $$$

rimantadine (*Flumadine*): Influenza A: 100 mg PO bid x 7 days. Peds: 5 mg/kg PO daily up to 150 mg/day. [Trade: Tabs 100 mg, syrup 50 mg/5 ml.] ▶LK ♀C ▶- $$

zanamivir (*Relenza*): Influenza treatment: 2 puffs bid x 5 days. [Trade: Rotadisk inhaler 5 mg/puff (20 puffs).] ▶K ♀C ▶? $$

Antiviral Agents - Other

adefovir (*Hepsera*): Chronic hepatitis B: 10 mg PO daily. Nephrotoxic; lactic acidosis and hepatic steatosis; discontinuation may exacerbate hepatitis B; HIV resistance in untreated HIV infection. [Trade: Tabs 10 mg.] ▶K ♀C ▶- $$$$$

entecavir (**Baraclude**): Chronic hepatitis B: 0.5 mg PO once daily if treatment naïve; 1 mg if lamivudine-resistant or history of viremia despite lamivudine treatment. Give 2h before or after meals. [Trade: 0.5, 1 mg tabs.] ▶K ♀C ▶- $$$$$

interferon alfa-2b (**Intron A**): Chronic hepatitis B: 5 million units/day or 10 million units 3 times/week SC/IM x 4 mo. Chronic hepatitis C: 3 million units SC/IM 3 times/week x 4 mo. Continue for 18-24 mo if ALT normalized. [Trade: Powder/soln for injection 3,5,10 million units/vial. Soln for injection 18,25 million units/multidose vial. Multidose injection pens 3,5,10 million units/dose (6 doses/pen).] ▶K ♀C ▶?+ $$$$$

interferon alfacon-1 (**Infergen**): Chronic hepatitis C: 9 mcg SC 3 times/week x 24 weeks. If relapse/no response, increase to 15 mcg SC 3 times/week. If intolerable adverse effects, reduce to 7.5 mcg SC 3 times/week. [Trade: Vials injectable soln 9,15 mcg.] ▶Plasma ♀C ▶? $$$$$

palivizumab (**Synagis**): Prevention of respiratory syncytial virus pulmonary disease in high-risk children: 15 mg/kg IM q month during RSV season. ▶L ♀C ▶? $$$$$

peginterferon alfa-2a (**Pegasys**): Chronic hepatitis C: 180 mcg SC in abdomen or thigh once weekly for 48 weeks +/- PO ribavirin. Hepatitis B: 180 mcg SC in abdomen or thigh once weekly for 48 weeks. May cause or worsen severe autoimmune, neuropsychiatric, ischemic, & infectious diseases. Frequent clinical & lab monitoring. [Trade: 180 mcg/1 mL solution in single-use vial, 180 mcg/0.5 mL pre-filled syringe.] ▶LK ♀C ▶- $$$$$

peginterferon alfa-2b (**PEG-Intron**): Chronic hepatitis C: Give SC once weekly for 1 year. Monotherapy 1 mcg/kg/week. In combo oral ribavirin: 1.5 mcg/kg/week. May cause or worsen severe autoimmune, neuropsychiatric, ischemic, & infectious diseases. Frequent clinical & lab monitoring. [Trade: 50,80,120,150 mcg/0.5 ml single-use vials with diluent, 2 syringes, and alcohol swabs. Disposable single-dose Redipen 50,80,120,150 mcg.] ▶K? ♀C ▶- $$$$$

Rebetron (interferon alfa-2b + ribavirin): Chronic hepatitis C: Interferon alfa-2b 3 million units SC 3 times/week and ribavirin (Rebetol) 600 mg PO bid if >75 kg; 400 mg q am and 600 q pm if ≤75 kg. Ribavirin dose adjusted according to hemoglobin level. Contraindicated in pregnant women or their male partners. [Trade: Each kit contains a 2-week supply of interferon alfa-2b, ribavirin caps 200 mg. Rebetol oral soln also 40 mg/mL available.] ▶K ♀X ▶- $$$$$

ribavirin - inhaled (**Virazole**): Severe respiratory syncytial virus infection in children: Aerosol 12-18 h/day x 3-7 days. Beware of sudden pulmonary deterioration; ventilator dysfunction due to drug precipitation. ▶Lung ♀X ▶- $$$$$

ribavirin - oral (**Rebetol, Copegus**): Hepatitis C. Rebetol: In combo with interferon alfa 2b (Intron A): 600 mg PO bid if >75 kg; 400 mg q am and 600 q pm if ≤75 kg. In combo with peginterferon alfa 2b (PEG-Intron): 400 mg PO bid. Copegus: In combo with peginterferon alfa 2a (Pegasys): For genotype 1/4, 1200 mg/day if ≥75 kg; 1000 mg/day if <75 kg. For genotype 2/3, 800 mg/day PO. For patients coinfected with HIV, Copegus dose is 800 mg/day regardless of genotype. Give bid with food. Decrease ribavirin dose if Hb decreases. [Trade: Caps 200 mg (Rebetol), tabs 200,400 mg (Copegus). Generic: Caps 200 mg (Ribasphere, others). Trade: Rebetol oral soln 40 mg/ml (100ml).] ▶Cellular, K ♀X ▶- $$$$$

Carbapenems

ertapenem (**Invanz**): 1 g IV/IM q24h. Peds: 15 mg/kg IV/IM q12h (max 1 g/day). Infuse IV over 30 minutes. ▶K ♀B ▶? $$$$$

imipenem-cilastatin (**Primaxin**): 250-1000 mg IV q6-8h. Peds >3 mo: 15-25 mg/kg IV q6h. ▶K ♀C ▶? $$$$$

OVERVIEW OF BACTERIAL PATHOGENS (selected)

Gram Positive Aerobic Cocci: *Staph epidermidis* (coagulase negative), *Staph aureus* (coagulase positive), Streptococci: *S pneumoniae* (pneumococcus), *S pyogenes* (Group A), *S agalactiae* (Group B), enterococcus

Gram Positive Aerobic / Facultatively Anaerobic Bacilli: *Bacillus, Corynebacterium diphtheriae, Erysipelothrix rhusiopathiae, Listeria monocytogenes, Nocardia*

Gram Negative Aerobic Diplococci: *Moraxella catarrhalis, Neisseria gonorrhoeae, Neisseria meningitidis*

Gram Negative Aerobic Coccobacilli: *Haemophilus ducreyi, Haemoph. influenzae*

Gram Negative Aerobic Bacilli: *Acinetobacter, Bartonella species, Bordetella pertussis, Brucella, Burkholderia cepacia, Campylobacter, Francisella tularensis, Helicobacter pylori, Legionella pneumophila, Pseudomonas aeruginosa, Stenotrophomonas maltophilia, Vibrio cholerae, Yersinia*

Gram Neg Facultatively Anaerobic Bacilli: *Aeromonas hydrophila, Eikenella corrodens, Pasteurella multocida,* Enterobacteriaceae: *E coli, Citrobacter, Shigella, Salmonella, Klebsiella, Enterobacter, Hafnia, Serratia, Proteus, Providencia*

Anaerobes: *Actinomyces, Bacteroides fragilis, Clostridium botulinum, Clostridium difficile, Clostridium perfringens, Clostridium tetani, Fusobacterium, Lactobacillus, Peptostreptococcus*

Defective Cell Wall Bacteria: *Chlamydia pneumoniae, Chlamydia psittaci, Chlamydia trachomatis, Coxiella burnetii, Myocoplasma pneumoniae, Rickettsia prowazekii, Rickettsia rickettsii, Rickettsia typhi, Ureaplasma urealyticum*

Spirochetes: *Borrelia burgdorferi, Leptospira, Treponema pallidum*

Mycobacteria: *M avium complex, M kansasii, M leprae, M tuberculosis*

meropenem (***Merrem IV***): Complicated skin infections 10 mg/kg up to 500 mg IV q8h. Intra-abdominal infections: 20 mg/kg up to 1 g IV q8h. Peds meningitis: 40 mg/kg IV q8h for age ≥3 mo; 2 g IV q8h if >50 kg. ▶K ♀B ▶? $$$$$

Cephalosporins - 1st Generation

cefadroxil (***Duricef***): 1-2 g/day PO divided daily-bid. Peds: 30 mg/kg/day divided bid. [Generic/Trade: Tabs 1 g, caps 500 mg. Trade: Susp 125,250, & 500 mg/5 ml.] ▶K ♀B ▶+ $$

cefazolin (***Ancef, Kefzol***): 0.5-1.5 g IM/IV q6-8h. Peds: 25-50 mg/kg/day divided q6-8h, severe infections 100 mg/kg/day. ▶K ♀B ▶+ $$$

cephalexin (***Keflex, Keftab, Panixine DisperDose***): 250-500 mg PO qid. Peds 25-50 mg/kg/day. Not for otitis media, sinusitis. [Generic/Trade: Caps 250,500 mg, tabs 500 mg, susp 125 & 250 mg/5 ml. Generic: Tabs 250 mg. Keftab: 500 mg. Panixine DisperDose 125, 250 mg scored tabs for oral susp.] ▶K ♀B ▶? $

Cephalosporins - 2nd Generation

cefaclor (***Ceclor, Raniclor***): 250-500 mg PO tid. Peds: 20-40 mg/kg/day PO divided tid. Otitis media: 40 mg/kg/day PO divided bid. Group A streptococcal pharyngitis: 20 mg/kg/day PO divided bid. Extended release (Ceclor CD): 375-500 mg PO bid. Serum sickness-like reactions with repeated use. [Generic/Trade: Caps 250,500 mg, susp 125,187,250, 375 mg/5 ml. Extended release 500 mg. Trade only (Ceclor CD): 375 mg. Generic: Chew tabs 125,187,250,375 mg.] ▶K ♀B ▶? $$$

cefotetan (***Cefotan***): 1-2 g IM/IV q12h. Peds: 20-40 mg/kg IV q12h. ▶K/Bile ♀B ▶? $$$$$

cefoxitin (**Mefoxin**): 1-2 g IM/IV q6-8h. Peds: 80-160 mg/kg/day IV divided q4-8h. ▶K **9**B ▶+ $$$$$

cefprozil (**Cefzil**): 250-500 mg PO bid. Peds otitis media: 15 mg/kg/dose PO bid. Peds group A streptococcal pharyngitis (2nd-line to penicillin): 7.5 mg/kg/dose PO bid x 10d. [Trade: Tabs 250,500 mg, susp 125 & 250 mg/5 ml.] ▶K **9**B ▶+ $$$$

cefuroxime (**Zinacef, Ceftin, Kefurox**): 750-1500 mg IM/IV q8h. Peds: 50-100 mg/kg/day IV divided q6-8h, not for meningitis. 250-500 mg PO bid. Peds: 20-30 mg/kg/day susp PO divided bid. [Generic/trade: Tabs 250,500 mg. Generic: 125 mg tab. Trade: Susp 125 & 250 mg/5 ml.] ▶K **9**B ▶? $$$$

loracarbef (**Lorabid**): 200-400 mg PO bid. Peds: 30 mg/kg/day for otitis media (15 mg/kg/day for other infections) divided bid. [Trade: Caps 200,400 mg, susp 100 & 200 mg/5 ml.] ▶K **9**B ▶? $$$$

Cephalosporins - 3rd Generation

cefdinir (**Omnicef**): 14 mg/kg/day up to 600 mg/day PO divided daily or bid. [Trade: Cap 300 mg, susp 125 & 250 mg/5 ml.] ▶K **9**B ▶? $$$

cefditoren (**Spectracef**): 200-400 mg PO bid with food. [Trade: Tabs 200 mg.] ▶K **9**B ▶? $$$

cefixime (**Suprax**): 400 mg PO once daily. Gonorrhea: 400 mg PO single-dose. Peds: 8 mg/kg/day divided daily-bid. [Trade: Tabs 400 mg, susp 100 mg/5 ml.] ▶K/Bile **9**B ▶? $

cefoperazone (**Cefobid**): Usual dose 2-4 g/day IM/IV given q12h. Maximum dose: 6-12 g/day IV given q6-12 h. Possible clotting impairment. ▶Bile/K **9**B ▶? $$$$$

cefotaxime (**Claforan**): Usual dose: 1-2 g IM/IV q6-8h. Peds: 50-180 mg/kg/day IM/IV divided q4-6h. AAP dose for pneumococcal meningitis: 225-300 mg/kg/day IV divided q6-8h. ▶KL **9**B ▶+ $$$$$

cefpodoxime (**Vantin**): 100-400 mg PO bid. Peds: 10 mg/kg/day divided bid. [Generic/trade: Tabs 100,200 mg. Trade: susp 50 & 100 mg/5 ml.] ▶K **9**B ▶? $$$$

ceftazidime (**Ceptaz, Fortaz, Tazicef**): 1 g IM/IV or 2 g IV q8-12h. Peds: 30-50 mg/kg IV q8h. ▶K **9**B ▶+ $$$$$

ceftibuten (**Cedax**): 400 mg PO daily. Peds: 9 mg/kg up to 400 mg PO daily. [Trade: Cap 400 mg, susp 90 mg/5 ml.] ▶K **9**B ▶? $$$$

ceftizoxime (**Cefizox**): 1-2 g IV q8-12h. Peds: 50 mg/kg/dose IV q6-8h. ▶K **9**B ▶? $$$$$

ceftriaxone (**Rocephin**): 1-2 g IM/IV q24h. Meningitis: 2 g IV q12h. Gonorrhea: single dose 125 mg IM (250 mg if PID). Peds: 50-75 mg/kg/day up to 2 g divided q12-24h. Meningitis: 100 mg/kg/day up to 4 g/day. Otitis media: 50 mg/kg up to 1 g IM single dose. Dilute in 1% lidocaine for IM. ▶K/Bile **9**B ▶+ $$$$$

Cephalosporins - 4th Generation

cefepime (**Maxipime**): 0.5-2 g IM/IV q12h. Peds: 50 mg/kg IV q8-12h. ▶K **9**B ▶? $$$$$

CEPHALOSPORINS – GENERAL ANTIMICROBIAL SPECTRUM

1st generation: gram positive (including Staph aureus); basic gram neg. coverage
2nd generation: diminished Staph aureus, improved gram negative coverage compared to 1st generation; some with anaerobic coverage
3rd generation: further diminished Staph aureus, further improved gram negative coverage compared to 1st & 2nd generation; some with Pseudomonal coverage & diminished gram positive coverage
4th generation: same as 3rd generation plus coverage against Pseudomonas

SEXUALLY TRANSMITTED DISEASES & VAGINITIS*

Bacterial vaginosis: 1) metronidazole 5 g of 0.75% gel intravaginally qd for 5 days. 2) metronidazole 500 mg PO bid for 7 days . 3) clindamycin 5 g of 2% cream intravaginally qhs for 7 days. In pregnancy: 1) metronidazole 250 mg PO tid for 7 days. 2) clindamycin 300 mg PO bid for 7 days.

Candidal vaginitis: 1) intravaginal clotrimazole, miconazole, terconazole, nystatin, tioconazole, or butoconazole. 2) fluconazole 150 mg PO single dose.

Chlamydia: 1) azithromycin 1 g PO single dose. 2) doxycycline 100 mg PO bid for 7 days. 3) ofloxacin 300 mg PO bid for 7 days. 4) levofloxacin 500 mg PO qd for 7 days. 5) erythromycin base 500 mg PO qid for 7 days.

Chlamydia (in pregnancy): 1) erythromycin base 500 mg PO qid for 7 days or 250 mg PO qid for 14 days. 2) amoxicillin 500 mg PO tid for 7 days). 3) azithromycin 1 g PO single dose.

Epididymitis: 1) ceftriaxone 250 mg IM single dose + doxycycline 100 mg PO bid x 10 days. 2) ofloxacin 300 mg PO bid or levofloxacin 500 mg PO qd for 10 days if enteric organisms suspected, cephalosporin/doxycycline allergic, or >35 yo.

Gonorrhea: Single dose of: 1) ceftriaxone 125 mg IM 2) cefixime 400 mg PO single dose 3) ciprofloxacin 500 mg PO 4) ofloxacin 400 mg PO or 5) levofloxacin 250 mg PO. Treat chlamydia empirically. Due to high resistance rates, quinolones not recommended for infections acquired in Hawaii, California, Asia, or Pacific islands, or in men who have sex with men.

Herpes simplex (genital, first episode): 1) acyclovir 400 mg PO tid for 7-10 days. 2) famciclovir 250 mg PO tid for 7-10 days. 3) valacyclovir 1 g PO bid for 7-10 days.

Herpes simplex (genital, recurrent): 1) acyclovir 400 mg PO tid for 5 days. 2) famciclovir 125 mg PO bid for 5 days. 3) valacyclovir 500 mg PO bid for 3-5 days. 4) valacyclovir 1 g PO qd for 5 days.

Herpes simplex (suppressive therapy): 1) acyclovir 400mg PO bid. 2) famciclovir 250 mg PO bid. 3) valacyclovir 500-1000 mg PO qd.

Herpes simplex (genital, recurrent in HIV infection): 1) Acyclovir 400 mg PO tid for 5-10 days. 2) famciclovir 500 mg PO bid for 5-10 days. 3) Valacyclovir 1 g PO bid for 5-10 days.

Herpes simplex (suppressive therapy in HIV infection): 1) Acyclovir 400-800 mg PO bid-tid. 2) Famciclovir 500 mg PO bid. 3) Valacyclovir 500 mg PO bid.

Herpes simplex (prevention of transmission in immunocompetent patients with ≤9 recurrences/year): Valacyclovir 500 mg PO qd by source partner, in conjunction with safer sex practices.†

Pelvic inflammatory disease (PID), outpatient treatment: 1) ceftriaxone 250 mg IM single dose + doxycycline 100 mg PO bid +/- metronidazole 500 mg PO bid for 14 days. 2) ofloxacin 400 mg PO bid/ levofloxacin 500 mg PO qd +/- metronidazole 500 mg PO bid for 14 days.

Sexual assault prophylaxis: ceftriaxone 125 mg IM single dose + metronidazole 2 g PO single dose + azithromycin 1 g PO single dose/doxycycline 100 mg PO bid for 7 days. Consider giving antiemetic.

Syphilis (primary and secondary): 1) benzathine penicillin 2.4 million units IM single dose. 2) doxycycline 100 mg PO bid for 2 weeks if penicillin allergic.

Trichomonal vaginitis: metronidazole 2 g PO single dose or 500 mg bid for 7days. Can use 2 g single dose in pregnant women.

Urethritis, Cervicitis: Test for chlamydia and gonorrhea. Treat based on test results or treat for both if testing not available or if patient unlikely to return for follow-up.

---

* MMWR 2002;51:RR-6 or http://www.cdc.gov/std/.   †NEJM 2004;350:11.
Treat sexual partners for all except herpes, candida, and bacterial vaginosis.

Ketolides

telithromycin (**Ketek**): 800 mg PO daily x 5 days for acute exacerbation of chronic bronchitis or acute sinusitis, x 7 days for community-acquired pneumonia. [Trade: 300,400 mg tabs. Ketek Pak: #10, 400 mg tabs.] ▶LK ♀C ▶? $$$

Macrolides

azithromycin (**Zithromax, Zmax**): 500 mg IV daily. PO: 10 mg/kg up to 500 mg on day 1, then 5 mg/kg up to 250 mg daily to complete 5 days. Group A streptococcal pharyngitis (second-line to penicillin): 12 mg/kg up to 500 mg PO daily x 5 d. Short regimens for peds otitis media (30 mg/kg PO single dose or 10 mg/kg PO daily x 3 days) and sinusitis (10 mg/kg PO daily x 3 days). Short regimen for adult acute sinusitis or exacerbation of chronic bronchitis: 500 mg PO daily x 3 days. Chlamydia, chancroid: 1 g PO single dose. Prevention of disseminated Mycobacterium avium complex disease: 1200 mg PO q week. Acute sinusitis in children: 10 mg/kg PO daily x 3 days. [Generic/Trade: Tab 250,500,600 mg. Trade only: Packet 1000 mg, susp 100 & 200 mg/5 ml. Tri-Pak: #3, 500 mg tab. Zmax extended release oral susp: 2 g in 60 ml single dose bottle.] ▶L ♀B ▶? $$$

clarithromycin (**Biaxin, Biaxin XL**): 250-500 mg PO bid. Peds: 7.5 mg/kg PO bid. H pylori: See table in GI section. See table for prophylaxis of bacterial endocarditis. Mycobacterium avium complex disease prevention: 7.5 mg/kg up to 500 mg PO bid. Biaxin XL: 1000 mg PO daily with food. [Generic/trade: Tab 250,500 mg. Extended release 500 mg. Trade only: susp 125, 250 mg/5 ml. Biaxin XL-Pak: #14, 500 mg tabs. Generic only: Extended release 1000 mg.] ▶KL ♀C ▶? $$$

erythromycin base (**Eryc, E-mycin, Ery-Tab, ✦Erybid, Erythromid, P.C.E.**): 250-500 mg PO qid, 333 mg PO tid, or 500 mg PO bid. Peds: 30-50 mg/kg/day PO divided qid. [Generic/Trade: Tab 250, 333, 500 mg, delayed-release cap 250.] ▶L ♀B ▶+ $

erythromycin ethyl succinate (**EES, Eryped**): 400 mg PO qid. Peds: 30-50 mg/kg/day divided qid. [Generic/Trade: Tab 400 tab, susp 200 & 400 mg/5 ml. Trade (EryPed): Susp 100 mg/2.5mL.] ▶L ♀B ▶+ $

erythromycin lactobionate, **✦Erythrocin IV**: 15-20 mg/kg/day (max 4g) IV divided q6h. Peds: 15-50 mg/kg/day IV divided q6h. ▶L ♀B ▶+ $$$$

Pediazole (erythromycin ethyl succinate + sulfisoxazole): 50 mg/kg/day (based on EES dose) PO divided tid-qid. [Generic/Trade: Susp, erythromycin ethyl succinate 200 mg + sulfisoxazole 600 mg/5 ml.] ▶KL ♀C ▶- $$$

PENICILLINS - GENERAL ANTIMICROBIAL SPECTRUM

1st generation: Most streptococci; oral anaerobic coverage
2nd generation: Most streptococci; Staph aureus
3rd generation: Most streptococci; basic gram negative coverage
4th generation: Pseudomonas

Penicillins - 1st generation - Natural

benzathine penicillin (**Bicillin L-A, ✦Megacillin**): 1.2 million units IM. Peds <27 kg 0.3-0.6 MU IM, ≥27 kg 0.9 MU IM. Doses last 2-4 wks. [Trade: for IM use, 600,000 units/ml; 1, 2, and 4 ml syringes.] ▶K ♀B ▶? $$

benzylpenicilloyl polylysine (**Pre-Pen**): Skin test for penicillin allergy: 1 drop in needle scratch, then 0.01-0.02 ml intradermally if no reaction. ▶K ♀? ▶? $$

Bicillin C-R (procaine penicillin + benzathine penicillin): For IM use. Not for treatment of syphilis. [Trade: for IM use 300/300 thousand units procaine/benzathine penicillin; 1, 2, and 4 ml syringes.] ▶K ♀B ▶? $$$

penicillin G: Pneumococcal pneumonia & severe infections: 250,000-400,000 units/kg/day (8-12 million in adult) IV divided q4-6h. Pneumococcal meningitis: 250,000 units/kg/day (24 million U in an adult) IV divided q2-4h. ▶K ♀B ▶? $$$

penicillin V (**Pen-Vee K, Veetids, ✚PVF-K, Nadopen-V**): Adults: 250-500 mg PO qid. Peds: 25-50 mg/kg/day divided bid-qid. AHA doses for pharyngitis: 250 mg (peds) or 500 mg (adults) PO bid-tid x 10 days. [Generic/Trade: Tabs 250,500 mg, oral soln 125 & 250 mg/5 ml.] ▶K ♀B ▶? $

procaine penicillin (**Wycillin**): 0.6-1.0 million units IM daily (peak 4h, lasts 24h). ▶K ♀B ▶? $$$$

Penicillins - 2nd generation - Penicillinase-Resistant

dicloxacillin (**Dynapen**): 250-500 mg PO qid. Peds: 12.5-25 mg/kg/day divided qid. [Generic: Caps 250,500 mg. Trade: Susp 62.5 mg/5 ml.] ▶KL ♀B ▶? $$

nafcillin: 1-2 g IM/IV q4h. Peds: 50-200 mg/kg/day divided q4-6h. ▶L ♀B ▶? $$$$$

oxacillin (**Bactocill**): 1-2 g IM/IV q4-6h. Peds 150-200 mg/kg/day IM/IV divided q4-6h. ▶KL ♀B ▶? $$$$$

Penicillins - 3rd generation - Aminopenicillins

amoxicillin (**Amoxil, DisperMox, Polymox, Trimox, ✚Novamoxin**): 250-500 mg PO tid, or 500-875 mg PO bid. Acute sinusitis with antibiotic use in past month &/or drug-resistant S pneumoniae rate >30%: 3-3.5 g/day PO. High-dose for community-acquired pneumonia: 1 g PO tid. Peds AAP otitis media: 80-90 mg/kg/day divided bid-tid. AAP recommends 5-7 days of therapy for older (≥6 yo) children with non-severe otitis media, and 10 days for younger children and those with severe disease. Peds non-otitis: 40 mg/kg/day PO divided tid or 45 mg/kg/day divided bid. [Generic/Trade: Caps 250,500 mg, tabs 500,875 mg, chews 125,200, 250,400mg, susp 125, 250 mg/5 ml, susp 200 & 400 mg/5 ml. Trade: Infant drops 50 mg/ml (Amoxil). DisperMox 200,400,600 mg tabs for oral susp.] ▶K ♀B ▶+ $

PROPHYLAXIS FOR BACTERIAL ENDOCARDITIS*

For dental, oral, respiratory tract, or esophageal procedures	
Standard regimen	amoxicillin[1] 2 g PO 1h before procedure
Unable to take oral meds	ampicillin[1] 2 g IM/IV within 30 minutes before procedure
Allergic to penicillin	clindamycin[2] 600 mg PO; or cephalexin[1] or cefadroxil[1] 2 g PO; or azithromycin[3] or clarithromycin[3] 500 mg PO 1h before procedure
Allergic to penicillin and unable to take oral meds	clindamycin[2] 600 mg IV; or cefazolin[4] 1 g IM/IV within 30 minutes before procedure
For genitourinary and gastrointestinal (excluding esophageal) procedures	
High-risk patients	ampicillin[1] 2 g IM/IV plus gentamicin 1.5 mg/kg (max 120 mg) within 30 min of starting procedure; 6h later ampicillin[1] 1 g IM/IV or amoxicillin[1] 1 g PO.
High-risk patients allergic to ampicillin	vancomycin[2] 1 g IV over 1-2h plus gentamicin 1.5 mg/kg IV/IM (max 120 mg) complete within 30 minutes of starting procedure
Moderate-risk patients	amoxicillin[1] 2 g PO or ampicillin[1] 2 g IM/IV within 30 minutes of starting procedure
Moderate-risk patients allergic to ampicillin	vancomycin[2] 1 g IV over 1-2h complete within 30 minutes of starting procedure

*JAMA 1997; 277:1794-1801 or http://www.americanheart.org
Footnotes for pediatric doses: 1 = 50 mg/kg; 2 = 20 mg/kg; 3 = 15 mg/kg; 4 = 25 mg/kg. Total pediatric dose should not exceed adult dose.

amoxicillin-clavulanate (*Augmentin, Augmentin ES-600, Augmentin XR, ♣Clavulin*): 500-875 mg PO bid or 250-500 mg tid. Augmentin XR: 2 tabs PO q12h with meals. Peds AAP otitis media: Augmentin ES 90 mg/kg/day divided bid. AAP recommends 5-7 days of therapy for older (≥6 yo) children with non-severe otitis media, and 10 days for younger children and those with severe disease. Peds: 45 mg/kg/day PO divided bid or 40 mg/kg/day divided tid for otitis, sinusitis, pneumonia; 25 mg/kg/day divided bid or 20 mg/kg/day divided tid for less severe infections. [Generic/Trade: (amoxicillin + clavulanate) Tabs 500+125, 875+125 mg, chewables and susp 200+28.5, 400+57, mg per tab or 5 mL, (ES) susp 600+ 42.9 mg/5mL Trade only: Tabs 250+125 mg, chewables and susp 125+31.25, 250+62.5 mg per tab or 5 mL. Extended-release tabs (Augmentin XR) 1000+62.5 mg.] ▶K ♀B ▶? $$$

ampicillin (*Principen, ♣Penbritin*): Usual dose: 1-2 g IV q4-6h. Sepsis, meningitis: 150-200 mg/kg/day IV divided q3-4h. Peds: 50-400 mg/kg/day IM/IV divided q4-6h. [Generic/Trade: Caps 250,500 mg, susp 125 & 250 mg/5 ml.] ▶K ♀B ▶? $ PO $$$$$ IV

ampicillin-sulbactam (*Unasyn*): 1.5-3 g IM/IV q6h. Peds: 100-400 mg/kg/day of ampicillin divided q6h. ▶K ♀B ▶? $$$$$

pivampicillin (*Pondocillin*): Canada only. Adults: 500-1000 mg PO bid. Infants, 3-12 mo: 40-60 mg/kg/day PO divided BID. Peds, 1-10 yo: 25-35 mg/kg/day PO divided bid up to 525 mg PO bid. [Trade: Tabs 500 mg (377 mg ampicillin), # 20, oral susp 35 mg/ml (26 mg ampicillin), 100,150,200 ml bottles.] ▶K ♀? ▶? $

Penicillins - 4th generation - Extended Spectrum

piperacillin: 3-4 g IM/IV q4-6h. ▶K/Bile ♀B ▶? $$$$$

piperacillin-tazobactam (*Zosyn, ♣Tazocin*): 3.375-4.5 g IV q6h. Peds: 240 mg/kg/day of piperacillin IV divided q8h. ▶K ♀B ▶? $$$$$

ticarcillin (*Ticar*): 3-4 g IM/IV q4-6h. Peds: 200-300 mg/kg/d divided q4-6h. ▶K ♀B ▶+ $$$$$

ticarcillin-clavulanate (*Timentin*): 3.1 g IV q4-6h. Peds: 50 mg/kg up to 3.1 g IV q4-6h. ▶K ♀B ▶? $$$$$

Quinolones - 1st Generation

nalidixic acid (*NegGram*): 1 g PO qid. [Trade: Tabs 0.25,0.5,1 g.] ▶KL ♀C ▶? $$$$

Quinolones - 2nd Generation

ciprofloxacin (*Cipro, Cipro XR, Proquin XR*): 200-400 mg IV q8-12h. 250-750 mg PO bid. Simple UTI: 250 mg bid x 3d or Cipro XR/Proquin XR 500 mg PO daily x 3d. Give Proquin XR with main meal of day. Cipro XR for pyelonephritis or complicated UTI: 1000 mg PO daily x 7-14 days. Gonorrhea: 500 mg PO single dose (not for infections acquired in California, Hawaii, Asia, or Pacific islands, or in men who have sex with men). [Generic/Trade: Susp 250 & 500 mg/5 ml. Tabs 100,250,500,750 mg. Trade: Extended release tabs (Cipro XR) 500, 1000 mg.] ▶LK ♀C but teratogenicity unlikely ▶?+ $$$$

lomefloxacin (*Maxaquin*): 400 mg PO daily. Take at night. Photosensitivity. [Trade: Tabs 400 mg.] ▶LK ♀C ▶? $$$

norfloxacin (*Noroxin*): Simple UTI: 400 mg PO bid x 3 days. [Trade: Tabs 400 mg.] ▶LK ♀C ▶? $$$

ofloxacin (*Floxin*): 200-400 mg IV/PO q12h. [Generic/Trade: Tabs 200,300,400 mg.] ▶LK ♀C ▶?+ $$$

QUINOLONES- GENERAL ANTIMICROBIAL SPECTRUM

1st generation: gram negative (excluding Pseudomonas), urinary tract only, no atypicals

2nd generation: gram negative (including Pseudomonas); Staph aureus but not pneumococcus; some atypicals

3rd generation: gram negative (including Pseudomonas); gram positive (including Staph aureus and pneumococcus); expanded atypical coverage

4th generation: same as 3rd generation plus enhanced coverage of pneumococcus, decreased activity vs. Pseudomonas.

Quinolones - 3rd Generation

levofloxacin (**Levaquin**): 250-750 mg PO/IV daily. [Generic/Trade: Tabs 250,500,750 mg. Trade: oral sol'n 25 mg/mL. Leva-Pak: #5, 750 mg tabs.] ▶KL ♀C ▶? $$$

Quinolones - 4th Generation

gatifloxacin (**Tequin**): 400 mg IV/PO daily. Simple UTI: 400 mg PO single dose or 200 mg PO daily x 3 d. Gonorrhea: 400 mg PO single dose (not for infections acquired in California, Hawaii, Asia, or Pacific islands, or in men who have sex with men). [Trade: Tabs 200,400 mg. Susp 200 mg/5 mL. Teq-Paq: #5, 400 mg tabs.] ▶K ♀C ▶- $$$

gemifloxacin (**Factive**): 320 mg PO daily x 5-7 days. [Trade: Tabs 320 mg.] ▶Feces, K ♀C ▶- $$$

moxifloxacin (**Avelox**): 400 mg PO/IV daily x 5 days (chronic bronchitis exacerbation), 7 days (uncomplicated skin infections), 10 days (acute sinusitis), 7-14 days (community acquired pneumonia), 7-21 days (complicated skin infections). [Trade: Tabs 400 mg.] ▶LK ♀C ▶- $$$

Sulfonamides

sulfadiazine: CNS toxoplasmosis in AIDS. 1000 mg (<60 kg) to 1500 mg (≥60 kg) PO qid for acute tx; 500-1000 mg PO qid for secondary prevention. Give with pyrimethamine + leucovorin. [Generic: Tab 500 mg.] ▶K ♀C ▶+ $$$$

trimethoprim-sulfamethoxazole (**Bactrim, Septra, Sulfatrim, cotrimoxazole**): One tab PO bid, double strength (DS, 160 mg/800 mg) or single strength (SS, 80 mg/400 mg). Pneumocystis treatment: 15-20 mg/kg/day (based on TMP) IV divided q6-8h or PO divided tid x 21 days total. Pneumocystis prophylaxis: 1 DS tab PO daily. Peds: 5 ml susp/10 kg (up to 20 ml)/dose PO bid. [Generic/Trade: Tabs 80 mg TMP/400 mg SMX (single strength), 160 mg TMP/800 mg SMX (double strength; DS), susp 40 mg TMP/200 mg SMX per 5 ml. 20 ml susp = 2 SS tabs = 1 DS tab.] ▶K ♀C ▶+ $

Tetracyclines

doxycycline (**Adoxa, Vibramycin, Doryx, Monodox, Periostat, ✚Doxycin**): 100 mg PO bid on first day, then 50 mg bid or 100 mg daily. 100 mg PO/IV bid for severe infections. Periostat for periodontitis: 20 mg PO bid. [Generic/Trade: Tabs 75,100 mg, caps 50,100 mg. Trade: Susp 25 mg/5 ml, syrup 50 mg/5 ml, Periostat: Tabs 20 mg.] ▶LK ♀D ▶?+ $

minocycline (**Minocin, Dynacin**): 200 mg IV/PO initially, then 100 mg q12h. [Generic/Trade: Caps, tabs 50,75,100 mg. Trade: Susp 50 mg/5 ml.] ▶LK ♀D ▶?+ $

tetracycline (**Sumycin**): 250-500 mg PO qid. [Generic/Trade: Caps 250,500 mg. Trade: Tabs 250, 500 mg, susp 125 mg/5 ml.] ▶LK ♀D ▶?+ $

Other Antimicrobials

aztreonam (Azactam): 0.5-2 g IM/IV q6-12h. Peds: 30 mg/kg q6-8h. ▶K ♀B ▶+ $$$$$

chloramphenicol (Chloromycetin): 50-100 mg/kg/day IV divided q6h. Aplastic anemia. ▶LK ♀C ▶- $$$$$

clindamycin (Cleocin, ✚Dalacin C): 600-900 mg IV q8h. Each IM injection should be ≤600 mg. 150-450 mg PO qid. Peds: 20-40 mg/kg/day IV divided q6-8h or 8-25 mg/kg/day PO divided tid-qid. [Generic/Trade: Cap 75,150,300 mg. Trade: Oral soln 75 mg/5 ml.] ▶L ♀B ▶?+ $$$

daptomycin (Cubicin, Cidecin): 4 mg/kg IV daily infused over 30 min x 7-14 days. ▶K ♀B ▶? $$$$$

drotrecogin (Xigris): To reduce mortality in sepsis: 24 mcg/kg/h IV x 96 h. ▶Plasma ♀C ▶? $$$$$

fosfomycin (Monurol): Simple UTI: One 3 g packet PO single-dose. [Trade: 3 g packet of granules.] ▶K ♀B ▶? $$

linezolid (Zyvox, ✚Zyvoxam): 400-600 mg IV/PO q12 h. Infuse over 30-120 minutes. Peds: 10 mg/kg IV/PO q8h. Uncomplicated skin infections: 10 mg/kg PO q8h if <5 yo, q12h if 5-11 yo. Myelosuppression. MAO inhibitor. [Trade: Tabs 600 mg, susp 100 mg/5 ml.] ▶Oxidation/K ♀C ▶? $$$$$

metronidazole (Flagyl, ✚Florazole ER, Trikacide, Nidazol): Bacterial vaginosis: 500 mg PO bid x 7 days or Flagyl ER 750 mg PO daily x 7 days. H pylori: See table in GI section. Anaerobic bacterial infections: Load 1 g or 15 mg/kg IV, then 500 mg or 7.5 mg/kg IV/PO q6h, each IV dose over 1h (not to exceed 4 g/day). Peds: 7.5 mg/kg IV q6h. C difficile diarrhea: 500 mg (10-15 mg/kg/dose for peds) PO tid. [Generic/Trade: Tabs 250,500 mg, ER tabs 750 mg, Caps 375 mg.] ▶KL ♀B ▶?- $

nitrofurantoin (Furadantin, Macrodantin, Macrobid): 50-100 mg PO qid. Peds: 5-7 mg/kg/day divided qid. Sustained release: 100 mg PO bid. [Macrodantin: Caps 25,50,100 mg. Generic: Caps 50,100 mg. Furadantin: Susp 25 mg/5 ml. Macrobid: Caps 100 mg.] ▶KL ♀B ▶+? $$

rifampin (Rimactane, Rifadin, ✚Rofact): Neisseria meningitidis carriers: 600 mg PO bid x 2 days. Peds: age ≥1 mo, 10 mg/kg up to 600 mg PO bid x 2 days. Age <1 mo, 5 mg/kg PO bid x 2 days. IV & PO doses are the same. [Generic/Trade: Caps 150,300 mg. Pharmacists can make oral suspension.] ▶L ♀C ▶+ $$$$

rifaximin (Xifaxan): Travelers diarrhea: 200 mg PO tid x 3 days. [Trade: Tab 200 mg.] ▶Feces, no GI absorption ♀C ▶? $$$

Synercid (quinupristin + dalfopristin): 7.5 mg/kg IV q8-12 h, each dose over 1 h. Not active against E. faecalis. ▶Bile ♀B ▶? $$$$$

tigecycline (Tygacil): Complicated skin or intra-abdominal infections: 100 mg IV first dose, then 50 mg IV q12h. Infuse over 30-60 minutes. ▶Bile, K ♀D ▶?+ ?

trimethoprim (Primsol, ✚Proloprim): 100 mg PO bid or 200 mg PO daily. [Generic: Tabs 100,200 mg. Primsol: Oral soln 50 mg/5 ml.] ▶K ♀C ▶- $

vancomycin (Vancocin): 1g IV q12h, each dose over 1h. Peds: 10-15 mg/kg IV q6h. Clostridium difficile diarrhea: 40-50 mg/kg/day up to 500 mg/day PO divided qid x 7-10 days. IV administration ineffective for this indication. [Trade: Caps 125, 250 mg] ▶K ♀C ▶? $$$$$

CARDIOVASCULAR

ACE Inhibitors

NOTE: See also antihypertensive combos. Hyperkalemia possible. Renoprotection and decreased cardiovascular morbidity/mortality seen with some ACE inhibitors are most likely a class effect.

ACE INHIBITOR DOSING	Hypertension		Heart Failure		
	Initial	Max/day	Initial	Target	Max
benazepril (*Lotensin*)	10 mg qd*	80 mg	-	-	-
captopril (*Capoten*)	25 mg bid/tid	450 mg	6.25-12.5 mg tid	50 mg bid	150 mg tid
enalapril (*Vasotec*)	5 mg qd*	40 mg	2.5 mg bid	10 mg bid	20 mg bid
fosinopril (*Monopril*)	10 mg qd*	80 mg	10 mg qd	20 mg qd	40 mg qd
lisinopril (*Zestril/Prinivil*)	10 mg qd*	80 mg	5 mg qd	20 mg qd	40 mg qd
moexipril (*Univasc*)	7.5 mg qd*	30-60 mg	-	-	-
perindopril (Aceon)	4 mg qd*	16 mg	-	-	-
quinapril (*Accupril*)	10-20 mg qd*	80 mg	5 mg bid	10 mg bid	20 mg bid
ramipril (*Altace*)	2.5 mg qd*	20 mg	2.5 mg bid	5 mg bid	10 mg bid
trandolapril (*Mavik*)	1-2 mg qd*	8 mg	1 mg qd	4 mg qd	4 mg qd

Data taken from prescribing information.   *May require bid dosing for 24-hour BP control.*

benazepril (*Lotensin*): HTN: Start 10 mg PO daily, usual maintenance dose 20-40 mg PO daily or divided bid, max 80 mg/day. [Generic/Trade: Tabs, non-scored 5,10,20,40 mg.] ▶LK ♀C (1st trimester) D (2nd & 3rd) ▶? $$

captopril (*Capoten*): HTN: Start 25 mg PO bid-tid, usual maintenance dose 25-150 mg bid-tid, max 450 mg/day. Heart failure: Start 6.25-12.5 mg PO tid, usual dose 50-100 mg PO tid, max 450 mg/day. Diabetic nephropathy: 25 mg PO tid. [Generic/Trade: Tabs, scored 12.5,25,50,100 mg.] ▶LK ♀C (1st trimester) D (2nd & 3rd) ▶+ $

cilazapril (♣*Inhibace*): Canada only. HTN: 1.25-10 mg PO daily. [Trade: Scored tabs 1, 2.5, 5 mg.] ▶LK ♀C (1st trimester) D (2nd & 3rd) ▶? $

enalapril (*enalaprilat, Vasotec*): HTN: Start 5 mg PO daily, usual maintenance dose 10-40 mg PO daily or divided bid, max 40 mg/day. If oral therapy not possible, can use 1.25 mg IV q6h over 5 minutes, and increase up to 5 mg IV q6h if needed. Renal impairment or concomitant diuretic therapy: Start 2.5 mg PO daily. Heart failure: Start 2.5 mg PO daily, usual 10-20 mg PO bid, max 40 mg/day. [Generic/Trade: Tabs, scored 2.5,5, non-scored 10, 20 mg.] ▶LK ♀C (1st trimester) D (2nd & 3rd) ▶+ $

fosinopril (*Monopril*): HTN: Start 10 mg PO daily, usual maintenance dose 20-40 mg PO daily or divided bid, max 80 mg/day. Heart failure: Start 10 mg PO daily, usual dose 20-40 mg PO daily, max 40 mg/day. [Generic/Trade: Tabs, scored 10, non-scored 20,40 mg.] ▶LK ♀C (1st trimester) D (2nd & 3rd) ▶? $$

lisinopril (*Prinivil, Zestril*): HTN: Start 10 mg PO daily, usual maintenance dose 20-40 mg PO daily, max 80 mg/day. Heart failure, acute MI: Start 2.5-5 mg PO daily, usual dose 5-20 mg PO daily, max dose 40 mg. [Generic/Trade: Tabs, non-scored 2.5,10,20,30,40, scored 5 mg.] ▶K ♀C (1st trimester) D (2nd & 3rd) ▶? $$

moexipril (*Univasc*): HTN: Start 7.5 mg PO daily, usual maintenance dose 7.5-30 mg PO daily or divided bid, max 30 mg/day. [Generic/Trade: Tabs, scored 7.5, 15 mg.] ▶LK ♀C (1st trimester) D (2nd & 3rd) ▶? $

perindopril (*Aceon*, ♣*Coversyl*): HTN: Start 4 mg PO daily, usual maintenance dose 4-8 mg PO daily or divided bid, max 16 mg/day. [Trade: Tabs, scored 2,4,8 mg.] ▶K ♀C (1st trimester) D (2nd & 3rd) ▶? $$

quinapril (*Accupril*): HTN: Start 10-20 mg PO daily (start 10 mg/day if elderly), usual maintenance dose 20-80 mg PO daily or divided bid, max 80 mg/day. Heart failure: Start 5 mg PO daily, usual 10-20 mg bid. [Generic/Trade: tabs, scored 5, non-scored 10,20,40 mg.] ▶LK ♀C (1st trimester) D (2nd & 3rd) ▶? $$

ramipril (*Altace*): HTN: 2.5 mg PO daily, usual maintenance dose 2.5-20 mg PO daily or divided bid, max 20 mg/day. Heart failure post-MI: Start 2.5 mg PO bid, usual maintenance dose 5 mg PO bid. Reduce risk of MI, stroke, death from cardiovascular causes: 2.5 mg PO daily x 1 week, then 5 mg daily x 3 weeks, increase as tolerated to max 10 mg/day. [Trade: Caps, 1.25,2.5,5,10 mg] ▶LK ♀C (1st trimester) D (2nd & 3rd) ▶? $$

trandolapril (*Mavik*): HTN: Start 1 mg PO daily, usual maintenance dose 2-4 mg PO daily or divided bid, max 8 mg/day. Heart failure/post-MI: Start 0.5-1 mg PO daily, usual maintenance dose 4 mg PO daily. [Trade: Tabs, scored 1, non-scored 2,4 mg.] ▶LK ♀C (1st trimester) D (2nd & 3rd) ▶? $$

Aldosterone Antagonists

eplerenone (*Inspra*): HTN: Start 50 mg PO daily; max 50 mg bid. Improve survival of stable patients with left ventricular systolic dysfunction (EF ≤40%) and heart failure post-MI: Start 25 mg PO daily; titrate to target dose 50 mg daily within 4 weeks, if tolerated. [Trade: Tabs non-scored 25, 50 mg] ▶L ♀B ▶? $$$$

spironolactone (*Aldactone*): HTN: 50-100 mg PO daily or divided bid. Edema: 25-200 mg/day. Hypokalemia: 50-100 mg PO daily. Primary hyperaldosteronism, maintenance: 100-400 mg PO daily. Cirrhotic ascites: Start 100 mg once daily or in divided doses. Maintenance 25-200 mg/day. [Generic/Trade: Tabs, non-scored 25; scored 50,100 mg.] ▶LK ♀D ▶+ $

Angiotensin Receptor Blockers (ARBs)

candesartan (*Atacand*): HTN: Start 16 mg PO daily, maximum 32 mg/day. Reduce cardiovascular death and hospitalizations from heart failure (NYHA II-IV and ejection fraction ≤40%): Start 4 mg PO daily, maximum 32 mg/day; has added effect when used with ACE inhibitor. [Trade: Tabs, non-scored 4,8,16,32 mg.] ▶K ♀C (1st trimester) D (2nd & 3rd) ▶? $$

eprosartan (*Teveten*): HTN: Start 600 mg PO daily, maximum 800 mg/day given daily or divided bid. [Trade: tabs non-scored 400, 600 mg.] ▶Fecal excretion ♀C (1st trimester) D (2nd & 3rd) ▶? $$

irbesartan (*Avapro*): HTN: Start 150 mg PO daily, maximum 300 mg/day. Type 2 diabetic nephropathy: Start 150 mg PO daily, target dose 300 mg daily. [Trade: Tabs, non-scored 75,150,300 mg.] ▶L ♀C (1st trimester) D (2nd & 3rd) ▶? $$

losartan (*Cozaar*): HTN: Start 50 mg PO daily, max 100 mg/day given daily or divided bid. Stroke risk reduction in patients with HTN & left ventricular hypertrophy (may not occur in Blacks): Start 50 mg PO daily. If need more BP reduction: add HCTZ 12.5 mg PO daily; then increase losartan to 100 mg, then increase HCTZ to 25 mg/day. Type 2 diabetic nephropathy: Start 50 mg PO daily, target dose 100 mg daily. [Trade: Tabs, non-scored 25,50,100 mg.] ▶L ♀C (1st trimester) D (2nd & 3rd) ▶? $$

olmesartan (*Benicar*): HTN: Start 20 mg PO daily, max 40 mg/day. [Trade: Tabs, non-scored 5,20,40 mg.] ▶K ♀C (1st trimester) D (2nd & 3rd) ▶? $$

telmisartan (*Micardis*): HTN: Start 40 mg PO daily, maximum 80 mg/day. [Trade: Tabs, non-scored 20,40,80 mg.] ▶L ♀C (1st trimester) D (2nd & 3rd) ▶? $$

valsartan (*Diovan*): HTN: Start 80-160 mg PO daily, max 320 mg/day. Heart failure: Start 40 mg PO bid, target dose 160 mg bid; provides no added effect when used with adequate dose of ACE inhibitor. Reduce mortality/morbidity post-MI with LV systolic dysfunction/failure: Start 20 mg PO bid, target dose 160 mg bid. [Trade: Tabs, nonscored 80, 160, 320 mg.] ▶L ♀C (1st trimester) D (2nd & 3rd) ▶? $$$

Antiadrenergic Agents

clonidine (*Catapres*, ♥*Dixarit*): HTN: Start 0.1 mg PO bid, usual maintenance dose 0.2 to 1.2 mg/day divided bid-tid, max 2.4 mg/day. Rebound HTN with abrupt discontinuation, especially at doses ≥0.8 mg/d. Transdermal (Catapres-TTS): Start 0.1 mg/24 hour patch q week, titrate to desired effect, max effective dose 0.6 mg/24 hour (two, 0.3 mg/24 hour patches). [Generic/Trade: Tabs, non-scored 0.1, 0.2, 0.3 mg. Trade only: transdermal weekly patch 0.1 mg/day (TTS-1), 0.2 mg/day (TTS-2), 0.3 mg/day (TTS-3).] ▶LK ♀C ▶? $

doxazosin (*Cardura, Cardura XL*): HTN: Start 1 mg PO qhs, max 16 mg/day. Take first dose at bedtime to minimize orthostatic hypotension. See urology section. Extended release form is not FDA approved for HTN. [Generic/Trade: Tabs, scored 1,2,4,8 mg. Trade only: XL tabs 4,8 mg.] ▶L ♀C ▶? $

guanfacine (*Tenex*): HTN: Start 1 mg PO qhs, increase to 2-3 mg qhs if needed after 3-4 weeks, max 3 mg/day. ADHD in children: Start 0.5 mg PO daily, titrate by 0.5 mg q3-4 days as tolerated to 0.5 mg PO tid. [Generic/Trade: Tabs, non-scored 1,2 mg.] ▶K ♀B ▶? $

methyldopa (*Aldomet*): HTN: Start 250 mg PO bid-tid, maximum 3000 mg/day. May cause hemolytic anemia. [Generic/Trade: Tabs, non-scored 500 mg. Generic: Tabs, non-scored 125, 250 mg.] ▶LK ♀B ▶+ $

prazosin (*Minipress*): HTN: Start 1 mg PO bid-tid, max 40 mg/day. Take first dose at bedtime to minimize orthostatic hypotension. [Generic/Trade: Caps 1,2,5 mg.] ▶L ♀C ▶? $

terazosin (*Hytrin*): HTN: Start 1 mg PO qhs, usual effective dose 1-5 mg PO daily or divided bid, max 20 mg/day. Take first dose at bedtime to minimize orthostatic hypotension. [Generic (Caps, Tabs)/Trade (Caps): 1,2,5,10 mg.] ▶LK ♀C ▶? $$

Anti-Dysrhythmics / Cardiac Arrest

adenosine (*Adenocard*): PSVT conversion (not A-fib): Adult and peds ≥50 kg: 6 mg rapid IV & flush, preferably through a central line. If no response after 1-2 mins then 12 mg. A third dose of 12 mg may be given prn. Peds <50 kg: initial dose 50-100 mcg/kg, subsequent doses 100-200 mcg/kg q1-2 min prn up to a max single dose of 300 mcg/kg or 12 mg. Half-life is <10 seconds. Give doses by rapid IV push followed by normal saline flush. Need higher dose if on theophylline or caffeine, lower dose if on dipyridamole or carbamazepine. ▶Plasma ♀C ▶? $$$

amiodarone (*Cordarone, Pacerone*): Life-threatening ventricular arrhythmia without cardiac arrest: Load 150 mg IV over 10 min, then 1 mg/min x 6h, then 0.5 mg/min x 18h. Mix in D5W. Oral loading dose 800-1600 mg PO daily for 1-3 weeks, reduce to 400-800 mg PO daily for 1 month when arrhythmia is controlled, reduce to lowest effective dose thereafter, usually 200-400 mg PO daily. Photosensitivity with oral therapy. Pulmonary & hepatic toxicity. Hypo or hyperthyroidism possible. Co-administration of fluoroquinolones, macrolides, or azoles may prolong QTc. May increase digoxin levels; discontinue digoxin or decrease dose by 50%. May increase INR with warfarin by 100%; decrease warfarin dose by 33-50%. Do not use with grapefruit juice. Caution with simvastatin >20 mg/day or lovastatin >40 mg/day; may cause myopathy and rhabdomyolysis. Caution with beta blockers and calcium channel blockers. IV therapy may cause hypotension. Contraindicated with marked sinus bradycardia and second or third degree heart block in the absence of a functioning pacemaker. [Generic: Tabs, scored 300 mg. Generic/Trade: Tabs, scored 200; unscored 100,400 mg.] ▶L ♀D ▶- $$$$

atropine: Bradyarrhythmia/CPR: 0.5-1.0 mg IV q3-5 min to max 0.04 mg/kg. Peds: 0.02 mg/kg/dose; minimum single dose, 0.1 mg; max cumulative dose, 1 mg. ▶K ♀C ▶- $

bicarbonate: Severe acidosis: 1 mEq/kg IV up to 50-100 mEq/dose. Prevention of contrast-induced nephropathy: Administer sodium bicarbonate 154 mEq/L soln at 3 ml/kg/hr IV x 1h before contrast, followed by infusion of 1 ml/kg/hr x 6 hrs post-procedure. If >110 kg dose based on 110 kg weight. ▶K ♀C ▷? $

digoxin (**Lanoxin, Lanoxicaps, Digitek, digitalis**): Atrial fibrillation/Systolic heart failure: 0.125-0.25 mg PO daily. Rapid A-fib: Load 0.5 mg IV, then 0.25 mg IV q6h x 2 doses, maintenance 0.125-0.375 mg IV/PO daily. [Generic/Trade: Tabs, scored (Lanoxin, Digitek) 0.125,0.25 mg; elixir 0.05 mg/mL. Trade only: Caps (Lanoxicaps), 0.05,0.1,0.2 mg.] ▶KL ♀C ▷+ $

digoxin immune Fab (**Digibind, Digifab**): Digoxin toxicity: 2-20 vials IV, one formula is: Number vials = (serum drug level in ng/mL) x (kg) / 100. ▶K ♀C ▷? $$$$$

disopyramide (**Norpace, Norpace CR, ✤Rythmodan, Rythmodan-LA**): Rarely indicated, consult cardiologist. Ventricular arrhythmia: 400-800 mg PO daily in divided doses (immediate-release, q6h or extended-release, q12h). Proarrhythmic. [Generic/Trade: Caps, immediate-release, 100,150 mg; extended-release 150 mg. Trade only: extended-release 100 mg.] ▶KL ♀C ▷+ $$$$

flecainide (**Tambocor**): Proarrhythmic. Prevention of paroxysmal atrial fib/flutter or PSVT, with symptoms & no structural heart disease: Start 50 mg PO q12h, may increase by 50 mg bid q4 days, max 300 mg/day. Use with AV nodal slowing agent (beta blocker, verapamil, diltiazem) to minimize risk of 1:1 atrial flutter. Life-threatening ventricular arrhythmias without structural heart disease: Start 100 mg PO q12h, may increase by 50 mg bid q 4 days, max 400 mg/day. With severe renal impairment (CrCl<35 mL/min): Start 50 mg PO bid. [Generic/Trade: Tabs, non-scored 50, scored 100,150 mg.] ▶K ♀C ▷- $$$$$

ibutilide (**Corvert**): Recent onset A-fib/flutter: 0.01 mg/kg up to 1 mg IV over 10 mins, may repeat once if no response after 10 additional minutes. Keep on cardiac monitor ≥4 hours. ▶K ♀C ▷? $$$$$

isoproterenol (**Isuprel**): Refractory bradycardia or third degree AV block: 0.02-0.06 mg IV bolus or infusion 2 mg in 250 ml D5W (8 mg/mL) at 5 mcg/min. 5 mcg/min = 37 mL/h. Peds: 0.05-2 mcg/kg/min. 10 kg: 0.1 mcg/kg/min = 8 mL/h. ▶LK ♀C ▷? $$

lidocaine (**Xylocaine, Xylocard**): Ventricular arrhythmia: Load 1 mg/kg IV, then 0.5 mg/kg q8-10min as needed to max 3 mg/kg. IV infusion: 4 gm in 500 mL D5W (8 mg/ml) at 1-4 mg/min. Peds: 20-50 mcg/kg/min. ▶LK ♀B ▷? $

mexiletine (**Mexitil**): Rarely indicated, consult cardiologist. Ventricular arrhythmia: Start 200 mg PO q8h with food or antacid, max dose 1,200 mg/day. Proarrhythmic. [Generic/Trade: Caps, 150,200,250 mg.] ▶L ♀C ▷- $$$

procainamide (**Procanbid, Pronestyl**): Ventricular arrhythmia: 500-1250 mg PO q6h or 50 mg/kg/day. Extended-release: 500-1000 mg PO q12h. Load 100 mg IV q10min or 20 mg/min (150 mL/h) until: 1) QRS widens >50%, 2) dysrhythmia suppressed, 3) hypotension, or 4) total of 17 mg/kg or 1000 mg. Infusion 2g in 250 ml D5W (8 mg/mL) at 2-6 mg/min (15-45 mL/h). Proarrhythmic. [Generic/Trade: Caps, immediate-release 250 mg; tabs, sustained-release, non-scored (Pronestyl SR). Generic only: tabs, sustained-release, non-scored (generic procainamide SR, q6h dosing) 750,1000 mg; caps, immediate-release 500 mg. Trade only: Tabs, immediate-release, non-scored (Pronestyl) 250,375,500 mg, extended-release, non-scored (Procanbid, q12h dosing) 500,1000 mg.] ▶LK ♀C ▷? $$$

propafenone (**Rythmol, Rythmol SR**): Proarrhythmic. Prevention of paroxysmal atrial fib/flutter or PSVT, with symptoms & no structural heart disease; or life-threatening ventricular arrhythmias: Start (immediate release) 150 mg PO q8h; may increase after 3-4 days to 225 mg PO q8h; max 900 mg/day. Prolong time to recurrence of symptomatic atrial fib without structural heart disease: 225 mg SR PO q12h, may increase ≥5 days to 325 mg PO q12h, max 425 mg q12h. Use with AV nodal slowing agent (beta blocker, verapamil, diltiazem) to minimize risk of 1:1 atrial flutter. [Generic/Trade: Tabs (immediate release), scored 150,225,300 mg; Trade: SR, capsules 225,325,425 mg.] ▸L ♀C ▸? $$$$

quinidine (**♣Biquin durules**): Arrhythmia: gluconate, extended-release: 324-648 mg PO q8-12h; sulfate, immediate-release: 200-400 mg PO q6-8h; sulfate, extended-release: 300-600 mg PO q8-12h. Proarrhythmic. [Generic gluconate: Tabs, extended-release non-scored 324 mg; Generic sulfate: Tabs, scored immediate-release 200,300 mg. Generic sulfate: Tabs, extended-release 300 mg.] ▸LK ♀C ▸? $$-gluconate, $-sulfate

sotalol (**Betapace, Betapace AF**, **♣Rylosol, Sotacor, Sotamol**): Ventricular arrhythmia (Betapace), A-fib/A-flutter (Betapace AF): Start 80 mg PO bid, max 640 mg/d. Proarrhythmic. [Generic/Trade: Tabs, scored 80,120,160,240 mg. Trade only: 80,120,160 mg (Betapace AF).] ▸K ♀B ▸- $$$$

Anti-Hyperlipidemic Agents - Bile Acid Sequestrants

cholestyramine (**Questran, Questran Light, Prevalite, LoCHOLEST, LoCHOLEST Light**): Elevated LDL cholesterol: Powder: Start 4 g PO daily-bid before meals, increase up to max 24 g/day. [Generic/Trade: Powder for oral suspension, 4 g cholestyramine resin / 9 g powder (Questran, LoCHOLEST), 4 g cholestyramine resin / 5 g powder (Questran Light), 4 g cholestyramine resin / 5.5 g powder (Prevalite, LoCHOLEST Light).] ▸Not absorbed ♀C ▸+ $

colesevelam (**Welchol**): Elevated LDL cholesterol: 3 Tabs bid with meals or 6 Tabs once daily with a meal, max dose 7 Tabs/day. [Trade: Tabs, non-scored, 625 mg.] ▸Not absorbed ♀B ▸+ $$$$

colestipol (**Colestid, Colestid Flavored**): Elevated LDL cholesterol: Tabs: Start 2 g PO daily-bid, max 16 g/day. Granules: Start 5 g daily-bid, max 30 g/day. [Trade: Tab 1 g. Granules for oral susp, 5 g / 7.5 g powder.] ▸Not absorbed ♀B ▸+ $$$

Anti-Hyperlipidemic Agents - HMG-CoA Reductase Inhibitors ("Statins")

NOTE: Hepatotoxicity - monitor LFTs initially, approximately 12 weeks after starting therapy, then annually or more frequently if indicated. Evaluate muscle symptoms & creatine kinase before starting therapy. Evaluate muscle symptoms 6-12 weeks after starting therapy & at each follow-up visit. Obtain creatine kinase when patient complains of muscle soreness, tenderness, weakness, or pain. These factors increase risk of myopathy: advanced age (especially >80, women >men); multisystem disease (eg, chronic renal insufficiency, especially due to diabetes); multiple medications; perioperative periods; alcohol abuse; grapefruit juice (>1 quart/day); specific concomitant medications: fibrates (especially gemfibrozil), nicotinic acid (rare), cyclosporine, erythromycin, clarithromycin, itraconazole, ketoconazole, protease inhibitors, nefazodone, verapamil, amiodarone. Weigh potential risk of combination therapy against potential benefit.

Advicor (lovastatin + niacin): Hyperlipidemia: 1 tab PO qhs with a low-fat snack. Establish dose using extended-release niacin first, or if already on lovastatin substitute combo product with lowest niacin dose. Aspirin or ibuprofen 30 min prior may decrease niacin flushing reaction. [Trade: Tabs, non-scored extended-release niacin/lovastatin 500/20, 750/20, 1000/20 mg.] ▸LK ♀X ▸- $$$

atorvastatin (**Lipitor**): Hyperlipidemia/prevention of cardiovascular disease: Start 10-40 mg PO daily, max 80 mg PO daily. [Trade: Tabs, non-scored 10,20,40,80 mg.] ▸L ♀X ▸- $$$

Caduet (amlodipine + atorvastatin): Simultaneous treatment of HTN and hypercholesterolemia: Establish dose using component drugs first. Dosing interval: daily [Trade: Tabs, 2.5/10, 2.5/20, 2.5/40, 5/10, 5/20, 5/40, 5/80, 10/10, 10/20, 10/40, 10/80 mg.] ▸L ♀X ▸- $$$$

fluvastatin (Lescol, Lescol XL): Hyperlipidemia: Start 20-80 mg PO qhs, max 80 mg daily or divided bid. Post percutaneous coronary intervention: 80 mg of extended release PO qhs, max 80 mg daily. [Trade: Caps, 20,40 mg; tab, extended-release, non-scored 80 mg.] ▶L ♀X ▶- $$$

lovastatin (Mevacor, Altocor, Altoprev): Reduced cardiovascular morbidity, hyperlipidemia: Start 20 mg PO q pm, max 80 mg/day daily or divided bid. [Generic/Trade: Tabs, non-scored 10,20,40 mg. Trade only: Tabs, extended-release (Altocor, Altoprev) 20,40,60 mg.] ▶L ♀X ▶- $$$

pravastatin (Pravachol): Primary/secondary prevention of coronary events, hyperlipidemia: Start 40 mg PO daily, max 80 mg/day. [Trade: Tabs, non-scored 10,20, 40,80 mg.] ▶L ♀X ▶- $$$

STATINS*

Minimum Dose for 30-40% LDL Reduction	LDL	LFT Monitoring**
atorvastatin 10 mg	-39%	B, 12 wk, semiannually
fluvastatin 40 mg bid	-36%	B, 8 wk
fluvastatin XL 80 mg	-35%	B, 8 wk
lovastatin 40 mg	-31%	B, 6 & 12 wk, semiannually
pravastatin 40 mg	-34%	B, prior to dose increase
rosuvastatin 5 mg	-45%	B, 12 wk, semiannually
simvastatin 20 mg	-38%	B, ***

*Adapted from *Circulation* 2004;110:227-239. Data taken from prescribing information for primary hypercholesterolemia. B=baseline, LDL=low-density lipoprotein, LFT=liver function tests. Will get ~6% decrease in LDL with every doubling of dose. **From prescribing info. ACC/AHA/NHLBI schedule for LFT monitoring: baseline, ~12 weeks after starting therapy, annually, when clinically indicated. Stop statin therapy if LFTs are >3 times upper limit of normal. ***Get LFTs prior to & 3 months after dose increase to 80 mg, then semiannually for first year.

LDL CHOLESTEROL GOALS[1]

Risk Category	LDL Goal	Lifestyle Changes[2]	Also Consider Meds at LDL (mg/dL)[3]
High risk: CHD or equivalent risk,[4] 10-year risk >20%	<100 (optional < 70)*	LDL ≥100**	≥100 (<100: consider Rx options)#
Moderately-high risk: 2+ risk factors,[5] 10-year risk 10-20%	<130 mg/dL	LDL ≥130**	≥130 (100-129: consider Rx options)##
Moderate risk: 2+ risk factors,[5] 10-year risk <10%	<130 mg/dL	LDL ≥130	≥160
Lower risk: 0 to 1 risk factor[5]	<160 mg/dL	LDL ≥160	≥190 (160-189: Rx optional)

1. CHD=coronary heart disease. LDL=low density lipoprotein. Adapted from NCEP: *JAMA* 2001; 285:2486; NCEP Report: Circulation 2004;110:227-239. All 10-year risks based upon Framingham stratification; calculator available at: http://hin.nhlbi.nih.gov/atpiii/calculator.asp?usertype=prof. 2. Dietary modification, weight reduction, exercise. 3. When using LDL lowering therapy, achieve at least 30-40% LDL reduction. 4. Equivalent risk defined as diabetes, other atherosclerotic disease (peripheral artery disease, abdominal aortic aneurysm, symptomatic carotid artery disease), or ≥2 risk factors such that 10 year risk >20%. 5. Risk factors: Cigarette smoking, HTN (BP≥140/90 mmHg or on antihypertensive meds), low HDL (<40 mg/dL), family hx of CHD (1° relative: ♂ <55 yo, ♀ <65 yo), age (♂ ≥45 yo, ♀ ≥55 yo). * For very high risk patients (CVD with: acute coronary syndrome; diabetes; 2+ risk factors for metabolic syndrome; or severe/ poorly controlled risk factors), consider LDL goal <70. **Regardless of LDL, lifestyle changes are indicated when lifestyle-related risk factors (obesity, physical inactivity, ↑TG, ↓ HDL, or metabolic syndrome) are present. # If baseline LDL <100, starting LDL lowering therapy is an option based on clinical trials. With ↑TG or ↓HDL, consider combining fibrate or nicotinic acid with LDL lowering drug. ## At baseline or after lifestyle changes - initiating therapy to achieve LDL <100 is an option based on clinical trials.

rosuvastatin (***Crestor***): Hyperlipidemia: Start 10 mg PO daily, max 40 mg/d. [Trade: tabs non-scored 5, 10, 20, 40 mg]. ▶L ♀X ▶- $$$

simvastatin (***Zocor***): Hyperlipidemia: Start 20-40 mg PO q pm, max 80 mg/day. High risk for coronary heart disease event: Start 40 mg PO q pm, max 80 mg/day. [Trade: Tabs, non-scored 5,10,20,40,80 mg.] ▶L ♀X ▶- $$$$

Vytorin (simvastatin + ezetimibe): Hyperlipidemia: Start 10/20 mg PO q pm, max 10/80 mg/day. Start 10/40 if need >55% LDL reduction. [Trade: Tabs, non-scored ezetimibe/simvastatin 10/10, 10/20, 10/40, 10/80 mg.] ▶L ♀X ▶- $$$

Anti-Hyperlipidemic Agents - Other

bezafibrate (❤***Bezalip***): Canada only. Hyperlipidemia/hypertriglyceridemia: 200 mg immediate release PO bid-tid, or 400 mg of sustained release PO daily. [Trade: Immediate release tab: 200 mg. Sustained release tab: 400 mg.] ▶K ♀D ▶- $$$

ezetimibe (***Zetia***, ❤***Ezetrol***): Hyperlipidemia: 10 mg PO daily. [Trade: Tabs non-scored 10 mg] ▶L ♀C ▶? $$$

fenofibrate (***Tricor, Lofibra, Antara, Triglide***, ❤***Lipidil Micro, Lipidil Supra***): Hypertriglyceridemia: Tricor tablets: 48-145 mg PO daily, max 145 mg daily. Triglide: 50-160 mg PO daily, max 160 mg daily. Generic tablets: 54-160 mg, max 160 mg daily. Lofibra or generic micronized capsules: 67-200 mg PO daily; max 200 mg daily. Antara micronized capsules: 43-130 mg PO daily; max 130 mg daily. Hypercholesterolemia/mixed dyslipidemia: Tricor tablets: 145 mg PO daily. Triglide: 160 mg PO daily. Generic tablets: 160 mg daily. Lofibra or generic micronized capsules 200 mg PO daily. Antara, micronized capsules: 130 mg PO daily. Micronized capsules should be taken with food. [Trade: Tricor tabs, non-scored 48,145 mg. Triglide tabs, non-scored 50, 160 mg. Antara micronized caps 43, 87, 130 mg. Generic tabs, non-scored 54, 160 mg. Generic/Trade (Lofibra) micronized caps, 67, 134, 200 mg.] ▶LK ♀C ▶- $$$

gemfibrozil (***Lopid***): Hypertriglyceridemia / primary prevention of coronary artery disease: 600 mg PO bid 30 minutes before meals. [Generic/Trade: Tabs, scored 600 mg.] ▶LK ♀C ▶? $$$

niacin (***nicotinic acid, vitamin B3, Niacor, Nicolar, Niaspan***): Hyperlipidemia: Start 50-100 mg PO bid-tid with meals, increase slowly, usual maintenance range 1.5-3 g/day, max 6 g/day. Extended-release (Niaspan): Start 500 mg qhs, increase monthly as needed up to max 2000 mg. Extended-release formulations not listed here may have greater hepatotoxicity. Titrate slowly and use aspirin or ibuprofen 30 minutes before niacin doses to decrease flushing reaction. [Generic (OTC): Tabs, scored 25,50,100,150,500 mg. Trade: Tabs, immediate-release, scored (Niacor), 500 mg; extended-release, non-scored (Niaspan), 500,750 mg. Trade/Generic: Tabs, ext'd-release, non-scored (Niaspan) 1000 mg.] ▶K ♀C ▶? $

Antihypertensive Combinations (See components for ▶ ♀ ▶)

NOTE: Dosage should first be adjusted by using each drug separately.

BY TYPE: <u>ACE Inhibitor/Diuretic:</u> *Accuretic, Capozide, Inhibace Plus, Lotensin HCT, Monopril HCT, Prinzide, Uniretic, Vaseretic, Zestoretic.* <u>ACE Inhibitor/Calcium Channel Blocker:</u> *Lexxel, Lotrel, Tarka.* <u>Angiotensin Receptor Blocker/Diuretic:</u> *Atacand HCT, Avalide, Benicar HCT, Diovan HCT, Hyzaar, Micardis HCT, Teveten HCT.* <u>Beta-blocker/Diuretic:</u> *Corzide, Inderide, Lopressor HCT, Tenoretic, Timolide, Ziac.* <u>Diuretic combinations:</u> *Aldactazide, Dyazide, Maxzide, Maxzide-25, Moduretic, Triazide.* <u>Diuretic/miscellaneous antihypertensive:</u> *Aldoril, Apresazide, Chlorpres, Diutensin-R, Enduronyl, Minizide, Rauzide, Renese-R, Ser-Ap-Es.* <u>Other:</u> *BiDil.*

BY NAME: Accuretic (quinapril + hydrochlorothiazide): Generic/Trade: Tabs, 10/12.5, 20/12.5, 20/25. **Aldactazide** (spironolactone + hydrochlorothiazide): Generic/Trade: Tabs, non-scored 25/25, scored 50/50 mg. **Aldoril** (methyldopa + hydrochlorothiazide): Generic/Trade: Tabs, non-scored 250/15 (Aldoril-15), 250/25 mg (Aldoril-25). Trade: Tabs, non-scored, 500/30 (Aldoril D30), 500/50 mg (Aldoril D50). **Apresazide** (hydralazine + hydrochlorothiazide): Generic only: Caps 25/25, 50/50 mg. **Atacand HCT** (candesartan + hydrochlorothiazide, ✦*Atacand Plus*): Trade: tab, non-scored 16/12.5, 32/12.5 mg. **Avalide** (irbesartan + hydrochlorothiazide): Trade: Tabs, non-scored 150/12.5, 300/12.5, 300/25 mg. **Benicar HCT** (olmesartan + hydrochlorothiazide): Trade: Tabs, non-scored 20/12.5, 40/12.5, 40/25. **BiDil** (hydralazine + isosorbide): Trade: Tabs, scored 37.5/20. **Capozide** (captopril + hydrochlorothiazide): Generic/Trade: Tabs, scored 25/15, 25/25, 50/15, 50/25 mg. **Clorpres** (clonidine + chlorthalidone): Trade: Tabs, scored 0.1/15, 0.2/15, 0.3/15 mg. **Corzide** (nadolol + bendroflumethiazide): Trade: Tabs, scored 40/5, 80/5 mg. **Diovan HCT** (valsartan + hydrochlorothiazide): Trade: Tabs, non-scored 80/12.5, 160/12.5, 160/25 mg. **Diutensen-R** (reserpine + methyclothiazide): Trade: Tabs non-scored, 0.1/2.5 mg. **Dyazide** (triamterene + hydrochlorothiazide): Generic/Trade: Caps, (Dyazide) 37.5/25, (generic only) 50/25 mg. **Enduronyl** (deserpidine + methyclothiazide): Trade: Tabs, non-scored, 0.25/5 (Enduronyl), 0.5/5 mg (Enduronyl Forte). **Hyzaar** (losartan + hydrochlorothiazide): Trade: Tabs, non-scored 50/12.5, 100/25 mg. **Inderide** (propranolol + hydrochlorothiazide): Generic/Trade: Tabs, scored 40/25, 80/25. **Inhibace Plus** (cilazapril + hydrochlorothiazide): Trade: Scored tabs 5 mg cilazapril + 12.5 mg HCTZ. **Lexxel** (enalapril + felodipine): Trade: Tabs, non-scored 5/2.5, 5/5 mg. **Lopressor HCT** (metoprolol + hydrochlorothiazide): Generic/Trade: Tabs, scored 50/25, 100/25, 100/50 mg. **Lotensin HCT** (benazepril + hydrochlorothiazide): Trade: Tabs, scored 5/6.25, 10/12.5, 20/12.5, 20/25 mg. **Lotrel** (amlodipine + benazepril): Trade: cap, 2.5/10, 5/10, 5 /20 10/20 mg. **Maxzide** (triamterene + hydrochlorothiazide, ✦*Triazide*): Generic/Trade: Tabs, scored (Maxzide-25) 37.5/25 (Maxzide) 75/50 mg. **Maxzide-25** (triamterene + hydrochlorothiazide): Generic/Trade: Tabs, scored (Maxzide-25) 37.5/25 (Maxzide) 75/50 mg. **Micardis HCT** (telmisartan + hydrochlorothiazide, ✦*Micardis Plus*): Trade: Tabs, non-scored 40/12.5, 80/12.5, 80/25 mg. **Minizide** (prazosin + polythiazide): Trade: cap, 1/0.5, 2/0.5, 5/0.5 mg. **Moduretic** (amiloride + hydrochlorothiazide, ✦*Moduret*): Generic/Trade: Tabs, scored 5/50 mg. **Monopril HCT** (fosinopril + hydrochlorothiazide): Generic/Trade: Tabs, non-scored 10/12.5, scored 20/12.5 mg. **Prinzide** (lisinopril + hydrochlorothiazide): Generic/Trade: Tabs, non-scored 10/12.5, 20/12.5, 20/25 mg. **Rauzide** (rauwolfia + bendroflumethiazide): Trade: Tabs, non-scored 50/4 mg. **Renese-R** (reserpine + polythiazide): Trade: Tabs, scored, 0.25/2 mg. **Ser-Ap-Es** (hydralazine + hydrochlorothiazide + reserpine): Generic: Tabs, non-scored, 25/15/0.1 mg. **Tarka** (trandolapril + verapamil): Trade: Tabs, non-scored 2/180, 1/240, 2/240, 4/240 mg. **Tenoretic** (atenolol + chlorthalidone): Generic/Trade: Tabs, scored 50/25, non-scored 100/25 mg. **Teveten HCT** (eprosartan + hydrochlorothiazide): Trade: Tabs, non-scored 600/12.5, 600/25 mg. **Timolide** (timolol + hydrochlorothiazide): Trade: Tabs, non-scored 10/25 mg. **Uniretic** (moexipril + hydrochlorothiazide): Trade: Tabs, scored 7.5/12.5, 15/12.5, 15/25 mg. **Vaseretic** (enalapril + hydrochlorothiazide): Generic/Trade: Tabs, non-scored 5/12.5, 10/25 mg. **Zestoretic** (lisinopril + hydrochlorothiazide): Generic/Trade: Tabs, non-scored 10/12.5, 20/12.5, 20/25 mg. **Ziac** (bisoprolol + hydrochlorothiazide): Generic/Trade: Tabs, non-scored 2.5/6.25, 5/6.25, 10/6.25 mg.

Antihypertensives - Other

epoprostenol (*Flolan*): Specialized dosing for pulmonary arterial HTN. ▶Plasma ♀B ▶? $$$$$

fenoldopam (*Corlopam*): Severe HTN: 10 mg in 250 ml D5W (40 mcg/mL), start at 0.1 mcg/kg/min titrate q15 min, usual effective dose 0.1-1.6 mcg/kg/min. ▶LK ♀B ▶? $$$$$

hydralazine (*Apresoline*): Hypertensive emergency: 10-50 mg IM or 10-20 mg IV, repeat as needed. HTN: Start 10 mg PO bid-qid, max 300 mg/day. Headaches, peripheral edema, lupus syndrome. [Generic/Trade: Tabs, non-scored 10,25,50, 100 mg.] ▶LK ♀C ▶+ $

nitroprusside (*Nipride, Nitropress*): Hypertensive emergency: 50 mg in 250 mL D5W (200 mcg/mL), start at 0.3 mcg/kg/min (for 70 kg adult = 6 mL/h). Max 10 mcg/kg/min. Protect from light. Cyanide toxicity with high doses, hepatic/renal impairment, and prolonged infusions; check thiocyanate levels. ▶RBC's ♀C ▶- $

phentolamine (*Regitine, Rogitine*): Diagnosis of pheochromocytoma: 5 mg increments IV/IM. Peds 0.05-0.1 mg/kg IV/IM up to 5 mg per dose. Extravasation: 5-10 mg in 10 mL NS local injection. ▶Plasma ♀C ▶? $$

Antiplatelet Drugs

abciximab (*ReoPro*): Platelet aggregation inhibition, percutaneous coronary intervention: 0.25 mg/kg IV bolus via separate infusion line before procedure, then 0.125 mcg/kg/min (max 10 mcg/min) IV infusion for 12h. ▶Plasma ♀C ▶? $$$$$

Aggrenox (aspirin + dipyridamole): Platelet aggregation inhibition: 1 cap bid. [Trade Caps, 25 mg aspirin/ 200 mg extended-release dipyridamole.] ▶LK ♀D ▶? $$$$

aspirin (*Ecotrin, Empirin, Halfprin, Bayer, ASA, ✦Entrophen, Asaphen, Novasen*): Platelet aggregation inhibition: 81-325 mg PO daily. [Generic/Trade (OTC): tabs, 325,500 mg; chewable 81 mg; enteric-coated 81,162 mg (Halfprin), 81,325, 500 mg (Ecotrin), 650,975 mg. Trade only: tabs, controlled-release 650,800 mg (ZORpbin, Rx). Generic only (OTC): suppository 120,200,300,600 mg.] ▶K♀D▶? $

clopidogrel (*Plavix*): Reduction of thrombotic events: recent AMI/stroke, established peripheral arterial disease: 75 mg PO daily; acute coronary syndrome (unstable angina or non Q-wave MI): 300 mg loading dose, then 75 mg PO daily in combination with ASA x 9-12 months. [Trade: Tab non-scored 75 mg.] ▶LK ♀B ▶? $$$$

dipyridamole (*Persantine*): Antithrombotic: 75-100 mg PO qid. [Generic/Trade: Tabs, non-scored 25,50,75 mg.] ▶L ♀B ▶? $

eptifibatide (*Integrilin*): Acute coronary syndrome: Load 180 mcg/kg IV bolus, then infusion 2 mcg/kg/min for up to 72 hr. Discontinue infusion prior to CABG. Percutaneous coronary intervention: Load 180 mcg/kg IV bolus just before procedure, followed by infusion 2 mcg/kg/min and a second 180 mcg/kg IV bolus 10 min after the first bolus. Continue infusion for up to 18-24 hr (minimum 12 hr) after procedure. Reduce infusion dose with CrCl <50 ml/min; contraindicated in dialysis patients. ▶K ♀B ▶? $$$$$

ticlopidine (*Ticlid*): Due to high incidence of neutropenia and thrombotic thrombocytopenia purpura, other drugs preferred. Platelet aggregation inhibition/reduction of thrombotic stroke: 250 mg PO bid with food. [Generic/Trade: Tab, non-scored 250 mg.] ▶L ♀B ▶? $$$$

tirofiban (*Aggrastat*): Acute coronary syndromes: Start 0.4 mcg/kg/min IV infusion for 30 mins, then decrease to 0.1 mcg/kg/min for 48-108 hr or until 12-24 hr after coronary intervention. Half dose with CrCl <30 mL/min. Use concurrent heparin to keep PTT twice normal. ▶K ♀B ▶? $$$$$

Beta Blockers

NOTE: See also antihypertensive combinations. Abrupt discontinuation may precipitate angina, myocardial infarction, arrhythmias, or rebound hypertension; discontinue by tapering over 2 weeks. Avoid using nonselective beta-blockers and use agents with beta1 selectivity cautiously in asthma/COPD. Beta 1 selectivity diminishes at high doses. Avoid in decompensated heart failure.

acebutolol (*Sectral*, ✦*Rhotral, Monitan*): HTN: Start 400 mg PO daily or 200 mg PO bid, maximum 1200 mg/day. Beta1 receptor selective. [Generic/Trade: Caps, 200,400 mg.] ▶LK ♀B ▶- $

atenolol (*Tenormin*): Acute MI: 5 mg IV over 5 min, repeat in 10 min. HTN: Start 25-50 mg PO daily or divided bid, maximum 100 mg/day. Beta1 receptor selective. [Generic/Trade: Tabs, non-scored 25,100; scored, 50 mg.] ▶K ♀D ▶- $

betaxolol (*Kerlone*): HTN: Start 5-10 mg PO daily, max 20 mg/day. Beta1 receptor selective. [Trade: Tabs, scored 10, non-scored 20 mg.] ▶LK ♀C ▶? $$

bisoprolol (*Zebeta*, ✦*Monocor*): HTN: Start 2.5-5 mg PO daily, max 20 mg/day. Beta1 receptor selective. [Generic/Trade: Tabs, scored 5, non-scored 10 mg.] ▶LK ♀C ▶? $$

carvedilol (*Coreg*): Heart failure: Start 3.125 mg PO bid with food, double dose q2 weeks as tolerated up to max of 25 mg bid (if <85 kg) or 50 mg bid (if >85 kg). LV dysfunction following acute MI: Start 6.25 mg PO bid, double dose q 3-10 days as tolerated to max of 25 mg bid. HTN: Start 6.25 mg PO bid, double dose q7-14 days to max 50 mg/day. Alpha1, beta1, and beta2 receptor blocker. [Trade: Tabs, non-scored 3.125, 6.25, 12.5,25 mg.] ▶L ♀C ▶? $$$$

esmolol (*Brevibloc*): SVT/HTN emergency: Mix infusion 5 g in 500 mL (10 mg/mL), load with 500 mcg/kg over 1 minute (70 kg: 35 mg or 3.5 mL) then infusion 50-200 mcg/kg/min (70 kg: 100 mcg/kg/min = 40 mL/h). Half-life = 9 minutes. Beta1 receptor selective. ▶K ♀C ▶? $$$

labetalol (*Trandate*): HTN: Start 100 mg PO bid, max 2400 mg/day. HTN emergency: Start 20 mg IV slow injection, then 40-80 mg IV q10 min prn up to 300 mg or IV infusion 0.5-2 mg/min. Peds: Start 0.3-1 mg/kg/dose (max 20 mg). Alpha1, beta1, and beta2 receptor blocker. [Generic/Trade: Tabs, scored 100,200,300 mg.] ▶LK ♀C ▶+ $$$

metoprolol (*Lopressor, Toprol-XL*, ✦*Betaloc*): Acute MI: 5 mg increments IV q5-15 min up to 15 mg followed by oral therapy. HTN (immediate release): Start 100 mg PO daily or in divided doses, increase as needed up to 450 mg/day; may require multiple daily doses to maintain 24 hour BP control. HTN (extended release): Start 25-100 mg PO daily, increase as needed up to 400 mg/day. Heart failure: Start 12.5-25 mg (extended-release) PO daily, double dose every 2 weeks as tolerated up to max 200 mg/day. Angina: Start 50 mg PO bid (immediate release) or 100 mg PO daily (extended-release), increase as needed up to 400 mg/day. Beta1 receptor selective. [Generic/Trade: tabs, scored 50,100 mg. Trade only: tabs, extended-release (Toprol-XL) 25,50,100,200 mg.] ▶L ♀C ▶? $$$

nadolol (*Corgard*): HTN: Start 20-40 mg PO daily, max 320 mg/day. Beta1 and beta2 blocker. [Generic/Trade: Tabs, scored 20,40,80,120,160 mg.] ▶K ♀C ▶- $$

oxprenolol (✦*Trasicor, Slow-Trasicor*): Canada only. HTN: Regular release: Initially 20 mg PO tid, titrate upwards prn to usual maintenance 120-320 mg/day divided bid-tid. Alternatively, may substitute an equivalent daily dose of sustained release product; do not exceed 480 mg/day. [Trade: Regular release tabs: 40, 80 mg. Sustained release tabs: 80, 160 mg.] ▶L ♀D ▶- $$

penbutolol (*Levatol*): HTN: Start 20 mg PO daily, max 80 mg/day. [Trade: Tabs, scored 20 mg.] ▶LK ♀C ▶? $$$

pindolol, ✦*Visken*): HTN: Start 5 mg PO bid, max 60 mg/day. Beta1 and beta2 receptor blocker. [Generic: Tabs, scored 5,10 mg.] ▶K ♀B ▶? $$$

propranolol (***Inderal, Inderal LA, InnoPran XL***): HTN: Start 20-40 PO bid or 60-80 mg PO daily; extended-release (Inderal LA) max 640 mg/day; extended-release (InnoPran XL) 80 mg qhs (10 PM), max 120 mg qhs. Supraventricular tachycardia or rapid atrial fibrillation/flutter: 1 mg IV q2min. Max of 2 doses in 4 hours. Migraine prophylaxis: Start 40 mg PO bid or 80 mg PO daily (extended-release), max 240 mg/day. Beta1 and beta2 receptor blocker. [Generic/Trade: Tabs, scored 10,20,40,60,80. Generic only: Solution 20,40/5 mL. Concentrate 80 mg/mL. Trade: Caps, extended-release (Inderal LA daily) 60,80,120,160 mg, (InnoPran XL qhs) 80,120 mg.] ▶L ♀C ▶+ $$

timolol (***Blocadren***): HTN: Start 10 mg PO bid, max 60 mg/d. Beta1 and beta2 blocker. [Generic/Trade: Tabs, non-scored 5, scored 10,20 mg.] ▶LK ♀C ▶+ $$

Calcium Channel Blockers (CCBs) - Dihydropyridines

amlodipine (***Norvasc***): HTN: Start 2.5 to 5 mg PO daily, max 10 daily. [Trade: Tabs, non-scored 2.5,5,10 mg.] ▶L ♀C ▶? $$

felodipine (***Plendil, ✦Renedil***): HTN: Start 2.5-5 mg PO daily, maximum 10 mg/day. [Generic/Trade: Tabs, ext'd release, non-scored 2.5,5,10 mg.] ▶L ♀C ▶? $$

isradipine (***DynaCirc, DynaCirc CR***): HTN: Start 2.5 mg PO bid, max 20 mg/day (max 10 mg/day in elderly). Controlled-release: 5-10 mg PO daily. [Trade: Caps 2.5,5 mg; tab, controlled-release 5,10 mg.] ▶L ♀C ▶? $$$

nicardipine (***Cardene, Cardene SR***): HTN emergency: Begin IV infusion at 5 mg/h, titrate to effect, max 15 mg/h. HTN: Start 20 mg PO tid, max 120 mg/day. Sustained release: Start 30 mg PO bid, max 120 mg/day. [Generic/Trade: caps, immediate-release 20,30 mg. Trade only: caps sust'd release 30,45,60 mg.] ▶L ♀C ▶? $$

nifedipine (***Procardia, Adalat, Procardia XL, Adalat CC, ✦Adalat XL, Adalat PA***): HTN/angina: extended-release: 30-60 mg PO daily, max 120/d. Angina: immediate-release: Start 10 mg PO tid, max 120 mg/d. Avoid sublingual administration, may cause excessive hypotension, AMI, stroke. Do not use immediate-release caps for treating HTN. [Generic/Trade: Caps, 10,20 mg. Tabs, extended-release 30,60,90 mg.] ▶L ♀C ▶+ $$

nisoldipine (***Sular***): HTN: Start 20 mg PO daily, max 60 mg/day. [Trade: Tabs, extended-release 10,20,30,40 mg.] ▶L ♀C ▶? $$

Calcium Channel Blockers (CCBs) - Other

diltiazem (***Cardizem, Cardizem SR, Cardizem LA, Cardizem CD, Cartia XT, Dilacor XR, Diltiazem CD, Diltia XT, Tiazac, Taztia XT***): Atrial fibrillation/flutter, PSVT: bolus 20 mg (0.25 mg/kg) IV over 2 min. Rebolus 15 min later (if needed) 25 mg (0.35 mg/kg). Infusion 5-15 mg/h. Once daily, extended-release, HTN: Start 120-240 mg PO daily, max 540 mg/day. Once daily, graded extended-release (Cardizem LA), HTN: Start 180-240 mg PO daily, max 540 mg/day. Twice daily, sustained-release, HTN: Start 60-120 mg PO bid, max 360 mg/day. Immediate-release, angina: Start 30 mg PO qid, max 360 mg/day divided tid-qid; extended-release, Start 120-240 mg PO daily, max 540 mg/day. Once daily, graded extended-release (Cardizem LA), angina: Start 180 mg PO daily, doses >360 mg may provide no additional benefit. [Generic/Trade: Immediate-release tabs, non-scored (Cardizem) 30, scored 60, 90, 120 mg; extended-release caps (Cardizem CD, Taztia XT daily) 120, 180, 240, 300, 360 mg, (Cartia XT, Dilt-CD daily) 120, 180, 240, 300, (Tiazac daily) 120, 180, 240, 300, 360, 420 mg, (Dilacor XR, Diltia XT daily) 120, 180, 240 mg. Trade only: Sustained-release caps (Cardizem SR q12h) 60, 90, 120 mg; extended-release graded tabs (Cardizem LA daily) 120, 180, 240, 300, 360, 420 mg.] ▶L ♀C ▶+ $$

verapamil (*Isoptin, Calan, Covera-HS, Verelan, Verelan PM, ♣Chronovera, Veramil*): SVT: 5-10 mg IV over 2 min; peds (1-15 yo): 2-5 mg (0.1-0.3 mg/kg) IV, max dose 5 mg. Angina: immediate-release, start 40-80 mg PO tid-qid, max 480 mg/day; sustained-release, start 120-240 mg PO daily, max 480 mg/day (use bid dosing for doses >240 mg/day with Isoptin SR and Calan SR); (Covera-HS) 180 mg PO qhs, max 480 mg/day. HTN: same as angina, except (Verelan PM) 100-200 mg PO qhs, max 400 mg/day; immediate-release tabs should be avoided in treating HTN. [Generic/Trade: tabs, immediate-release, scored 40,80,120 mg; sustained-release, non-scored (Calan SR, Isoptin SR) 120, scored 180,240 mg; caps, sustained-release (Verelan) 120,180,240,360 mg. Trade only: tabs, extended-release (Covera HS) 180,240 mg; caps, extended-release (Verelan PM) 100,200,300 mg.] ▶L ♀C ▶+ $$

Diuretics - Carbonic Anhydrase Inhibitors

acetazolamide (*Diamox*): Acute mountain sickness: 125-250 mg PO bid-tid, beginning 1-2 days prior to ascent and continuing for ≥5 days at higher altitude. [Generic only: Tabs, 125,250 mg; Trade cap sust'd release 500 mg.] ▶LK ♀C ▶+ $

Diuretics - Loop

bumetanide (*Bumex, ♣Burinex*): Edema: 0.5-1 mg IV/IM; 0.5-2 mg PO daily. 1 mg bumetanide is roughly equivalent to 40 mg furosemide. [Generic/Trade: Tabs, scored 0.5,1,2 mg.] ▶K ♀C ▶? $

ethacrynic acid (*Edecrin*): Rarely used. May be useful in sulfonamide-allergic patients. Edema: 0.5-1.0 mg/kg IV, max 50 mg; 25-100 mg PO daily-bid. [Trade: Tabs, scored 25] ▶LK ♀B ▶? $$

furosemide (*Lasix*): Edema: Initial dose 20-80 mg IV/IM/PO, increase dose by 20-40 mg every 6-8h until desired response is achieved, max 600 mg/day. [Generic/Trade: Tabs, non-scored 20, scored 40,80 mg. Generic only: Oral solution 10 mg/mL, 40 mg/5 mL.] ▶K ♀C ▶? $

torsemide (*Demadex*): Edema: 5-20 mg IV/PO daily. [Generic/Trade: Tabs, scored 5,10,20,100 mg.] ▶LK ♀B ▶? $

Diuretics - Potassium Sparing

amiloride (*Midamor*): Diuretic-induced hypokalemia: Start 5 mg PO daily, max 20 mg/day. [Generic/Trade: Tabs, non-scored 5 mg.] ▶LK ♀B ▶? $$

Diuretics - Thiazide Type (See also antihypertensive combinations.)

chlorothiazide (*Diuril*): HTN: 125-250 mg PO daily or divided bid, max 1000 mg/day divided bid. Edema: 500-2000 mg PO/IV daily or divided bid. [Generic: Tabs, scored 250,500 mg.] ▶L ♀C, D if used in pregnancy-induced HTN ▶+ $

chlorthalidone (*Thalitone*): HTN: 12.5-25 mg PO daily, max 50 mg/day. Edema: 50-100 mg PO daily, max 200 mg/day. Nephrolithiasis (unapproved use): 25-50 mg PO daily. [Trade only: Tabs, non-scored (Thalitone) 15 mg. Generic only: Tabs non-scored 25,50 mg.] ▶L ♀B, D if used in pregnancy-induced HTN ▶+ $

hydrochlorothiazide (*HCTZ, Esidrix, Oretic, Microzide*): HTN: 12.5-25 mg PO daily, max 50 mg/day. Edema: 25-100 mg PO daily, max 200 mg/day. [Generic/Trade: Tabs, scored 25, 50 mg; Cap 12.5 mg.] ▶L ♀B, D if used in pregnancy-induced HTN ▶+ $

indapamide (*Lozol, ♣Lozide*): HTN: 1.25-5 mg PO daily, max 5 mg/day. Edema: 2.5-5 mg PO qam. [Generic/Trade: Tabs, non-scored 1.25, 2.5 mg.] ▶L ♀B, D if used in pregnancy-induced HTN ▶? $

metolazone (**Zaroxolyn**): Edema: 5-10 mg PO daily, max 10 mg/day in heart failure, 20 mg/day in renal disease. If used with loop diuretic, start with 2.5 mg PO daily. [Generic/Trade: tabs 2.5,5,10 mg.] ▶L ♀B, D if used in pregnancy-induced HTN ▶? $$$

Nitrates

isosorbide dinitrate (**Isordil, Dilatrate-SR, ✦Cedocard SR, Coronex**): Angina prophylaxis: 5-40 mg PO tid (7 am, noon, 5 pm), sustained-release: 40-80 mg PO bid (8 am, 2 pm). Acute angina, SL Tabs: 2.5-10 mg SL q5-10 min prn, up to 3 doses in 30 min. [Generic/Trade: Tabs, scored 5,10,20,30,40, chewable, scored 5,10, sublingual tabs, non-scored 2.5,5,10 mg. Trade only: cap, sustained-release (Dilatrate-SR) 40 mg. Generic only: tab, sustained-release 40 mg.] ▶L ♀C ▶? $

isosorbide mononitrate (**ISMO, Monoket, Imdur**): Angina: 20 mg PO bid (8 am and 3 pm). Extended-release: Start 30-60 mg PO daily, maximum 240 mg/day. [Generic/Trade: Tabs, non-scored (ISMO, bid dosing) 20, scored (Monoket, bid dosing) 10,20, extended-release, scored (Imdur, daily dosing) 30,60, non-scored 120 mg.] ▶L ♀C ▶? $$

nitroglycerin intravenous infusion (**Tridil**): Perioperative HTN, acute MI/Heart failure, acute angina: mix 50 mg in 250 mL D5W (200 mcg/mL), start at 10-20 mcg/min (3-6 mL/h), then titrate upward by 10-20 mcg/min as needed. [Brand name "Tridil" no longer manufactured, but retained herein for name recognition.] ▶L ♀C ▶? $

nitroglycerin ointment (**Nitrol, Nitro-BID**): Angina prophylaxis: Start 0.5 inch q8h, maintenance 1-2 inches q8h, maximum 4 inches q4-6h; 15 mg/inch. Allow for a nitrate-free period of 10-14 h to avoid nitrate tolerance. 1 inch ointment is approximately 15 mg. [Trade: Ointment, 2%, tubes 1,30,60g (Nitro-BID).] ▶L ♀C ▶? $

nitroglycerin spray (**Nitrolingual**): Acute angina: 1-2 sprays under the tongue prn, max 3 sprays in 15 min. [Trade: Solution, 0.4 mg/spray (200 sprays/canister).] ▶L ♀C ▶? $

nitroglycerin sublingual (**Nitrostat, NitroQuick**): Acute angina: 0.4 mg SL under tongue, repeat dose every 5 min as needed up to 3 doses in 15 min. [Generic/Trade: Sublingual tabs, non-scored 0.3,0.4,0.6 mg; in bottles of 100 or package of 4 bottles with 25 tabs each.] ▶L ♀C ▶? $

nitroglycerin sustained release: Angina prophylaxis: Start 2.5 or 2.6 mg PO bid-tid, then titrate upward prn. Allow for a nitrate-free period of 10-14 h to avoid nitrate tolerance. [Generic only: cap, extended-release 2.5, 6.5, 9 mg.] ▶L ♀C ▶? $

nitroglycerin transdermal (**Minitran, Nitro-Dur, ✦Trinipatch**): Angina prophylaxis: 1 patch 12-14 h each day. Allow for a nitrate-free period of 10-14 h each day to avoid nitrate tolerance. [Trade: Transdermal system, doses in mg/h: Nitro-Dur 0.1,0.2,0.3,0.4,0.6,0.8; Minitran 0.1,0.2,0.4,0.6. Generic only: Transdermal system, doses in mg/h: 0.1,0.2,0.4,0.6.] ▶L ♀C ▶? $$$

CARDIAC PARAMETERS AND FORMULAS	Normal
Cardiac output (CO) = heart rate x stroke volume	4-8 l/min
Cardiac index (CI) = CO/BSA	2.8-4.2 l/min/m2
MAP (mean arterial press) = [(SBP - DBP)/3] + DBP	80-100 mmHg
SVR (systemic vasc resis) = (MAP - CVP)x(80)/CO	800-1200 dyne/sec/cm5
PVR (pulm vasc resis) = (PAM - PCWP)x(80)/CO	45-120 dyne/sec/cm5
QTc = QT / square root of RR [calculate using both measures in sec]	≤0.44
Right atrial pressure (central venous pressure)	0-8 mmHg
Pulmonary artery systolic pressure (PAS)	20-30 mmHg
Pulmonary artery diastolic pressure (PAD)	10-15 mmHg
Pulmonary capillary wedge pressure (PCWP)	8-12 mmHg (post-MI ~16 mmHg)

nitroglycerin transmucosal (**Nitroguard**): Acute angina and prophylaxis: 1-3 mg PO, between lip and gum or between cheek and gum, q 3-5 hours while awake. [Trade: Tabs, controlled-release 2,3 mg.] ▶L ♀C ▷- $$$

Pressors / Inotropes

dobutamine (**Dobutrex**): Inotropic support: 2-20 mcg/kg/min. 70 kg: 5 mcg/kg/min with 1 mg/mL concentration (eg, 250 mg in 250 mL D5W) = 21 mL/h. ▶Plasma ♀D ▷- $

dopamine (**Intropin**): Pressor: Start at 5 mcg/kg/min, increase as needed by 5-10 mcg/kg/min increments at 10 min intervals, max 50 mcg/kg/min. 70 kg: 5 mcg/kg/min with 1600 mcg/mL concentration (eg, 400 mg in 250 mL D5W) = 13 mL/h. Doses in mcg/kg/min: 2-4 = (traditional renal dose, apparently ineffective) dopaminergic receptors; 5-10 = (cardiac dose) dopaminergic and beta1 receptors; >10 = dopaminergic, beta1, and alpha1 receptors. ▶Plasma ♀C ▷- $

ephedrine (**Pressor**): 10-25 mg slow IV, repeat q5-10 min prn. [Generic: Caps, 25,50 mg.] ▶K ♀C ▷? $

epinephrine (**EpiPen, EpiPen Jr, Twinject, adrenalin**): Cardiac arrest: 1 mg IV q3-5 minutes. Anaphylaxis: 0.1-0.5 mg SC/IM, may repeat SC dose q 10-15 minutes. Acute asthma & hypersensitivity reactions: Adults: 0.1 to 0.3 mg of 1:1,000 soln SC or IM; Peds: 0.01 mg/kg (up to 0.3 mg) of 1:1,000 soln SC or IM; Sustained release: 0.005 mg/kg (up to 0.15 mg) of 1:200 soln SC or IM. [Soln for injection: 1,10,000 (1 mg/ml in 10 ml syringe), 1:1,000 (1 mg/ml in 1 ml amps). Sust'd formulation (Sus-Phrine): 1:200 (5 mg/ml) in 0.3 ml amps or 5 ml multi-dose vials. EpiPen Auto-injector delivers 0.3 mg (1:1,000 soln) IM dose. EpiPen Jr. Autoinjector delivers 0.15 mg (1:2,000 solution) IM dose. Twinject Auto-injector delivers 0.15, 0.3 mg IM/SQ dose.] ▶Plasma ♀C ▷- $

inamrinone (**Amrinone**): Heart failure: 0.75 mg/kg bolus IV over 2-3 min, then infusion 100 mg in 100 mL NS (1 mg/mL) at 5-10 mcg/kg/min. 70 kg: 5 mcg/kg/min = 21 mL/h. ▶K ♀C ▷? $$$$$

midodrine (**Orvaten, ProAmatine, ✿ Amatine**): Orthostatic hypotension: 10 mg PO tid while awake. [Generic/Trade: Tabs, scored 2.5,5,10 mg.] ▶LK ♀C ▷? $$$$$

milrinone (**Primacor**): Systolic heart failure (NYHA class III,IV): Load 50 mcg/kg IV over 10 min, then begin IV infusion of 0.375-0.75 mcg/kg/min. ▶K ♀C ▷? $$$$$

norepinephrine (**Levophed**): Acute hypotension: 4 mg in 500 mL D5W (8 mcg/mL) start 8-12 mcg/min, adjust to maintain BP, average maintenance rate 2-4 mcg/min, ideally through central line. 3 mcg/min = 22.5 mL/h. ▶Plasma ♀C ▷? $

phenylephrine (**Neo-Synephrine**): Severe hypotension: 50 mcg boluses IV. Infusion: 20 mg in 250 mL D5W (80 mcg/mL), start 100-180 mcg/min (75-135 mL/h), usual dose once BP is stabilized 40-60 mcg/min. ▶Plasma ♀C ▷- $

Thrombolytics

alteplase (**tpa, t-PA, Activase, Cathflo, ✿ Activase rt-PA**): Acute MI: 15 mg IV bolus, then 50 mg over 30 min, then 35 mg over the next 60 min; (patient ≤67 kg) 15 mg IV bolus, then 0.75 mg/kg (max 50 mg) over 30 min, then 0.5 mg/kg (max 35 mg) over the next 60 min. Concurrent heparin infusion. Acute ischemic stroke: 0.9 mg/kg up to 90 mg infused over 60 min, with 10% of dose as initial IV bolus over 1 minute; start within 3 h of symptom onset. Acute pulmonary embolism: 100 mg IV over 2h, then restart heparin when PTT ≤twice normal. Occluded central venous access device: 2 mg/ml in catheter for 2 hr. May use second dose if needed. ▶L ♀C ▷? $$$$$

THROMBOLYTIC THERAPY FOR ACUTE MI (if high-volume cath lab unavailable)
Indications: Clinical history & presentation strongly suggestive of MI within 12 hours plus ≥1 of the following: 1 mm ST↑ in ≥2 contiguous leads; new left BBB; or 2 mm ST↓ in V1-4 suggestive of true posterior MI. *Absolute contraindications*: Previous cerebral hemorrhage, known cerebral aneurysm or arteriovenous malformation, known intracranial neoplasm, recent (<3 months) ischemic stroke (except acute ischemic stroke <3 hours), aortic dissection, active bleeding or bleeding diathesis (excluding menstruation), significant closed head or facial trauma (<3 months). *Relative contraindications*: Severe uncontrolled HTN (>180/110 mmHg) on presentation or chronic severe HTN; prior ischemic stroke (>3 months), dementia, other intracranial pathology; traumatic/prolonged (>10 minutes) cardiopulmonary resuscitation; major surgery (<3 weeks); recent (within 2-4 weeks) internal bleeding; puncture of non-compressible vessel; pregnancy; active peptic ulcer disease; current use of anticoagulants. For streptokinase/anistreplase: prior exposure (>5 days ago) or prior allergic reaction.   *Circulation* 2004;110:588-636

reteplase (**Retavase**): Acute MI: 10 units IV over 2 min; repeat in 30 min. ▶L ♀C ▶? $$$$$

streptokinase (**Streptase, Kabikinase**): Acute MI: 1.5 million units IV over 60 minutes. ▶L ♀C ▶? $$$$$

tenecteplase (**TNKase**): Acute MI: Single IV bolus dose over 5 seconds based on body weight; <60 kg, 30 mg; 60-69 kg, 35 mg; 70-79 kg, 40 mg; 80-89 kg, 45 mg; ≥90kg, 50 mg. ▶L ♀C ▶? $$$$$

urokinase (**Abbokinase, Abbokinase Open -Cath**): PE: 4400 units/kg IV loading dose over 10 min, followed by IV infusion 4400 units/kg/h for 12 hours. Occluded IV catheter: 5000 units instilled into catheter, remove after 5 min. ▶L ♀B ▶? $$$$$

Volume Expanders

albumin (**Albuminar, Buminate, Albumarc, ✦Plasbumin**): Shock, burns: 500 mL of 5% solution IV infusion as rapidly as tolerated, repeat in 30 min if needed. ▶L ♀C ▶? $$$$

dextran (**Rheomacrodex, Gentran, Macrodex**): Shock/hypovolemia: 20 mL/kg up to 500 mL IV. ▶K ♀C ▶? $$$$

hetastarch (**Hespan, Hextend**): Shock/hypovolemia: 500-1000 mL IV 6% solution. ▶K ♀C ▶? $$$

plasma protein fraction (**Plasmanate, Protenate, Plasmatein**): Shock/hypovolemia: 5% soln 250-500 mL IV prn. ▶L ♀C ▶? $$$$

Other

cilostazol (**Pletal**): Intermittent claudication: 100 mg PO bid on empty stomach. 50 mg PO bid with cytochrome P450 3A4 inhibitors (eg, ketoconazole, itraconazole, erythromycin, diltiazem) or cytochrome P450 2C19 inhibitors (eg, omeprazole). Avoid grapefruit juice. [Generic/Trade: Tabs 50, 100 mg.] ▶L ♀C ▶? $$$

nesiritide (**Natrecor**): Hospitalized patients with decompensated heart failure with dyspnea at rest: 2 mcg/kg IV bolus over 60 seconds, then 0.01 mcg/kg/min IV infusion for up to 48 hours. Do not initiate at higher doses. Limited experience with increased doses. 1.5 mg vial in 250mL D5W (6 mcg/mL). 70 kg: 2 mcg/kg bolus = 23.3 mL, 0.01 mcg/kg/min infusion = 7 mL/h. Symptomatic hypotension. May increase mortality. Not indicated for outpatient infusion, for scheduled repetitive use, to improve renal function, or to enhance diuresis. ▶K, plasma ♀C ▶? $$$$$

pentoxifylline (**Trental**): 400 mg PO tid with meals. [Generic/Trade: Tabs 400 mg.] ▶L ♀C ▶? $$$

CONTRAST MEDIA

MRI Contrast

gadodiamide (*Omniscan*): Non-iodinated, non-ionic IV contrast for MRI. ▶K ♀C ▶?
$$$$

gadopentetate (*Magnevist*): Non-iodinated IV contrast for MRI. ▶K ♀C ▶? $$$

Radiography Contrast

> NOTE: Beware of allergic or anaphylactoid reactions. Avoid IV contrast in renal insufficiency or dehydration. Hold metformin (Glucophage) prior to or at the time of iodinated contrast dye use and for 48 h after procedure. Restart after procedure only if renal function is normal.

barium sulfate: Non-iodinated GI (eg, oral, rectal) contrast. ▶Not absorbed ♀? ▶+ $

diatrizoate (*Hypaque, Renografin, Gastrografin, MD-Gastroview, Cystografin, ✦Renocal*): Iodinated, ionic, high osmolality IV or GI contrast. ▶K ♀C ▶? $

iodixanol (*Visipaque*): Iodinated, non-ionic, low osm IV contrast. ▶K ♀B ▶? $$$

iohexol (*Omnipaque*): Iodinated, non-ionic, low osmolality IV and oral/body cavity contrast. ▶K ♀B ▶? $$$

iopamidol (*Isovue*): Iodinated, non-ionic, low osmolality IV contrast. ▶K ♀? ▶? $$

iothalamate (*Conray, ✦Vascoray*): Iodinated, ionic, high osmolality IV contrast. ▶K ♀B ▶- $

ioversol (*Optiray*): Iodinated, non-ionic, low osmolality IV contrast. ▶K ♀B ▶? $$

ioxaglate (*Hexabrix*): Iodinated, ionic, low osmolality IV contrast. ▶K ♀B ▶- $$$

Ultrasound Contrast

perflexane (*Imagent*): Echocardiography contrast. ▶Respiratory ♀C ▶? ?

Other

acetylcysteine (*Mucomyst, ✦Parvolex*): Contrast nephropathy prophylaxis: 600 mg PO bid on the day before and on the day of contrast. [Generic/Trade: solution 10%, 20%.] ▶L ♀B ▶? $

DERMATOLOGY

Acne Preparations

adapalene (*Differin*): apply qhs. [Trade only: gel 0.1% (15,45 g) cream 0.1% (15,45 g), soln 0.1% pad (30 mL).] ▶Bile ♀C ▶? $$

azelaic acid (*Azelex, Finacea, Finevin*): apply bid. [Trade only: cream 20%, 30g, 50g (Azelex, Finevin), gel 15% 30g (Finacea).] ▶K ♀B ▶? $$$

BenzaClin (clindamycin + benzoyl peroxide): apply bid. [Trade only: gel clindamycin 1% + benzoyl peroxide 5%; 19.7 g.] ▶K ♀C ▶? $$$

Benzamycin (erythromycin + benzoyl peroxide): apply bid. [Trade only: gel erythromycin 3% + benzoyl peroxide 5%; 23.3, 46.6 g.] ▶LK ♀C ▶? $$$

benzoyl peroxide (*Benzac, Benzagel 10%, Desquam, Clearasil, ✦Acetoxyl, Solugel, Benoxyl, Oxyderm*): apply daily; increase to bid-tid if needed. [OTC and Rx generic: liquid 2.5,5,10%, bar 5,10%, mask 5%, lotion 5,5.5,10%, cream 5,10%, cleanser 10%, gel 2.5,4,5,6,10,20%.] ▶LK ♀C ▶? $

Clenia (sodium sulfacetamide + sulfur): apply 1-3 times daily. [Generic: lotion (sodium sulfacetamide 10% & sulfur 5%) 25 g. Trade only (sodium sulfacetamide 10% & sulfur 5%): cream 28 g, foaming wash 170,340 g.] ▶K ♀C ▶? $$

clindamycin (*Cleocin T, ClindaMax, Evoclin, ClindaMax, ✦Dalacin T*): apply daily (Evoclin) or bid (Cleocin T). [Generic/Trade: gel 1% 7.5, 30g, lotion 1% 60 ml, solution 1% 30,60 ml. Trade only: foam 1% 50 g (Evoclin).] ▶L ♀B ▶- $

Diane-35 (cyproterone + ethinyl estradiol): Canada only. 1 tab PO daily for 21 consecutive days, stop for 7 days, repeat cycle. [Rx: Trade: blister pack of 21 tabs 2 mg/0.035 mg cyproterone acetate/ethinyl estradiol.] ▶L ♀X ▶- $$

doxycycline (*Vibramycin, Doryx, Adoxa, ✦Doxycin*): Acne vulgaris: 100 mg PO bid. [Generic/Trade: Tabs 75, 100 mg, caps 20, 50,100 mg. Trade only: susp 25 mg/5 ml, syrup 50 mg/5 ml (contains sulfites).] ▶LK ♀D ▶+ $$

Duac (clindamycin + benzoyl peroxide, *✦Clindoxyl*): apply qhs. [Trade only: gel clindamycin 1% + benzoyl peroxide 5%; 45 g.] ▶K ♀C ▶+ $$$

erythromycin (*Eryderm, Erycette, Erygel, A/T/S, ✦Sans-Acne, Erysol*): apply bid. [Generic: solution 1.5% 60 ml, 2% 60,120 ml, pads 2%, gel 2% 30,60 g, ointment 2% 25 g.] ▶L ♀B ▶? $$

isotretinoin (*Accutane, Amnesteem, Sotret, ✦Isotrex*): 0.5-2 mg/kg/day PO divided bid for 15-20 weeks. Typical target dose is 1 mg/kg/day. Can only be prescribed by healthcare professionals who have undergone specific training. Potent teratogen; use extreme caution. May cause depression. Not for long-term use. [Trade/generic: caps 10,20,30,40 mg.] ▶LK ♀X ▶- $$$$$

Rosula (sodium sulfacetamide + sulfur): apply 1-3 times daily. [Generic: lotion (sodium sulfacetamide 10% & sulfur 5%) 25 g. Trade only: gel (sodium Sulfacetamide 10% & sulfur 5%) 45 ml, aqueous cleanser (sodium sulfacetamide 10% & sulfur 5%) 355 ml.] ▶K ♀C ▶? $$

sodium sulfacetamide (*Klaron*): apply bid. [Trade only: lotion 10% 59 ml.] ▶K ♀C ▶? $$

Sulfacet-R (sodium sulfacetamide + sulfur): apply 1-3 times daily. [Trade (Sulfacet-R) & generic: lotion (sodium sulfacetamide 10% & sulfur 5%) 25 g.] ▶K ♀C ▶? $$

tazarotene (*Tazorac, Avage*): Acne (Tazorac): apply 0.1% cream qhs. Psoriasis: apply 0.05% cream qhs, increase to 0.1% prn. [Trade (Tazorac): cream 0.05% 30,100g; 0.1% 30,100g. Trade (Avage): cream 0.1% 15,30g.] ▶L ♀X ▶? $$$

tretinoin (*Retin-A, Retin-A Micro, Renova, Retisol-A, ✦Stieva-A, Rejuva-A, Vitamin A Acid Cream*): Apply qhs. [Generic/Trade: cream 0.025% 20,45 g, 0.05% 20,45 g, 0.1% 20,45 g, gel 0.025% 15,45 g, 0.1% 15,45 g, liquid 0.05% 28 ml. Trade only: Renova cream 0.02%, 0.05% 40,60 g, Retin-A Micro gel 0.04%, 0.1% 20,45 g.] ▶LK ♀C ▶? $$

Actinic Keratosis Preparations

diclofenac (*Solaraze*): Actinic/solar keratoses: apply bid to lesions x 60-90 days. [Trade only: gel 3% 25, 50 g.] ▶L ♀B ▶? $$$$

fluorouracil (*5-FU, Carac, Efudex, Fluoroplex*): Actinic keratoses: apply bid x 2-6 wks. Superficial basal cell carcinomas: apply 5% cream/solution bid. [Trade only: cream 0.5% 30 g (Carac), 5% 25 g (Efudex), 1% 30 g (Fluoroplex), solution 1% 30 ml (Fluoroplex), 2% 10 ml (Efudex), 5% 10 ml (Efudex).] ▶L ♀X ▶- $$$$$

Antibacterials

bacitracin, *✦Baciguent*: apply daily-tid. [OTC Generic/Trade: ointment 500 units/g 1,15,30g.] ▶Not absorbed ♀C ▶? $

fusidic acid (*Fucidin*): Canada only. Apply tid-qid. [Trade: cream 2% fusidic acid 15,30 g, ointment 2% sodium fusidate 15,30 g.] ▶L ♀? ▶? $

gentamicin (*Garamycin*): apply tid-qid. [Generic/Trade: ointment 0.1% 15,30 g, cream 0.1% 15,30 g.] ▶K ♀D ▶? $

mafenide (*Sulfamylon*): Apply daily-bid. [Trade only: cream 37, 114, 411 g, 5% topical solution 50 g packets.] ▶LK ♀C ▶? $$$

metronidazole (*Noritate, MetroCream, MetroGel, MetroLotion, ✦Rosasol*): Rosacea: apply daily (1%) or bid (0.75%). [Trade only: gel (MetroGel) 0.75% 29 g, 1% 45 g, cream (Noritate) 1% 30, 60 g, lotion (MetroLotion) 0.75% 59 ml. Trade/Generic: cream 0.75% 45 g.] ▶KL ♀B(- in 1st trimester) ▶- $$$

mupirocin (*Bactroban, Centany*): Impetigo/infected wounds: apply tid. Nasal MRSA eradication: 0.5 g in each nostril bid x 5 days. [Trade/Generic: cream/ointment 2% 15, 22, 30 g. Trade only: 2% nasal ointment 1 g single-use tubes (for MRSA eradication).] ▶Not absorbed ♀B ▶? $$

Neosporin cream (neomycin + polymyxin): apply daily-tid. [OTC trade only: neomycin 3.5 mg/g + polymyxin 10,000 units/g 15 g & unit dose 0.94 g.] ▶K ♀C ▶? $

Neosporin ointment (bacitracin + neomycin + polymyxin): apply daily-tid. [OTC Generic/Trade: bacitracin 400 units/g + neomycin 3.5 mg/g + polymyxin 5,000 units/g 2.4,9.6,14.2,15, 30 g and unit dose 0.94 g.] ▶? $

Polysporin (bacitracin + polymyxin, ✦*Polytopic*): apply ointment/aerosol/powder daily-tid. [OTC trade only: ointment 15,30 g and unit dose 0.9 g, powder 10 g, aerosol 90 g.] ▶K ♀C ▶? $

silver sulfadiazine (*Silvadene, ✦Dermazin, Flamazine, SSD*): apply daily-bid. [Generic/Trade: cream 1% 20,50,85,400,1000g.] ▶LK ♀B ▶- $

Antifungals

butenafine (*Lotrimin Ultra, Mentax*): apply daily-bid. [Trade only: Rx: cream 1% 15,30 g (Mentax). OTC: cream 1% (Lotrimin Ultra).] ▶L ♀B ▶? $$$

ciclopirox (*Loprox, Penlac, ✦Stieprox shampoo*): Cream, lotion: apply bid. Nail solution: apply daily to affected nails; apply over previous coat; remove with alcohol every 7 days. Seborrheic dermatitis (Loprox shampoo): shampoo twice/week x 4 weeks. [Trade only: gel (Loprox) 0.77% 30,45 g, shampoo (Loprox) 1% 120 ml, nail solution (Penlac) 8% 6.6 ml. Trade/generic: cream (Loprox) 0.77% 15,30,90 g, lotion (Loprox) 0.77% 30,60 ml.] ▶K ♀B ▶? $$

clotrimazole (*Lotrimin, Mycelex, ✦Canesten, Clotrimaderm*): apply bid. [Note that Lotrimin brand cream, lotion, solution are clotrimazole, while Lotrimin powders and liquid spray are miconazole. OTC & Rx generic/Trade: cream 1% 15, 30, 45, 90 g, solution 1% 10,30 ml. Trade only: lotion 1% 30 ml.] ▶L ♀B ▶? $

econazole (*Spectazole, ✦Ecostatin*): Tinea pedis, cruris, corporis, tinea versicolor: apply daily. Cutaneous candidiasis: apply bid. [Trade/Generic: cream 1% 15, 30, 85g.] ▶Not absorbed ♀C ▶? $$

ketoconazole (*Nizoral, ✦Ketoderm*): Tinea/candidal infections: apply daily. Seborrheic dermatitis: apply cream daily-bid. Dandruff: apply 1% shampoo twice a week. Tinea versicolor: apply shampoo to affected area, leave on for 5 min, rinse. [Trade only: shampoo 1% (OTC), 2%, 120 ml. Trade/Generic: cream 2% 15,30,60 g.] ▶L ♀C ▶? $

miconazole (*Monistat-Derm, Micatin, Lotrimin*): Tinea, candida: apply bid. [Note that Lotrimin brand cream, lotion, solution are clotrimazole, while Lotrimin powders and liquid spray are miconazole. OTC generic: ointment 2% 29 g, spray 2% 105 ml, solution 2% 7.39, 30 ml. Generic/Trade: cream 2% 15,30,90 g, powder 2% 90 g, spray powder 2% 90,100 g, spray liquid 2% 105,113 ml.] ▶L ♀+ ▶? $

naftifine (*Naftin*): Tinea: apply daily (cream) or bid (gel). [Trade only: cream 1% 15,30,60 g, gel 1% 20,40, 60 g.] ▶LK ♀B ▶? $$$

nystatin (*Mycostatin, ✦Nilstat, Nyaderm, Candistatin*): Candidiasis: apply bid-tid. [Generic/Trade: cream 100,000 units/g 15,30,240 g, ointment 100,000 units/g 15,30 g, powder 100,000 units/g 15 g.] ▶Not absorbed ♀C ▶? $

oxiconazole (***Oxistat, Oxizole***): Tinea pedis, cruris, and corporis: apply daily-bid. Tinea versicolor (cream only): apply daily. [Trade only: cream 1% 15,30,60 g, lotion 1% 30 ml.] ▶? ♀B ▶? $$

sertaconazole (***Ertaczo***): Tinea pedis: apply bid. [Trade only: cream 2% 15,30g.] ▶Not absorbed ♀C ▶? $$

terbinafine (***Lamisil, Lamisil AT***): Tinea: apply daily-bid. [Trade only: cream 1% 15,30 g, gel 1% 5,15,30 g OTC Trade only (Lamisil AT): cream 1% 12,24 g, spray pump solution 1% 30 ml.] ▶L ♀B ▶? $$

tolnaftate (***Tinactin, ♣ZeaSorb AF***): apply bid. [OTC Generic/Trade: cream 1% 15,30 g, solution 1% 10,15 ml, powder 1% 45,90 g, spray powder 1% 100,105, 150 g, spray liquid 1% 60,120 ml. Trade only: gel 1% 15 g.] ▶? ♀? ▶? $

Antiparasitics (topical)

A-200 (pyrethrins + piperonyl butoxide, ***♣R&C***): Lice: Apply shampoo, wash after 10 min. Reapply in 5-7 days. [OTC Generic/Trade: shampoo (0.33% pyrethrins, 4% piperonyl butoxide) 60,120,240 ml.] ▶? ♀C ▶? $

crotamiton (***Eurax***): Scabies: apply cream/lotion topically from chin to feet, repeat in 24 hours, bathe 48 h later. Pruritus: massage prn. [Trade only: cream 10% 60 g, lotion 10% 60,480 ml.] ▶? ♀C ▶? $$

lindane (***♣Hexit***): Other drugs preferred. Scabies: apply 30-60 ml of lotion, wash after 8-12h. Lice: 30-60 ml of shampoo, wash off after 4 min. Can cause seizures in epileptics or if overused/misused in children. Not for infants. [Generic/Trade: lotion 1% 30,60,480 ml, shampoo 1% 30,60,480 ml.] ▶L ♀B ▶? $

malathion (***Ovide***): Lice: apply to dry hair, let dry naturally, wash off in 8-12 hrs. [Trade only: lotion 0.5% 59 ml.] ▶? ♀B ▶? $$

permethrin (***Elimite, Acticin, Nix, ♣Kwellada-P***): Scabies: apply cream from head (avoid mouth/ nose/eyes) to soles of feet & wash after 8-14h. 30 g is typical adult dose. Lice: Saturate hair and scalp with 1% rinse, wash after 10 min. Do not use in children <2 months old. May repeat therapy in 7 days, as necessary. [Trade only: cream (Elimite, Acticin) 5% 60 g. OTC Trade/generic: liquid creme rinse (Nix) 1% 60 ml.] ▶L ♀B ▶? $$

RID (pyrethrins + piperonyl butoxide): Lice: Apply shampoo/mousse, wash after 10 min. Reapply in 5-10 days. [OTC Generic/Trade: shampoo 60,120,240 ml. Trade only: mousse 5.5 oz.] ▶L ♀C ▶? $

Antipsoriatics

acitretin (***Soriatane***): 25-50 mg PO daily. Avoid pregnancy during therapy and for 3 years after discontinuation. [Trade only: cap 10,25 mg.] ▶L ♀X ▶- $$$$$

alefacept (***Amevive***): 7.5 mg IV or 15 mg IM once weekly x 12 doses. May repeat with 1 additional 12-week course after 12 weeks have elapsed since last dose. ▶? ♀B ▶? $$$$$

anthralin (***Anthra-Derm, Drithocreme, ♣Anthrascalp, Anthranol, Anthraforte***): Apply daily. Short contact periods (i.e. 15-20 minutes) followed by removal may be preferred. [Trade only: ointment 0.1% 42.5 g, 0.25% 42.5 g, 0.4% 60 g, 0.5% 42.5 g, 1% 42.5 g, cream 0.1% 50 g, 0.2% 50 g, 0.25% 50 g, 0.5% 50 g. Generic/Trade: cream 1% 50 g.] ▶? ♀C ▶- $$

calcipotriene (***Dovonex***): apply bid. [Trade only: ointment 0.005% 30,60,100 g, cream 0.005% 30,60,100 g, scalp solution 0.005% 60 ml.] ▶L ♀C ▶? $$$

efalizumab (***Raptiva***): 0.7 mg/kg SC x 1 then 1 mg/kg SC q week. [Trade only: single use vials, 125 mg.] ▶L ♀C ▶? $$$$$

Antivirals (topical)

acyclovir (**Zovirax**): Herpes genitalis: apply oint q3h (6 times/d) x 7 days. Recurrent herpes labialis: apply cream 5 times/day for 4 days. [Trade only: ointment 5% 3,15 g, cream 5% 2 g.] ▶K ♀C ▶? $$$

docosanol (**Abreva**): oral-facial herpes simplex: apply 5x/day until healed. [OTC: Trade only: cream 10% 2 g.] ▶Not absorbed ♀B ▶? $

imiquimod (**Aldara**): Genital/perianal warts: apply 3 times weekly during sleeping hours for up to 16 weeks. Wash off after 8 hours. Nonhyperkeratotic, nonhypertrophic actinic keratoses on face/scalp in immunocompetent adults: apply 2 times weekly during sleeping hours for 16 weeks. Wash off after 8 hours. Primary superficial basal cell carcinoma: apply 5 times weekly x 6 weeks. Wash off after 8h. [Trade only: cream 5% 250 mg single use packets.] ▶Not absorbed ♀C ▶? $$$$

penciclovir (**Denavir**): Herpes labialis: apply cream q2h while awake x 4 days. [Trade only: cream 1% 2 g tubes.] ▶Not absorbed ♀B ▶? $$$

CORTICOSTEROIDS – TOPICAL*

	Agent	Strength/Formulation*	Freq
Low Potency	alclometasone dipropionate (*Aclovate*)	0.05% C **O**	bid-tid
	clocortolone pivalate (*Cloderm*)	0.1% **C**	tid
	desonide (*DesOwen, Tridesilon*)	0.05% C **L O**	bid-tid
	hydrocortisone (*Hytone*, others)	0.25% **CL**; 0.5% **CLO**; 1% **CLOS**; 2% **L**; 2.5% **CLO**	bid-qid
	hydrocortisone acetate (*Cortaid, Corticaine*)	0.5% C **O**, 1% C **O**	bid-qid
Medium Potency	betamethasone valerate	0.1% **CLO**; 0.12% F(*Luxiq*)	qd-bid
	desoximetasone‡ (*Topicort*)	0.05% **C**	bid
	fluocinolone (*Synalar*)	0.01% C **S**; 0.025% C **O**	bid-qid
	flurandrenolide (*Cordran*)	0.025% C; 0.05% CLO; T	bid-tid
	fluticasone propionate (*Cutivate*)	0.005% **O**; 0.05% C	qd-bid
	hydrocortisone butyrate (*Locoid*)	0.1% C **O S**	bid-tid
	hydrocortisone valerate (*Westcort*)	0.2% C **O**	bid-tid
	mometasone furoate (*Elocon*)	0.1% C **L O**	qd
	triamcinolone‡ (*Aristocort, Kenalog*)	0.025% C **L O**; 0.1% C **L O**	bid-tid
High Potency	amcinonide (*Cyclocort*)	0.1% C **L O**	bid-tid
	betamethasone dipropionate‡ (*Maxivate*)	0.05% **CLO** (non-*Diprolene*)	qd-bid
	desoximetasone‡ (*Topicort*)	0.05% **G**; 0.25% C **O**	bid
	diflorasone diacetate‡ (*Maxiflor*)	0.05% **O** (*Maxiflor*)	bid
	fluocinonide (*Lidex*)	0.05% **C G O S**	bid-qid
	halcinonide (*Halog*)	0.1% C **O S**	bid-tid
	triamcinolone‡ (*Aristocort, Kenalog*)	0.5% C **O**	bid-tid
Very high	betamethasone dipropionate‡ (*Diprolene, Diprolene AF*)	0.05% C **G L O**	qd-bid
	clobetasol (*Temovate, Cormax, Olux*)	0.05% **C O L S F**	bid
	diflorasone diacetate‡ (*Psorcon*)	0.05% C **O** (*Psorcon*)	qd-tid
	halobetasol propionate (*Ultravate*)	0.05% C **O**	qd-bid

*C-cream, G-gel, L-lotion, O-ointment, S-solution, T-tape, F-foam; bolded items have available generics. Potency based on vasoconstrictive assays, which may not correlate with efficacy. Not all available products are listed, including those lacking potency ratings.
‡These drugs have formulations in more than once potency category.

podofilox (*Condylox*, ♣*Condyline, Wartec*): External genital warts (gel, soln) and perianal warts (gel only): apply bid for 3 consecutive days of a week and repeat for up to 4 wks. [Trade only: gel 0.5% 3.5 g, solution 0.5% 3.5 ml.] ▶? ♀C ▶? $$$

podophyllin (*Podocon-25, Podofin, Podofilm*): Warts: apply by physician. Not to be dispensed to patients. [Trade only: liquid 25% 15 ml.] ▶? ♀- ▶- $$

Atopic Dermatitis Preparations

pimecrolimus (*Elidel*): Atopic dermatitis: apply bid. [Trade: cream 1% 15, 30, 100 g.] ▶L ♀C ▶? $$$

tacrolimus (*Protopic*): Atopic dermatitis: apply bid. [Trade only: ointment 0.03% 30,60 g, 0.1% 30,60 g.] ▶Minimal absorption ♀C ▶? $$$$

Corticosteroid / Antimicrobial Combinations

Cortisporin (neomycin + polymyxin + hydrocortisone): apply bid-qid. [Generic/ Trade: cream 7.5 g, ointment 15 g.] ▶LK ♀C ▶? $

Fucidin H (fusidic acid + hydrocortisone): Canada only. apply tid. [Trade: cream 2% fusidic acid, 1% hydrocortisone acetate 30 g.] ▶L ♀? ▶? $

Lotrisone (clotrimazole + betamethasone, ♣*Lotriderm*): Apply bid. Do not use for diaper rash. [Trade/generic: cream (clotrimazole 1% + betamethasone 0.05%) 15,45 g, lotion (clotrimazole 1% + betamethasone 0.05%) 30 ml.] ▶L ♀C ▶? $$$

Mycolog II (nystatin + triamcinolone): apply bid. [Generic/Trade: cream 15,30,60, 120 g, ointment 15,30,60,120 g.] ▶L ♀C ▶? $

Hemorrhoid Care

dibucaine (*Nupercainal*): apply cream/ointment tid-qid prn. [OTC Generic/Trade: ointment 1% 30 g.] ▶L ♀? ▶? $

hydrocortisone (*Anusol-HC, Cortifoam*, ♣*Hemcort HC, Egozinc-HC*): apply cream tid-qid prn or supp bid or foam daily-bid. [Generic/Trade: cream 1% (Anusol HC-1), 2.5% 30 g (Anusol HC), suppository 25 mg (Anusol HC), 10% rectal foam (Cortifoam) 15g.] ▶L ♀? ▶? $

pramoxine (*Anusol Hemorrhoidal Ointment, Fleet Pain Relief, Proctofoam NS*): ointment/pads/foam up to 5 times/day prn. [OTC Trade only: ointment (Anusol Hemorrhoidal Ointment), pads (Fleet Pain Relief), aerosol foam (ProctoFoam NS).] ▶Not absorbed ♀+ ▶+ $

starch (*Anusol Suppositories*): 1 suppository up to 6 times/day prn. [OTC Trade only: suppositories (51% topical starch; soy bean oil, tocopheryl acetate).] ▶Not absorbed ♀+ ▶+ $

witch hazel (*Tucks*): Apply to anus/perineum up to 6 times/day prn. [OTC Generic/ Trade: pads, gel.] ▶? ♀+ ▶+ $

Other Dermatologic Agents

alitretinoin (*Panretin*): Apply bid-qid to cutaneous Kaposi's lesions [Trade only: gel 60 g.] ▶Not absorbed ♀D ▶- $$$$$

aluminum chloride (*Drysol, Certain Dri*): Apply qhs. [Rx: Trade/Generic: solution 20%: 37.5 ml bottle, 35, 60 ml bottle with applicator. OTC: Trade (Certain Dri): solution 12.5%: 36 ml bottle.] ▶K ♀? ▶? $

becaplermin (*Regranex*): Diabetic ulcers: apply gel daily. [Trade only: gel 0.01% 2, 15 g.] ▶Minimal absorption ♀C ▶? $$$$$

botulinum toxin (*Botox, Botox Cosmetic*): Dose varies based on indication. [Trade only: 100 unit single-use vials.] ▶Not absorbed ♀C ▶? $$$$$

calamine: apply lotion tid-qid prn for poison ivy/oak or insect bite itching. [OTC Generic: lotion 120, 240, 480 ml.] ▶? ♀? ▶? $

capsaicin (*Zostrix, Zostrix-HP***):** Arthritis, post-herpetic or diabetic neuralgia: apply cream up to tid-qid. [OTC Generic/Trade: cream 0.025% 45,60 g, 0.075% 30,60 g, lotion 0.025% 59 ml, 0.075% 59 ml, gel 0.025% 15,30 g, 0.05% 43 g, roll-on 0.075% 60 ml.] ▶? ♀? ▶? $

coal tar (*Polytar, Tegrin, Cutar, Tarsum***):** apply shampoo at least twice a week, or for psoriasis apply daily-qid. [OTC Generic/Trade: shampoo, conditioner, cream, ointment, gel, lotion, soap, oil.] ▶? ♀? ▶? $

doxepin (*Zonalon***):** Pruritus: apply qid for up to 8 days. [Trade only: cream 5% 30,45 g.] ▶L ♀B ▶- $

eflornithine (*Vaniqa***):** Reduction of facial hair: apply to face bid. [Trade only: cream 13.9% 30 g.] ▶K ♀C ▶? $$

EMLA (lidocaine + prilocaine): Topical anesthesia: apply 2.5g cream or 1 disc to region at least 1 hour before procedure. Cover cream with an occlusive dressing. [Trade only: cream (2.5% lidocaine + 2.5% prilocaine) 5 g, disc 1 g. Trade/generic: cream (2.5% lidocaine + 2.5% prilocaine) 30 g.] ▶LK ♀B ▶? $$

finasteride (*Propecia***):** Androgenetic alopecia in men: 1 mg PO daily. [Trade only: tab 1 mg.] ▶L ♀X ▶- $$

hyaluronic acid (*Restylane***):** Moderate to severe facial wrinkles: inject into wrinkle/fold. [Rx: 0.4 ml and 0.7 ml syringe.] ▶? ♀? ▶? $$$$$

hydroquinone (*Eldopaque, Eldoquin, Eldoquin Forte, EpiQuin Micro, Esoterica, Glyquin, Lustra, Melanex, Solaquin, ✿Ultraquin, Neostrata HQ***):** Hyperpigmentation: apply to area bid. [OTC Generic/Trade: cream 1.5%, lotion 2%. Rx Generic/Trade: solution 3%, gel 4%, cream 4%.] ▶? ♀C ▶? $$$

lactic acid (*Lac-Hydrin***):** apply lotion/cream bid. [Trade only: lotion 12% 150,360 ml. Trade/Generic: cream 12% 140,385 g.] ▶? ♀? ▶? $$

lidocaine (*Xylocaine, Lidoderm, Numby Stuff, ELA-Max***):** Apply prn. Dose varies with anesthetic procedure, degree of anesthesia required and individual patient response. Postherpetic neuralgia: Postherpetic neuralgia: apply up to 3 patches to affected area at once for up to 12h within a 24h period. Apply 30 min prior to painful procedure (ELA-Max 4%). Discomfort with anorectal disorders: apply prn (ELA-Max 5%). [For membranes of mouth and pharynx: spray 10%, ointment 5%, liquid 5%, solution 2,4%, dental patch. For urethral use: jelly 2%. Patch (Lidoderm) 5%. OTC: Trade: liposomal lidocaine 4%, 5% (ELA-Max).] ▶LK ♀B ▶+ $$

methylaminolevulinate: Apply cream to non-hyperkeratotic actinic keratoses lesion and surrounding area on face or scalp; cover with dressing for 3h; remove dressing and cream and perform illumination therapy. Repeat in 7 days. [Trade only: cream. 16.8%, 2 g.] ▶? ♀? ?

minoxidil (*Rogaine, Rogaine Forte, Rogaine Extra Strength, Minoxidil for Men, Theroxidil Extra Strength, ✿Minox, Apo-Gain***):** Androgenetic alopecia (men or women): 1 ml to dry scalp bid. [OTC Trade only: soln 2%, 60 ml, 5%, 60 ml, 5% (Rogaine Extra Strength, Theroxidil Extra Strength - men only) 60 ml] ▶K ♀C ▶- $$

monobenzone (*Benoquin***):** Extensive vitiligo: apply bid-tid. [Trade only: cream 20% 35.4 g.] ▶Minimal absorption ♀C ▶? $$$

oatmeal (*Aveeno***):** Pruritus from poison ivy/oak, varicella: apply lotion qid prn. Also bath packets for tub. [OTC Generic/Trade: lotion, packets] ▶Not absorbed ♀?▶? $

Panafil (papain + urea + chlorophyllin copper complex): Debridement of acute or chronic lesions: apply to clean wound and cover daily-bid. [Trade only: Ointment: 6, 30 g, spray 33 mL.] ▶? ♀? ▶? $$$

Pramosone (pramoxine + hydrocortisone, ✚*Pramox HC*): Inflammatory and pruritic manifestations of corticosteroid-responsive dermatoses: Apply tid-qid. [Trade only: 1% pramoxine/1% hydrocortisone acetate: cream 30, 60 g, oint 30 g, lotion 60, 120, 240 mL. 1% pramoxine/2.5% hydrocortisone acetate: cream 30, 60 g, oint 30 g, lotion 60, 120 mL.] ▶Not absorbed ♀C ▶? $$$

selenium sulfide (**Selsun, Exsel, Versel**): Dandruff, seborrheic dermatitis: apply 5-10 ml lotion/shampoo twice weekly x 2 weeks then less frequently, thereafter. Tinea versicolor: Apply 2.5% lotion/shampoo to affected area daily x 7 days. [OTC Generic/Trade: lotion/shampoo 1% 120,210,240, 330 ml, 2.5% 120 ml. Rx generic/trade: lotion/shampoo 2.5% 120 ml.] ▶? ♀C ▶? $

Solag (mequinol + tretinoin, ✚*Solagé*): Apply to solar lentigines bid. [Trade only: soln 30 ml (mequinol 2% + tretinoin 0.01%).] ▶Not absorbed ♀X ▶? $$$$

Synera (lidocaine + tetracaine): Apply 20-30 min prior to superficial dermatological procedure. [Trade only: patch lidocaine 70 mg + tetracaine 70 mg.] ▶Minimal absorption ♀B ▶?

Tri-Luma (fluocinolone + hydroquinone + tretinoin): Melasma of the face: apply qhs x 4-8 weeks. [Trade only: soln 30 g (fluocinolone 0.01% + hydroquinone 4% + tretinoin 0.05%).] ▶Minimal absorption ♀C ▶? $$$

ENDOCRINE & METABOLIC

Androgens / Anabolic Steroids (See OB/GYN section for other hormones.)

methyltestosterone (**Android, Methitest, Testred, Virilon**): Advancing inoperable breast cancer in women who are 1-5 years postmenopausal: 50-200 mg/day PO in divided doses. Hypogonadism in men: 10-50 mg PO daily. [Trade: Caps 10 mg. Generic/Trade: Tabs 10, 25 mg.] ▶L ♀X ▶? ©III $$$

nandrolone (**Deca-Durabolin**): Anemia of renal disease: women 50-100 mg IM q week, men 100-200 mg IM q week. [Generic/Trade: injection 100 mg/ml, 200 mg/ml. Trade only: injection 50 mg/ml.] ▶L ♀X ▶- ©III $$$

oxandrolone (**Oxandrin**): Weight gain: 2.5 mg PO bid-qid for 2-4 wks. [Trade: Tabs 2.5, 10 mg.] ▶L ♀X ▶? ©III $$$$$

testosterone (**Androderm, Androgel, Delatestryl, Depo-Testosterone, Depotest, Everone 200, Striant, Testim, Testopel, Testro AQ, Testro-L.A., Virilon IM, ✚*Andriol*): Injectable enanthate or cypionate: 50-400 mg IM q2-4 wks. Transdermal - Androderm: 5 mg patch to nonscrotal skin qhs. AndroGel 1%: 1 gel pack (5 g) daily to shoulders/upper arms/abdomen. Testim: One tube (5 g) daily to shoulders/upper arms. Pellet - Testopel: 2-6 (150-450 mg testosterone) pellets SC q 3-6 months. Buccal- Striant: 30 mg q 12 hours on upper gum above the incisor tooth; alternate sides for each application. [Trade only: Patch 2.5, 5 mg (Androderm). Gel 1% 2.5, 5 g (AndroGel). Gel 1%, 5 g (Testim). Pellet 75mg (Testopel). Buccal: blister packs - 30 mg (Striant). Injection 200 mg/ml (enanthate). Generic/Trade: injection 100, 200 mg/ml (cypionate).] ▶L ♀X ▶? ©III $$$$

Bisphosphonates

alendronate (**Fosamax, Fosamax Plus D**): Postmenopausal osteoporosis prevention (5 mg PO daily or 35 mg PO weekly) & treatment (10 mg daily, 70 mg PO weekly or 70 mg/vit D3 2800 IU PO weekly). Treatment of glucocorticoid-induced osteoporosis in men & women: 5 mg PO daily or 10 mg PO daily (postmenopausal women not taking estrogen). Treatment of osteoporosis in men: 10 mg PO daily, 70 mg PO weekly, or 70 mg/vit D3 2800 IU PO weekly. Paget's disease in men & women: 40 mg PO daily x 6 mon. May cause severe esophagitis. [Trade: Tabs 5,10,35,40,70 mg, 70mg/Vit D3 2800 I.U. (Fosamax Plus D). Oral soln 70 mg/75 mL (single dose bottle).] ▶K ♀C ▶- $$$

clodronate (❦*Ostac, Bonefos*): Canada only. IV single dose - 1500 mg slow infusion over ≥4 hours. IV multiple dose - 300 mg slow infusion daily over 2-6 hours up to 10 days. Oral - following IV therapy, maintenance 1600-2400 mg/day in single or divided doses. Max PO dose 3200 mg/day; duration of therapy is usually 6 months. [Trade: Capsules 400 mg.] ▶K ♀D ▶- $$$$

etidronate (*Didronel*): Hypercalcemia: 7.5 mg/kg in 250 ml NS IV over ≥2h daily x 3d. Paget's disease: 5-10 mg/kg PO daily x 6 months or 11-20 mg/kg daily x 3 months. [Generic/Trade: Tabs 200, 400 mg.] ▶K ♀C ▶? $$$$

ibandronate (*Boniva*): Treatment/Prevention of postmenopausal osteoporosis: 2.5 mg PO daily or 150 mg PO q month. [Trade: 2.5, 150 mg tabs.] ▶K ♀C ▶? $$$

pamidronate (*Aredia*): Hypercalcemia of malignancy: 60-90 mg IV over 2-24 h. Wait ≥7 days before considering retreatment. ▶K ♀D ▶? $$$$$

risedronate (*Actonel*): Paget's disease: 30 mg PO daily x 2 months. Prevention & treatment of postmenopausal osteoporosis: 5 mg PO daily or 35 mg PO weekly. Prevention & treatment of glucocorticoid-induced osteoporosis: 5 mg PO daily. May cause esophagitis. [Trade: Tabs 5, 30, 35 mg.] ▶K ♀C ▶? $$$

zoledronic acid (*Zometa*): Hypercalcemia: 4 mg IV infusion over ≥15 min. Wait ≥7 days before considering retreatment. Multiple myeloma / metastatic bone lesions from solid tumors: 4 mg IV infusion over ≥15 min q3-4 weeks. ▶K ♀D ▶? $$$$$

CORTICOSTEROIDS	Approximate equivalent dose (mg)	Relative anti-inflammatory potency	Relative mineralocorticoid potency	Biologic Half-life (hours)
betamethasone	0.6-0.75	20-30	0	36-54
cortisone	25	0.8	2	8-12
dexamethasone	0.75	20-30	0	36-54
fludrocortisone	--	10	125	18-36
hydrocortisone	20	1	2	8-12
methylprednisolone	4	5	0	18-36
prednisolone	5	4	1	18-36
prednisone	5	4	1	18-36
triamcinolone	4	5	0	12-36

Corticosteroids (See also dermatology, ophthalmology.)

betamethasone (*Celestone, Celestone Soluspan*, ❦*Betnesol, Betaject*): Anti-inflammatory/Immunosuppressive: 0.6-7.2 mg/day PO divided bid-qid; up to 9 mg/day IM. Fetal lung maturation, maternal antepartum: 12 mg IM q24h x 2 doses. [Trade: Syrup 0.6 mg/5 ml.] ▶L ♀C ▶- $$$$$

cortisone (*Cortone*): 25-300 mg PO daily. [Generic/Trade: Tabs 5, 10, 25 mg.] ▶L ♀D ▶- $

dexamethasone (*Decadron, Dexone, Dexpak*, ❦*Dexasone, Maxidex*): Anti-inflammatory/Immunosuppressive: 0.5-9 mg/day PO/IV/IM, divided bid-qid. Fetal lung maturation, maternal antepartum: 6 mg IM q12h x 4 doses. [Generic/Trade: Tabs 0.25, 0.5, 0.75, 1.0, 1.5, 2, 4, 6 mg. elixir/ solution 0.5 mg/5 ml. Trade only: oral solution 0.5 mg/ 0.5 ml. Decadron Unipak (0.75 mg-12 tabs). Dexpak (51 total 1.5 mg tabs for a 13 day taper).] ▶L ♀C ▶- $

fludrocortisone (*Florinef*): Mineralocorticoid activity: 0.1 mg PO 3 times weekly to 0.2 mg PO daily. [Generic/Trade: Tabs 0.1 mg.] ▶L ♀C ▶? $

hydrocortisone (*Cortef, Cortenema, Hydrocortone, Solu-Cortef*): 100-500 mg IV/

IM q2-6h prn (sodium succinate). 20-240 mg/day PO divided tid-qid. Ulcerative colitis: 100 mg retention enema qhs (laying on side for ≥1 hour) for 21 days. [Trade: Tabs 5 mg. Generic/Trade: Tabs 10, 20 mg. Enema 100 mg/60 mL.] ▶L ♀C ▶- $

methylprednisolone (**Solu-Medrol, Medrol, Depo-Medrol**): Oral (Medrol): dose varies, 4-48 mg PO daily. Medrol Dosepak tapers 24 to 0 mg PO over 7 days. IM/Joints (Depo-Medrol): dose varies, 4-120 mg IM q1-2 weeks. Parenteral (Solu-Medrol): dose varies, 10-250 mg IV/IM. Acute spinal cord injury: 30 mg/kg IV over 15 min, followed in 45 min by a 5.4 mg/kg/h IV infusion q 23-47h. Peds: 0.5-1.7 mg/kg PO/IV/IM divided q6-12h. [Trade only: Tabs 2, 8, 16, 24, 32 mg. Generic/Trade: Tabs 4 mg. Medrol Dosepak (4 mg-21 tabs).] ▶L ♀C ▶- $$$

prednisolone (**Delta-Cortef, Prelone, Pediapred, Orapred**): 5-60 mg PO/IV/IM daily. [Generic/Trade: Tabs 5 mg; syrup 5 mg/5 ml, 15 mg/5 ml (Prelone: wild cherry flavor). Generic/Trade: solution 5 mg/5 ml (Pediapred; raspberry flavor); solution 15 mg/5 ml (Orapred; grape flavor).] ▶L ♀C ▶+ $$$

prednisone (**Deltasone, Meticorten, Pred-Pak, Sterapred, ✦Winpred**): 1-2 mg/kg or 5-60 mg PO daily. [Generic/Trade: Tabs 1, 5, 10, 20, 50 mg. Trade only: Tabs 2.5 mg. Sterapred (5 mg tabs: tapers 30 to 5 mg PO over 6d or 30 to 10 mg over 12d), Sterapred DS (10 mg tabs: tapers 60 to 10 mg over 6d, or 60 to 20 mg PO over 12d) & Pred-Pak (5 mg 45 & 79 tabs) taper packs. Solution 5 mg/5 ml & 5 mg/ml (Prednisone Intensol).] ▶L ♀C ▶+ $

triamcinolone (**Aristocort, Kenalog, ✦Aristospan**): 4-48 mg PO/IM daily. [Generic/Trade: Tabs 4 mg. Trade only: injection 10,25,40 mg/ml.] ▶L ♀C ▶- $$$$

Diabetes-Related - Alphaglucosidase Inhibitors

acarbose (**Precose, ✦Prandase**): Start 25 mg PO tid with meals, and gradually increase as tolerated to maintenance 50-100 mg tid. [Trade: Tabs 25, 50, 100 mg.] ▶Gut/K ♀B ▶- $$

miglitol (**Glyset**): Start 25 mg PO tid with meals, maintenance 50-100 tid. [Trade: Tabs 25, 50, 100 mg.] ▶K ♀B ▶- $$$

DIABETES NUMBERS*	Criteria for diagnosis of diabetes
Self-monitoring glucose goals	(repeat to confirm on subsequent day)

Self-monitoring glucose goals		Criteria for diagnosis	
Preprandial	90-130 mg/dL	Fasting glucose	≥126 mg/dL
Postprandial	< 180 mg/dL	Random glucose with symptoms	≥200 mg/dL

Management schedule: Aspirin** (75–162 mg/day) in Type 1 and 2 adults for primary prevention (those with an increased cardio-vascular risk, including >40 yo or with additional risk factors and	Control	A1c
	Normal	<6%
	Goal	<7%

secondary prevention (those with any vascular disease) unless contraindicated; statin therapy to achieve 30% LDL reduction for >40 yo & total cholesterol ≥135mg/dL.‡ *At every visit:* Measure weight & BP (goal <130/80 mmHg); visual foot exam; review self-monitoring glucose record; review/adjust meds; review self-management skills, dietary needs, and physical activity; smoking cessation counseling. *Twice a year:* A1c in those meeting treatment goals with stable glycemia (quarterly if not); dental exam. *Annually:* Fasting lipid profile (goal LDL <100 mg/dL, cardiovascular disease consider LDL <70mg/dL, HDL >40 mg/dL, TG <150 mg/dL†) q2 years with low-risk lipid values; creatinine; albumin to creatinine ratio spot collection; dilated eye exam; flu vaccine; comprehensive foot exam.

*See recommendations at the Diabetes Care website (http://care.diabetesjournals.org)
†ADA. Diabetes Care 2005;28 (Suppl 1):S14-S36, Circulation. 2004; 110:235
**Avoid aspirin below the age of 21 due to Reye's Syndrome risk. Use in those <30 yo has not been studied.

Diabetes-Related - Biguanides & Combinations

NOTE: Metformin-containing products may cause life-threatening lactic acidosis, usually in setting of decreased tissue perfusion, hypoxia, hepatic dysfunction, or impaired renal clearance. Hold prior to IV contrast agents and for 48 h after. Avoid if ethanol abuse, heart failure (requiring treatment), hepatic or renal insufficiency (creat ≥1.4 mg/dl in women, ≥1.5 mg/dl in men), or hypoxic states (cardiogenic shock, septicemia, acute MI).

ACTOPLUS Met (pioglitazone + metformin): 1 tablet PO daily-bid. Max 45/2550 mg/day. [Trade: Tabs 15/500, 15/850 mg.] ▶KL LC ▶?

Avandamet (rosiglitazone+metformin): 1 tab PO bid. If inadequate control with metformin monotherapy, select tab strength based on adding 4 mg/day rosiglitazone to existing metformin dose. If inadequate control with rosiglitazone monotherapy, select tab strength based on adding 1000 mg/day metformin to existing rosiglitazone dose. Max 8/2000 mg/day. Obtain LFTs before therapy & periodically thereafter. [Trade: Tabs 1/500, 2/500, 4/500, 2/1000, 4/1000 mg.] ▶KL ♀C ▶? $$$$

Glucovance (glyburide + metformin): As initial therapy: Start 1.25/250 mg PO daily or bid with meals; max 10/2000 mg daily. As second-line therapy: Start 2.5/500 or 5/500 mg PO bid with meals; max 20/2000 mg daily. [Trade/Generic: Tabs 1.25/250, 2.5/500, 5/500 mg.] ▶KL ♀B ▶? $$

Metaglip (glipizide + metformin): As initial therapy: Start 2.5/250 mg PO daily to 2.5/500 mg PO bid with meals; max 10/2000 mg daily. As second-line therapy: Start 2.5/500 or 5/500 mg PO bid with meals; max 20/2000 mg daily. [Trade: Tabs 2.5/250, 2.5/500, 5/500 mg.] ▶KL ♀C ▶? $$$

metformin (**Glucophage, Glucophage XR, Glumetza, Fortamet, Riomet**): Diabetes: Start 500 mg PO daily-bid with meals, may gradually increase to max 2550 mg/day or 2000 mg/day (ext'd release). Polycystic ovary syndrome (unapproved): 500 mg PO tid. Glucophage XR: 500 mg PO daily with evening meal; increase by 500 mg q week to max 2000 mg/day (may divide 1000 mg PO bid). Fortamet: 500-1000 mg daily with evening meal; increase by 500 mg q week to max 2500 mg/day. [Generic/Trade: Tabs 500, 625, 750, 850,1000 mg, extended release 500, 750 mg. Trade only: 500, 1000 mg (Fortamet), extended release 1000 mg (Glumetza). Trade only: oral soln 500 mg/5 mL (Riomet).] ▶K ♀B ▶? $$

Diabetes-Related - "Glitazones" (Thiazolidinediones)

pioglitazone (**Actos**): Start 15-30 mg PO daily, max 45 mg/day. Monitor LFTs. [Trade: Tabs 15, 30, 45 mg.] ▶L ♀C ▶- $$$$

rosiglitazone (**Avandia**): Diabetes monotherapy or in combination with metformin, sulfonylurea or insulin: Start 4 mg PO daily or divided bid, max 8 mg/day monotherapy or in combination with metformin and/or sulfonylurea. Max 4 mg/day when used with insulin. Obtain LFTs before therapy & periodically thereafter. [Trade: Tabs 2, 4, 8 mg.] ▶L ♀C ▶- $$$

Diabetes-Related - Meglitinides

nateglinide (**Starlix**): 120 mg PO tid ≤30 min before meals; use 60 mg PO tid in patients who are near goal A1C. [Trade: Tabs 60, 120 mg.] ▶L ♀C ▶? $$$

repaglinide (**Prandin**, ✢**Gluconorm**): Start 0.5- 2 mg PO tid before meals, maintenance 0.5-4 mg tid-qid, max 16 mg/day. [Trade: Tabs 0.5,1,2 mg.] ▶L ♀C ▶? $$$

Diabetes-Related - Sulfonylureas

gliclazide (**Diamicron, Diamicron MR**): Canada only. Immediate release: Start 80-160 mg PO daily, max 320 mg PO daily (≥160 mg in divided doses). Modified release: Start 30 mg PO daily, max 120 mg PO daily. [Generic/Trade: Tab 80 mg (Diamicron). Trade only: Tab 30 mg (Diamicron MR).] ▶KL ♀C ▶? $

glimepiride (**Amaryl**): Start 1-2 mg PO daily, usual 1-4 mg/day, max 8 mg/day. [Trade: Tabs 1, 2, 4 mg.] ▶LK ♀C ▶- $

glipizide (**Glucotrol, Glucotrol XL**): Start 5 mg PO daily, usual 10-20 mg/day, max 40 mg/day (divide bid if >15 mg/day). Extended release: Start 5 mg PO daily, usual 5-10 mg/day, max 20 mg/day. [Generic/Trade: Tabs 5, 10 mg; ext'd release tabs 5,10 mg. Trade only: Ext'd release tabs (Glucotrol XL) 2.5 mg.] ▶LK ♀C ▶? $

glyburide (**Micronase, DiaBeta, Glynase PresTab, ♥Euglucon**): Start 1.25-5 mg PO daily, usual 1.25-20 mg daily or divided bid, max 20 mg/day. Micronized tabs: Start 1.5-3 mg PO daily, usual 0.75-12 mg/day divided bid, max 12 mg/d. [Generic/Trade: Tabs (scored) 1.25, 2.5, 5 mg. micronized Tabs (scored) 1.5, 3, 4.5, 6 mg.] ▶LK ♀B ▶? $

Diabetes-Related Agents - Other

A1C home testing (**Metrika A1CNow**): Fingerstick blood. ▶None ♀+ $

dextrose (**Glutose, B-D Glucose, Insta-Glucose**): Hypoglycemia: 0.5-1 g/kg (1-2 ml/kg) up to 25 g (50 ml) of 50% soln IV. Dilute to 25% for pediatric administration. [OTC/Trade only: chew Tabs 5 g. gel 40%.] ▶L ♀C ▶? $

diazoxide (**Proglycem**): Hypoglycemia: 3-8 mg/kg/day divided q8-12h, max 10- 15 mg/kg/day. [Trade: susp 50 mg/ ml.] ▶L ♀C ▶- $$$$$

exenatide (**Byetta**): Type 2 DM who are receiving metformin, sulfonylurea or both: 5 mcg SC bid (within 1 h before the morning and evening meals). May increase to 10 mcg SC bid after 1 month. [Trade only: prefilled pen (60 doses each) 5 mcg/ dose, 1.2 mL; 10 mcg/dose, 2.4 mL.] ▶K ♀C ▶? $$$$$

glucagon (**Glucagon, GlucaGen**): Hypoglycemia: 1 mg IV/IM/SC, onset 5-20 min. Diagnostic aid: 1 mg IV/IM/SC. [Trade: injection 1 mg.] ▶LK ♀B ▶? $$$

glucose home testing (**Accu-Chek Active, Accu-Check Advantage, Accu-Check Compact, Ascencia, FreeStyle, GlucoWatch, OneTouch InDuo, OneTouch**

INSULIN*	Preparation	Onset (h)	Peak (h)	Duration (h)
Rapid-acting:	Insulin aspart (Novolog)	<0.2	1-3	3-5
	Insulin glulisine (Apidra)	0.30-0.4	1	4-5
	Insulin lispro (Humalog)	0.25-0.5	0.5-2.5	≤ 5
Short-acting:	Regular	0.5-1	2-3	3-6
Intermediate-acting:	NPH (Novolin N, Humulin N)	2-4	4-10	10-16
	Lente (Humulin L)†	3-4	4-12	12-18
Long-acting:	Ultralente (Humulin U) †	6-10	10-16	18-20
	Insulin detemir (Levemir)	not available	flat action profile	up to 23¶
	Insulin glargine (Lantus)	2-4	peakless	24
Mixtures:	Insulin aspart protamine suspension/insulin aspart (Novolog Mix 70/30)	0.25	1-4 (biphasic)	up to 24
	Insulin lispro protamine suspension/insulin lispro (Humalog Mix 75/25)	<0.25	1-3 (biphasic)	10-20
	NPH/Reg (Humulin 70/30, Humulin 50/50, Novolin 70/30))	0.5-1	2-10 (biphasic)	10-20

*These are general guidelines, as onset, peak, and duration of activity are affected by the site of injection, physical activity, body temperature, and blood supply.
† Products discontinued, expect stock depletion by end of 2005. Switch to alternative.
¶ Dose dependent duration of action, range from 6-23 hours.

Ultra, OneTouch UltraSmart, Precision Sof-Tact, Precision QID, Precision Xtra, True Track Smart System, Clinistix, Clinitest, Diastix, Tes-Tape, GlucoWatch): Use for home glucose monitoring. ▶None ♀+ ▶+ $$

insulin (*Apidra, Novolin, NovoLog, Humulin, Humalog, Lantus, Levemir, ✦NovoRapid*): Diabetes: Doses vary, but typically 0.3-0.5 unit/kg/day SC in divided doses (Type 1), and 1-1.5 unit/kg/day SC in divided doses (Type 2). Generally, 50-70% of insulin requirements are provided by rapid or short-acting insulin and the remainder from intermediate- or long-acting insulin. Administer rapid-acting insulin (Humalog, NovoLog, Apidra) within 15 min before or immediately after a meal. Administer regular insulin 30 minutes before meals. Lantus: Start 10 units SC daily (same time everyday) in insulin naïve patients, adjust to achieve glycemic control. Levemir: Type 2 DM (inadequately controlled on oral meds): Start 0.1-0.2 units/kg once daily in evening or 10 units SC daily or BID; adjust to achieve glycemic control. Severe hyperkalemia: 5-10 units regular insulin plus concurrent dextrose IV. Profound hyperglycemia (eg, DKA): 0.1 unit regular/kg IV bolus, then initial infusion 100 units regular in 100 ml NS (1 unit/ml), at 0.1 units/kg/hr. 70 kg: 7 units/h (7 ml/h). [Trade: injection NPH, regular, insulin glulisine (Apidra), insulin lispro (Humalog), insulin lispro protamine suspension/ insulin lispro (Humalog Mix 75/25), insulin glargine (Lantus), insulin aspart (NovoLog), insulin aspart protamine/insulin aspart (Novolog Mix 70/30) NPH and regular mixtures (Humulin 70/30, Novolin 70/30 or Humulin 50/50). Insulin available in pen form: Novolog, Novolin R, Novolin N, Novolog Mix 70/30, Novolog Mix 70/30 Humalog, Humulin N, Humulin 70/30, Humalog Mix 75/25, Lantus.] ▶LK ♀B/C ▶+ $$

pramlintide (*Symlin*): Type 1 DM with mealtime insulin therapy: Initiate 15 mcg SC immediately before major meals & titrate by 15 mcg increments (if significant nausea has not occurred for ≥3 days) to maintenance 30-60 mcg as tolerated. Type 2 DM with mealtime insulin therapy: Initiate 60 mcg SC immediately before major meals and increase to 120 mcg as tolerated (if significant nausea has not occurred for 3-7 days). [Trade only: 5 ml vials, 0.6 mg/mL.] ▶K ♀C ▶? $$$$

Gout-Related

allopurinol (*Aloprim, Zyloprim, ✦Purinol*): Mild gout or recurrent calcium oxalate stones: 200-300 mg PO daily-bid, max 800 mg/day. [Generic/Trade: Tabs 100, 300 mg.] ▶K ♀C ▶+ $

Colbenemid (colchicine + probenecid): 1 tab PO daily x 1 week, then 1 tab PO bid. [Generic/Trade: Tabs 0.5 mg colchicine + 500 mg probenecid.] ▶KL ♀C ▶? $$

colchicine: Rapid treatment of acute gouty arthritis: 0.6 mg PO q1h for up to 3h (max 3 tabs). Gout prophylaxis: 0.6 mg PO bid if CrCl ≥50 ml/min, 0.6 mg PO daily if CrCl 35-49 ml/min, 0.6 mg PO q2-3 days if CrCl 10-34 ml/min. [Generic/Trade: Tabs 0.6 mg.] ▶L ♀C ▶? $

probenecid (*✦Benuryl*): Gout: 250 mg PO bid x 7 days, then 500 bid. Adjunct to penicillin injection: 1-2 g PO. [Generic: Tabs 500 mg.] ▶KL ♀B ▶? $

Minerals

calcium acetate (*PhosLo*): Hyperphosphatemia: Initially 2 tabs/caps PO with each meal. [Trade only: Tab/Cap 667 mg (169 mg elem Ca).] ▶K ♀+ ▶? $

calcium carbonate (*Tums, Os-Cal, Caltrate, Viactiv, ✦Calsan*): 1-2 g elem Ca/day or more PO with meals divided bid-qid. [OTC Generic/Trade: tab 650,667, 1250,1500 mg, chew tab 750,1250 mg, cap 1250 mg, susp 1250 mg/5 ml. Calcium carbonate is 40% elem Ca and contains 20 mEq of elem Ca/g calcium car-

INTRAVENOUS SOLUTIONS	(ions in mEq/l)							
Solution	*Dextrose*	*Cal/l*	*Na*	*K*	*Ca*	*Cl*	*Lactate*	*Osm*
0.9 NS	0 g/l	0	154	0	0	154	0	310
LR	0 g/l	9	130	4	3	109	28	273
D5 W	50 g/l	170	0	0	0	0	0	253
D5 0.2 NS	50 g/l	170	34	0	0	34	0	320
D5 0.45 NS	50 g/l	170	77	0	0	77	0	405
D5 0.9 NS	50 g/l	170	154	0	0	154	0	560
D5 LR	50 g/l	179	130	4	3	109	28	527

bonate. Not more than 500-600 mg elem Ca/dose. Os-Cal 250 + D contains 125 units vitamin D/tab, Os-Cal 500 + D contains 200 units vitamin D/tab, Caltrate 600 + D contains 200 units vitamin D/tab. Viactiv (chew candy) 500 +100 units vitamin D + 40 mcg vitamin K/tab.] ▶K ♀+ ▶+ $

calcium chloride: 500-1000 mg slow IV q1-3 days. [Generic: injectable 10% (1000 mg/10 ml) 10 ml ampules, vials, syringes.] ▶K ♀+ ▶+ $

calcium citrate (*Citracal*): 1-2 g elem Ca/day or more PO with meals divided bid-qid. [OTC: Trade (mg elem Ca): tab 200 mg, 250 mg with 125 units vitamin D, 315 mg with 200 units vitamin D, 250 mg with 62.5 units magnesium stearate vitamin D, effervescent tab 500 mg.] ▶K ♀+ ▶+ $

calcium gluconate: 2.25-14 mEq slow IV. 500-2000 mg PO bid-qid. [Generic: injectable 10% (1000 mg/10 ml, 4.65mEq/10 ml) 10,50,100,200 ml. OTC generic: tab 500,650,975,1000 mg.] ▶K ♀+ ▶+ $

ferrous gluconate (*Fergon*): 800-1600 mg ferrous gluconate PO divided tid. [OTC Generic/Trade: tab (ferrous gluconate) 240,300,324,325 mg.] ▶K ♀+ ▶+ $

ferrous sulfate (*Fer-in-Sol, FeoSol Tabs, ♥Ferodan, Slow-Fe, Fero-Grad*): 500-1000 mg ferrous sulfate (100-200 mg elem iron) PO divided tid. Liquid: Adults 5-10 ml tid, non-infant children 2.5-5 ml tid. Many other available formulations. [OTC Generic/Trade: tab (mg ferrous sulfate) 324,325 mg, liquid 220 mg/5 ml, drops 75 mg/0.6 ml.] ▶K ♀+ ▶+ $

fluoride (*Luride, ♥Fluor-A-Day, Fluotic*): Adult dose: 10 ml of fluoride rinse swish and spit daily. Peds daily dose based on fluoride content of drinking water (table). [Generic: chew tab 0.5,1 mg, tab 1 mg, drops 0.125 mg, 0.25 mg, and 0.5 mg/dropperful, lozenges 1 mg, solution 0.2 mg/ml, gel 0.1%, 0.5%, 1.23%, rinse (sodium fluoride) 0.05,0.1,0.2%).] ▶K ♀? ▶? $

Peds qd dose is based on drinking water fluoride (shown in ppm)

Age	<0.3	0.3-0.6	>0.6
(years)	*ppm*	*ppm*	*ppm*
0-0.5	none	none	none
0.5-3	0.25mg	none	none
3-6	0.5mg	0.25mg	none
6-16	1 mg	0.5 mg	none

iron dextran (*InFed, DexFerrum, Infufer*): 25-100 mg IM daily prn. Equations available to calculate IV dose based on weight & Hb. ▶KL ♀- ▶? $$$$

iron polysaccharide (*Niferex, Niferex-150, Nu-Iron, Nu-Iron 150*): 50-200 mg PO divided daily-tid. [OTC Trade only: tab 50 mg (Niferex). Trade/Generic: cap 150 mg (Niferex-150, Nu-Iron 150), liquid 100 mg/5 ml (Niferex, Nu-Iron). 1 mg iron polysaccharide = 1 mg elemental iron.] ▶K ♀+ ▶+ $

iron sucrose (*Venofer*): Iron deficiency with hemodialysis: 5 ml (100 mg elem iron) IV over 5 min or diluted in 100 ml NS IV over ≥15 min. Iron deficiency in non-dialysis chronic kidney disease: 10 ml (200 mg elem iron) IV over 5 minutes. ▶KL ♀B ▶? $$$$$

magnesium chloride (*Slow-Mag*): 2 tabs PO daily. [OTC Trade: enteric coated tab 64 mg. 64 mg tab Slow-Mag = 64 mg elem magnesium.] ▶K ♀A ▶+ $

magnesium gluconate (*Almora, Magtrate, Maganate, ❦Magulcate*): 500-1000 mg PO divided tid. [OTC Generic: tab 500 mg, liquid 54 mg elem Mg/5 ml] ▶K♀A▶+ $

magnesium oxide (*Mag-200, Mag-Ox 400*): 400-800 mg PO daily. [OTC Generic/Trade: cap 140,250,400,420,500 mg.] ▶K♀A▶+ $

magnesium sulfate: Hypomagnesemia: 1 g of 20% soln IM q6h x 4 doses, or 2 g IV over 1 h (monitor for hypotension). Peds: 25-50 mg/kg IV/IM q4-6h for 3-4 doses, max single dose 2g. ▶K♀A▶+ $

phosphorus (*Neutra-Phos, K-Phos*): 1 cap/packet PO qid. 1-2 tabs PO qid. Severe hypophosphatemia (eg, <1 mg/dl): 0.08-0.16 mmol/kg IV over 6h. [OTC: Trade: (Neutra-Phos, Neutra-Phos K) tab/cap/packet 250 mg (8 mmol) phosphorus. Rx: Trade: (K-Phos) tab 250 mg (8 mmol) phosphorus.] ▶K♀C▶? $

potassium (*Cena-K, Effer-K, K+8, K+10, Kaochlor, Kaon, Kaon Cl, Kay Ciel, Kaylixir, K+Care, K+Care ET, K-Dur, K-G Elixir, K-Lease, K-Lor, Klor-con, Klorvess, Klorvess Effervescent, Klotrix, K-Lyte, K-Lyte Cl, K-Norm, Kolyum, K-Tab, K-vescent, Micro-K, Micro-K LS, Slow-K, Ten-K, Tri-K*): IV infusion 10 mEq/h (diluted). 20-40 mEq PO daily-bid. [Injectable, many different products in a variety of salt forms (i.e. chloride, bicarbonate, citrate, acetate, gluconate), available in tabs, caps, liquids, effervescent tabs, and packets. Potassium gluconate is available OTC.] ▶K♀C▶? $

sodium ferric gluconate complex (*Ferrlecit*): 125 mg elem iron IV over 10 min or diluted in 100 ml NS over 1 h. Peds ≥6 yo: 1.5 mg/kg (max 125 mg) elem iron diluted in 25 ml NS & administered IV over 1h. ▶KL♀B▶? $$$$$

POTASSIUM, oral forms

| Effervescent Granules: 20 mEq (*Klorvess Effervescent, K-vescent*) |
| Effervescent Tablets: 20 mEq (*K+Care ET, Klorvess*), 25 mEq (*Effer-K, K+Care ET, K-Lyte, K-Lyte/Cl, Klor-Con/EF*), 50 mEq (*K-Lyte DS, K-Lyte/Cl 50*) |
| Liquids: 20 mEq/15 ml (*Cena-K, Kaochlor S-F, K-G Elixir, Kaochlor 10%, Kay Ciel, Kaon, Kaylixir, Klorvess,Kolyum, Potasalan, Twin-K*), 30 mEq/15 ml (*Rum-K*), 40 mEq/15 ml (*Cena-K, Kaon-Cl 20%*), 45 mEq/15 ml (*Tri-K*) |
| Powders: 15 mEq/pack (*K+Care*), 20 mEq/pack (*Gen-K, K+Care, Kay Ciel, K-Lor, Klor-Con, Klorvess, Micro-K LS*), 25 mEq/pack (*K+Care, Klor-Con 25*) |
| Tablets/Capsules: 6.7 mEq (*Kaon-CL*), 8 mEq (*K+8, Kaon CL 8, Slow-K, Micro-K*), 10 mEq (*K+10, K-Lease, K-Norm, Kaon-Cl 10, Klor-Con 10, Klotrix, K-Tab, K-Dur 10, Micro-K 10,Ten-K*), 20 mEq (*K-Dur 20*) |

Nutritionals

banana bag, rally pack: Alcoholic malnutrition (one formula): Add thiamine 100 mg + folic acid 1 mg + IV multivitamins to 1 liter NS and infuse over 4h. Magnesium sulfate 2g may be added. "Banana bag" and "rally pack" are jargon and not valid drug orders; specify individual components. ▶KL♀+▶+ $

fat emulsion (*Intralipid, Liposyn*): dosage varies. ▶L♀C▶? $$$$$

formulas - infant (*Enfamil, Similac, Isomil, Nursoy, Prosobee, Soyalac, Alsoy, Nutramigen Lipil*): Infant meals. [OTC: Milk-based (Enfamil, Similac, SMA) or soy-based (Isomil, Nursoy, ProSobee, Soyalac, Alsoy).] ▶♀+▶+ $

levocarnitine (*Carnitor*): 10-20 mg/kg IV at each dialysis session. ▶KL♀B▶? $$$$$

omega-3 fatty acid (*fish oil, Promega, Cardio-Omega 3, Sea-Omega, Marine Lipid Concentrate, MAX EPA, Omacor, SuperEPA 1200*): Hypertriglyceridemia: 2-4 g EPA+DHA content daily; Omacor: 4 capsules PO daily or divided bid. Marine Lipid Concentrate, Super EPA 1200 mg cap contains EPA 360 mg + DHA 240 mg, daily dose = 4-8 caps. Omacor is only FDA approved fish oil. [Trade/Generic: cap, shown as EPA+DHA mg content, 240 (Promega Pearls), 300 (Cardi-Omega 3, Max EPA), 320 (Sea-Omega), 400 (Promega), 500 (Sea-Omega), 600 (Marine Lipid Concentrate, SuperEPA 1200), 740 mg (Omacor), 875 mg (Super-EPA 2000).] ▶L ♀? $$

PEDIATRIC REHYDRATION SOLUTIONS (ions in mEq/l)

Brand	Glucose	Cal/l	Na	K	Cl	Citrate	Phos	Ca	Mg
CeraLyte 50*	0 g/l	160	50	20	40	30	0	0	0
CeraLyte 70*	0 g/l	160	70	20	60	30	0	0	0
CeraLyte 90*	0 g/l	160	90	20	80	30	0	0	0
Infalyte	30 g/l	140	50	25	45	34	0	0	0
Kao Lectrolyte*	20 g/l	90	50	20	40	30	0	0	0
Lytren†	20 g/l	80	50	25	45	30	0	0	0
Naturalyte	25 g/l	0	45	20	35	48	0	0	0
Pedialyte‡	25 g/l	100	45	20	35	30	0	0	0
Rehydralyte	25 g/l	100	75	20	65	30	0	0	0
Resol	20 g/l	80	50	20	50	34	5	4	4

*Available in premeasured powder packet. †Canada. ‡and Pedialyte Freezer Pops

Thyroid Agents

levothyroxine (**L-Thyroxine, Levolet, Levo-T, Levothroid, Levoxyl, Novothyrox, Synthroid, Thyro-Tabs, Unithroid, T4, ♥Eltroxin**): Start 100-200 mcg PO daily (healthy adults) or 12.5-50 mcg PO daily (elderly or CV disease), increase by 12.5-25 mcg/day at 3-8 week intervals. Usual maintenance dose 100-200 mcg/day, max 300 mcg/d. [Generic/Trade: Tabs 25, 50, 75, 88, 100, 112, 125, 150, 175, 200, 300 mcg. Trade only: Tabs 137mcg.] ▶L ♀A ▶+ $

liothyronine (**T3, Cytomel**): Start 25 mcg PO daily, max 100 mcg/day. [Trade only: Tabs 5 mcg. Generic/Trade: Tabs 25, 50 mcg.] ▶L ♀A ▶? $

methimazole (**Tapazole**): Start 5-20 mg PO tid or 10-30 mg PO daily, then adjust. [Generic: Tabs 5, 10, 15, 20 mg. Trade: tabs 5, 10 mg.] ▶L ♀D ▶+ $$$

propylthiouracil (**PTU, ♥Propyl Thyracil**): Start 100 mg PO tid, then adjust. Thyroid storm: 200-300 mg PO qid, then adjust. [Generic: Tabs 50 mg.] ▶L ♀D (but preferred over methimazole) ▶+ $

sodium iodide I-131 (**Iodotope, Sodium Iodide I-131 Therapeutic**): Specialized dosing for hyperthyroidism and thyroid carcinoma. [Generic/Trade: Capsules & oral solution: radioactivity range varies at the time of calibration.] ▶K ♀X ▶- $$$$$

Vitamins

ascorbic acid (**vitamin C, ♥Redoxon**): 70-1000 mg PO daily. [OTC: Generic: tab 25,50,100,250,500,1000 mg, chew tab 100,250,500 mg, time-released tab 500 mg, 1000,1500 mg, time-released cap 500 mg, lozenge 60 mg, liquid 35 mg/0.6 ml, oral solution 100 mg/ml, syrup 500 mg/5 ml.] ▶K ♀C ▶? $

calcitriol (**Rocaltrol, Calcijex**): 0.25-2 mcg PO daily. [Generic/Trade: Cap 0.25, 0.5 mcg. Oral soln 1 mcg/ml. Injection 1,2 mcg/ml.] ▶L ♀C ▶? $$

cyanocobalamin (**vitamin B12, Nascobal, B12**): Deficiency states: 100-200 mcg IM q month or 1000-2000 mcg PO daily for 1-2 weeks followed by 1000 mcg PO daily or 500 mcg intranasal weekly. [OTC Generic: tab 100,500,1000,5000 mcg; lozenges 100,250,500 mcg. Rx Trade only: nasal gel 500 mcg/0.1 ml, nasal spray 500 mcg/spray.] ▶K ♀C ▶+ $

Diatx (folic acid + niacinamide + cobalamin + pantothenic acid + pyridoxine + d-biotin + thiamine + vitamin C + riboflavin): 1 tab PO daily. [Trade: Each tab contains folic acid 5 mg + niacinamide 20 mg + cobalamin 1 mg + pantothenic acid 10 mg + pyridoxine 50 mg + d-biotin 300 mcg + thiamine 1.5 mg + vitamin C 60 mg + riboflavin 1.5 mg. Diatx Fe: adds 100 mg ferrous fumarate per tab.] ▶LK ♀? ▶? $$

dihydrotachysterol (vitamin D, DHT): 0.2-1.75 mg PO daily. [Generic: tab 0.125,0.2, 0.4 mg, cap 0.125 mg, oral solution 0.2 mg/ml.] ▶L ♀C ▶? $$

doxercalciferol (Hectorol): Secondary hyperparathyroidism on dialysis: Oral: 10 mcg PO 3x/ week. May increase q8 weeks by 2.5 mcg/dose; max 60 mcg/week. IV: 4 mcg IV 3x/ week. May increase dose q8 weeks by 1-2 mcg/dose; max 18 mcg/week. Secondary hyperparathyroidism not on dialysis: Start 1 mcg PO daily, may increase by 0.5 mcg/dose q 2 weeks. Max 3.5 mcg/day. [Trade only: Caps 0.5, 2.5 mcg.] ▶L ♀B ▶? $$$$

Folgard (folic acid + cyanocobalamin + pyridoxine): 1 tab PO daily. [Trade: folic acid 0.8 mg + cyanocobalamin 0.115 mg + pyridoxine 10 mg tab.] ▶K ♀? ▶? $

folic acid (folate, Folvite): 0.4-1 mg IV/IM/PO/SC daily. [OTC Generic: Tab 0.4,0.8 mg. Rx Generic 1 mg.] ▶K ♀A ▶+ $

Foltx (folic acid + cyanocobalamin + pyridoxine): 1 tab PO daily. [Trade: folic acid 2.5 mg/ cyanocobalamin 2 mg/ pyridoxine 25 mg tab.] ▶K ♀A ▶+ $

multivitamins (MVI): Dose varies with product. Tabs come with and without iron. [OTC & Rx: Many different brands and forms available with and without iron (tab, cap, chew tab, drops, liquid).] ▶LK ♀+ ▶+ $

Nephrocap (vitamin C + folic acid + niacin + thiamine + riboflavin + pyridoxine + pantothenic acid + biotin + cyanocobalamin): 1 cap PO daily. If on dialysis, take after treatment. [Trade/Generic: vitamin C 100 mg/folic acid 1 mg/ niacin 20 mg/ thiamine 1.5 mg/ riboflavin 1.7 mg/ pyridoxine 10 mg/ pantothenic acid 5 mg/ biotin 150 mcg/ cyanocobalamin 6 mcg] ▶K ♀? ▶? $

Nephrovite (vitamin C + folic acid + niacin + thiamine + riboflavin + pyridoxine + pantothenic acid + biotin + cyanocobalamin): 1 tab PO daily. If on dialysis, take after treatment. [Trade/Generic: vitamin C 60 mg/folic acid 1 mg/ niacin 20 mg/ thiamine 1.5 mg/ riboflavin 1.7 mg/ pyridoxine 10 mg/ pantothenic acid 10 mg/ biotin 300 mcg/ cyanocobalamin 6 mcg] ▶K ♀? ▶? $

niacin (vitamin B3, Niacor, Slo-Niacin, Niaspan): 10-500 mg PO daily. See cardiovascular section for lipid-lowering dose. [OTC: Generic: tab 50,100,250,500 mg, timed-release cap 125,250,400 mg, timed-release tab 250,500 mg, liquid 50 mg/5 ml. Trade: 250,500,750 mg (Slo-Niacin). Rx: Trade only: tab 500 mg (Niacor), timed-release cap 500 mg (Slo-Niacin), timed-release tab 500,750,1000 mg (Niaspan, $$).] ▶K ♀C ▶? $

paricalcitol (Zemplar): Prevention/treatment of secondary hyperparathyroidism with renal insufficiency: 1-2 mcg PO daily or 2-4 mcg PO 3 times/wk; increase dose by 1 mcg/day or 2 mcg/week until desired PTH level is achieved. Prevention/treatment of secondary hyperparathyroidism with renal failure (CrCl<15 mL/min): 0.04-0.1 mcg/kg (2.8-7 mcg) IV 3 times/wk at dialysis; increase dose by 2-4 mcg q 2-4 weeks until desired PTH level is achieved. Max dose 0.24 mcg/kg (16.8 mcg). [Trade only: Caps 1, 2, 4 mcg.] ▶L ♀C ▶? $$$$$

phytonadione (vitamin K, Mephyton, AquaMephyton): Single dose of 0.5-1 mg IM within 1h after birth. Excessive oral anticoagulation: Dose varies based on INR. INR 5-9: 1-2.5 mg PO (=<5 mg PO may be used if rapid reversal necessary); INR >9 with no bleeding: 5-10 mg PO; Serious bleeding & elevated INR: 10 mg slow IV infusion. Adequate daily intake 120 mcg (males) and 90 mcg (females). [Trade only: Tab 5 mg.] ▶K ♀C ▶+ $

pyridoxine (*vitamin B6, B6*): 10-200 mg PO daily. INH overdose: 1 g IV/IM q 30 min, total dose of 1 g for each gram of INH ingested. [OTC Generic: Tab 25,50, 100 mg, timed-release tab 100 mg.] ▶K ♀A ▶+ $

riboflavin (*vitamin B2*): 5-25 mg PO daily. [OTC Generic: tab 25,50,100 mg.] ▶K ♀A ▶+ $

thiamine (*vitamin B1*): 10-100 mg IV/IM/PO daily. [OTC Generic: tab 50,100,250, 500 mg, enteric coated tab 20 mg.] ▶K ♀A ▶+ $

tocopherol (*vitamin E*, ♣*Aquasol E*): RDA is 22 units (natural, d-alpha-tocopherol) or 33 units (synthetic, d,l-alpha-tocopherol) or 15 mg (alpha-tocopherol). Max recommended 1000 units (alpha-tocopherol). Antioxidant: 400-800 units PO daily. [OTC Generic: tab 200,400 units, cap 73.5, 100, 147, 165, 200, 330, 400, 500, 600, 1000 units, drops 50 mg/ml.] ▶L ♀A ▶? $

vitamin A: RDA: 900 mcg RE (retinol equivalents) (males), 700 mcg RE (females). Treatment of deficiency states: 100,000 units IM daily x 3 days, then 50,000 units IM daily for 2 weeks. 1 RE = 1 mcg retinol or 6 mcg beta-carotene. Max recommended daily dose 3000 mcg. [OTC: Generic: cap 10,000, 15,000 units. Trade: tab 5,000 units. Rx: Generic: 25,000 units. Trade: soln 50,000 units/ml.] ▶L ♀A (C if exceed RDA, X in high doses) ▶+ $

vitamin D (*vitamin D2, ergocalciferol, Calciferol, Drisdol*, ♣*Osteoforte*): Familial hypophosphatemia (Vitamin D Resistant Rickets): 12,000-500,000 units PO daily. Hypoparathyroidism: 50,000-200,000 units PO daily. Adequate daily intake adults: 19-50 yo: 5 mcg (200 units) ergocalciferol; 51-70 yo: 10 mcg (400 units); >70 yo: 15 mcg (600 units). [OTC: Trade: soln 8000 units/ml. Rx: cap 50,000 units, inj 500,000 units/ml.] ▶L ♀A (C if exceed RDA) ▶+ $

Other

bromocriptine (*Parlodel*): Start 1.25-2.5 mg PO qhs with food. Hyperprolactinemia: Usual effective dose 2.5-15 mg/day, max 40 mg/day. Acromegaly: Usual effective dose 20-30 mg/day, max 100 mg/day. [Generic/Trade: Tabs 2.5 mg. Caps 5 mg.] ▶L ♀B ▶- $$$$

cabergoline (*Dostinex*): Hyperprolactinemia: 0.25-1 mg PO twice/wk. [Trade: Tabs 0.5 mg.] ▶L ♀B ▶- $$$$$

calcitonin (*Calcimar, Miacalcin*, ♣*Caltine*): Skin test before using injectable product: 1 unit intradermally and observe for local reaction. Osteoporosis: 100 units SC/IM or 200 units nasal spray daily (alternate nostrils). Paget's disease: 50-100 units SC/IM daily. Hypercalcemia: 4 units/kg SC/IM q12h. May increase after 2 days to max of 8 units/kg q6h. [Trade: nasal spray 100 units/ activation in 2 ml bottle (minimum of 14 doses/bottle).] ▶Plasma ♀C ▶? $$$

cinacalcet (*Sensipar*): Treatment of secondary hyperparathyroidism in dialysis patients: 30 mg PO daily. May titrate q 2-4 weeks through sequential doses of 60, 90, 120 & 180 mg daily to target intact parathyroid hormone level of 150-300 pg/mL. Treatment of hypercalcemia in parathyroid carcinoma: 30 mg PO bid. May titrate q 2-4 weeks through sequential does of 30 mg bid, 60 mg bid, 90 mg bid & 90 mg tid-qid as necessary to normalize serum calcium levels. [Trade: tab 30, 60, 90 mg] ▶LK ♀C ▶? $$$$$

cosyntropin (*Cortrosyn*, ♣*Synacthen*): Rapid screen for adrenocortical insufficiency: 0.25 mg (0.125 mg if <2 yo) IM/ IV over 2 min; measure serum cortisol before and 30-60 min after. ▶L ♀C ▶? $

demeclocycline (*Declomycin*): SIADH: 600-1200 mg/day PO given in 3-4 divided doses. [Trade only: Tabs 150, 300 mg] ▶K, feces ♀D ▶- $$$$$

desmopressin (**DDAVP, Stimate, ✦Minirin**): Diabetes insipidus: 10-40 mcg intranasally daily-tid, 0.05-1.2 mg/day PO or divided bid-tid, or 0.5-1 ml/day SC/IV in 2 divided doses. [Trade only: nasal solution 1.5 mg/ml (150 mcg/ spray). Generic/ Trade: Tabs 0.1, 0.2 mg. Nasal solution 0.1 mg/ml (10 mcg/ spray). Note difference in concentration of nasal solutions.] ▶LK ♀B ▶? $$$$

growth hormone human (**Protropin, Genotropin, Norditropin, Norditropin Nordi-Flex, Nutropin, Nutropin AQ, Humatrope, Serostim LQ, Saizen, Somatropin, Tev-Tropin, Zorbtive**): Dosages vary by product. [Single dose vials (powder for injection with diluent). Tev-Tropin: 5mg vial (powder for injection with diluent, stable for 14 days when refrigerated). Genotropin: 1.5, 5.8, 13.8 mg cartridges. Humatrope: 6, 12, 24 mg per cartridges. Nutropin AQ: 10 mg multiple dose vial & 10 mg/per cartridges. Norditropin: 5,10,15 mg per cartridges. Norditropin NordiFlex: 5, 10, 15 mg prefilled pens. Saizen: pre-assembled reconstitution device with autoinjector pen. Serostim LQ: 6 mg cartridge (packages come in 1 or 7 cartridges)] ▶LK ♀B/C ▶? $$$$$

hyaluronidase (**Amphadase**): Absorption and dispersion of injected drugs: Add 50-300 U (typically 150 U) to the injection solution. Hypodermoclysis: Administer 50-300 U after clysis or 150 U under the skin prior to clysis which will facilitate absorption of >1 L of solution. Subcutaneous urography: 75 U injected SC over each scapula, followed by injection of contrast media. [Trade only: 2 mL vial; 150 U/mL] ▶Serum ♀C ▶? ?

lanthanum carbonate (**Fosrenol**): Treatment of hyperphosphatemia in end stage renal disease: Start 750-1500 mg/day PO in divided doses with meals. Titrate dose every 2-3 weeks in increments of 750 mg/day until acceptable serum phosphate is reached. Most will require 1500-3000 mg/day to reduce serum phosphate <6.0 mg/dL. [Trade only: chewable tabs 250, 500 mg] ▶Not absorbed ♀C ▶? ?

sevelamer (**Renagel**): Hyperphosphatemia: 800-1600 mg PO tid with meals. [Trade: Tabs 400, 800 mg.] ▶Not absorbed ♀C ▶? $$$$

sodium polystyrene sulfonate (**Kayexalate**): Hyperkalemia: 1 g/kg up to 15-60 g PO or 30-50 g retention enema (in sorbitol) q6h prn. Irrigate with tap water after enema to prevent necrosis. [Generic: Suspension 15 g/ 60 ml. Powdered resin.] ▶Fecal excretion ♀C ▶? $$$$

teriparatide (**Forteo**): Treatment of postmenopausal women or men with primary or hypogonadal osteoporosis & high fracture risk: 20 mcg SC daily in thigh or abdomen for ≤2 years. [Trade only: 28-dose pen injector (20 mcg/dose).] ▶LK ♀C ▶- $$$$$

vasopressin (**Pitressin, ADH, ✦Pressyn AR**): Diabetes insipidus: 5-10 units IM/ SC bid-qid prn. Cardiac arrest: 40 units IV; may repeat if no response after 3 minutes. Septic shock: 0.01-0.1 units/min IV infusion, usual dose <0.04 units/min. Variceal bleeding: 0.2-0.4 units/min initially (max 0.9 units/min). ▶LK ♀C ▶? $$$$$

ENT

Antihistamines - Nonsedating

desloratadine (**Clarinex, ✦Aerius**): Adults & children ≥12 yo: 5 mg PO daily. 6-11 yo: 1 teaspoonful (2.5 mg) PO daily. 12 mo – 5 yo: ½ teaspoonful (1.25 mg) PO daily. 6-11 mo: 2 ml (1 mg) PO daily. [Trade: Tabs 5 mg. Fast-dissolve RediTabs 5 mg. Syrup 0.5 mg/ml] ▶LK ♀C ▶+ $$$

fexofenadine (**Allegra**): 60 mg PO bid or 180 mg daily. 6-12 yo: 30 mg PO bid. [Trade: Tabs 30, 60, & 180 mg. Generic/trade: Caps 60 mg.] ▶LK ♀C ▶+ $$$

loratadine (**Claritin, Claritin Hives Relief, Claritin RediTabs, Alavert, Tavist ND**):

ENT COMBINATIONS (selected)	Decongestant	Antihistamine	Antitussive	Typical Adult Doses
OTC				
Actifed Cold & Allergy	PS	TR	-	1 tab or 10 mL q4-6h
Actifed Cold & Sinus¶	PS	CH	-	2 tabs q 6h
Allerfrim, Aprodine	PS	TR	-	1 tab or 10 mL q4-6h
Benadryl Allergy/Cold¶	PS	DPH	-	2 tabs q 6h
Benadryl-D Allergy/Sinus Tablets	PS	DPH	-	1 tab q 4-6 h
Claritin-D 12 hour	PS	LO	-	1 tab q12h
Claritin-D 24 hour	PS	LO	-	1 tab daily
Dimetapp Cold & Allergy Elixir	PS	BR	-	20mL q 4h
Dimetapp Multi-Symp Cold & Allergy¶	PE	CH	-	2 tabs q4h
Mucinex-DM Extended-Release	-	-	GU,DM	1-2 tab q12h
Robitussin CF	PS	-	GU, DM	10 mL q4h*
Robitussin DM, Mytussin DM	-	-	GU, DM	10 mL q4h*
Robitussin PE, Guaituss PE	PS	-	GU	10 mL q4h*
Drixoral Cold & Allergy	PS	DBR	-	1 tab q12h
Drixoral Cold & Flu¶	PS	DBR	-	2 tab q 12h
Triaminic Cold & Allergy	PS	CH	-	20 mL q4-6h‡
Triaminic Cough	PS	-	DM	20 mL q4h‡
Rx Only				
Allegra-D12- hour	PS	FE	-	1 tab q12h
Allegra-D24- hour	PS	FE	-	1 tab daily
Bromfenex	PS	BR	-	1 cap q12h
Clarinex-D24-hour	PS	DL	-	1 tab daily
Deconamine	PS	CH	-	1 tab or 10 mL tid-qid
Codeprex	-	CH	CO	10 mL q12h
Deconamine SR, Chlordrine SR	PS	CH	-	1 tab q12h
Deconsal II	PS	-	GU	1-2 tabs q12h
Dimetane-DX	PS	BR	DM	10 mL PO q4h
Duratuss	PS	-	GU	1 tab q12h
Duratuss HD©III	PS	-	GU, HY	10mL q4-6h
Entex PSE, Guaifenex PSE 120	PS	-	GU	1 tab q12h
Histussin D ©III	PS	-	HY	5 mL qid
Histussin HC ©III	PE	CH	HY	10 mL q4h
Humibid DM	-	-	GU, DM	1 tab q12h
Hycotuss©III	-	-	GU, HY	5mL pc & qhs
Phenergan/Dextromethorphan	-	PR	DM	5 mL q4-6h
Phenergan VC	PE	PR	-	5 mL q4-6h
Phenergan VC w/codeine©V	PE	PR	CO	5 mL q4-6h
Poly-Histine Elixir	-	PT/PY/PH	-	10 mL q4h*
Robitussin AC ©V	-	-	GU, CO	10 mL q4h*
Robitussin DAC ©V	PS	-	GU, CO	10 mL q4h*
Rondec Syrup	PS	BR	-	5 mL qid*
Rondec DM Syrup	PS	BR	DM	5 mL qid*
Rondec Oral Drops	PS	CX	-	0.25 to 1 mL qid†
Rondec DM Oral Drops	PS	CX	DM	0.25 to 1 mL qid†
Rynatan	PE	CH	-	1-2 tabs q12h
Rynatan-P Pediatric	PE	CH, PY	-	2.5-5 mL q12h*
Semprex-D	PS	AC	-	1cap q4-6h
Tanafed	PS	CH	-	10-20 mL q12h*
Triacin-C, Actifed w/codeine©V	PS	TR	CO	10 mL q4-6h
Tussionex©III	-	CH	HY	5 mL q12h

Abbreviations and footnotes on next page

Adults & children ≥6 yo: 10 mg PO daily. 2-5 yo: 5 mg PO daily. [OTC: Generic/ Trade: Tabs 10 mg. Fast-dissolve tabs (Alavert, Claritin RediTabs) 10 mg. Syrup 1 mg/ml.] ▶LK ♀B ▶+ $

Antihistamines - Other

azatadine (*Optimine*): 1-2 mg PO bid. [Trade: Tabs 1 mg, scored.] ▶LK ♀B ▶- $$$

cetirizine (*Zyrtec*, ✦*Reactine, Aller-Relief*): Adults & children ≥6 yo: 5-10 mg PO daily. 2-5 yo: 2.5 mg PO daily-bid. 6-23 mo: 2.5 mg PO daily. [Trade: Tabs 5, 10 mg. Syrup 5 mg/5 ml. Chewable tabs, grape-flavored 5, 10 mg.] ▶LK ♀B ▶- $$$

chlorpheniramine (*Chlor-Trimeton, Chlo-Amine, Aller-Chlor*): 4 mg PO q4-6h. Max 24 mg/day. [OTC: Generic/Trade: Tabs chew 2 mg. Generic/Trade: Tabs 4 mg. Syrup 2 mg/5 ml. Generic/Trade: Tabs, Timed-release 8 mg. Trade only: Tabs, Timed-release 12 mg.] ▶LK ♀B ▶- $

clemastine (*Tavist*): 1.34 mg PO bid. Max 8.04 mg/day. [OTC: Generic/Trade: Tabs 1.34 mg. Rx: Generic/Trade: Tabs 2.68 mg. Trade only: Syrup 0.67 mg/5 ml.] ▶LK ♀B ▶- $

cyproheptadine (*Periactin*): Start 4 mg PO tid. Max 32 mg/day. [Generic/Trade: Tabs 4 mg (trade scored). Syrup 2 mg/5 ml.] ▶LK ♀B ▶- $

dexchlorpheniramine (*Polaramine*): 2 mg PO q4-6h. Timed release tabs: 4 or 6 mg PO at qhs or q8-10h. [Trade: Tabs, Immediate Release 2 mg. Syrup 2 mg/5 ml. Generic/Trade: Tabs, Timed Release: 4, 6 mg.] ▶LK ♀? ▶- $$$

diphenhydramine (*Benadryl*, ✦*Allerdryl, Allernix, Nytol*): 25-50 mg IV/IM/PO q4-6h. Peds: 5 mg/kg/day divided q4-6h. [OTC: Trade: Tabs 25, 50 mg, chew tabs 12.5 mg. OTC & Rx: Generic/Trade: Caps 25, 50 mg, softgel cap 25 mg. OTC: Generic/Trade: Liquid 6.25 mg/5 ml & 12.5 mg/5 ml.] ▶LK ♀B ▶- $

hydroxyzine (*Atarax, Vistaril*): 25-100 mg IM/PO daily-qid or prn. [Generic/Trade: Tabs 10, 25, 50 mg. Trade only: 100 mg. Generic/Trade: Caps 25, 50, 100 mg. Syrup 10 mg/5 ml (Atarax). Trade: Suspension 25 mg/5 ml (Vistaril).] ▶L ♀C ▶- $

promethazine (*Phenergan*): Adults: 12.5-25 mg PO/IM/IV/PR daily-qid. Peds: 6.25-12.5 mg PO/IM/IV/PR daily-qid. [Generic/Trade: Tabs 12.5 mg, scored. Generic/Trade: Tabs 25,50 mg. Syrup 6.25 mg/5 ml. Trade only: Phenergan Fortis Syrup 25 mg/5 ml. Trade: Supp 12.5 & 25 mg. Generic/Trade: Supp 50 mg.] ▶LK ♀C ▶- $

Antitussives / Expectorants

benzonatate (*Tessalon, Tessalon Perles*): 100-200 mg PO tid. Swallow whole. Do not chew. Numbs mouth, possible choking hazard. [Generic/Trade: Softgel caps: 100, 200 mg.] ▶L ♀C ▶? $

dextromethorphan (*Benylin, Delsym, Vick's*): 10-20 mg PO q4h or 30 mg PO q6-8h. Sustained action liquid 60 mg PO q12h. [OTC: Trade: Caps 30 mg. Lozenges 2.5, 5, 7.5, 15 mg. Liquid 3.5, 5, 7.5, 10, 12.5, 15 mg/5 ml; 10 & 15 mg/15 ml (Generic/Trade). Trade (Delsym): Sustained action liquid 30 mg/5 ml.] ▶L ♀+ ▶+ $

ENT COMBINATIONS abbreviations and footnotes

AC=acrivastine	DL=desloratadine	GU=guaifenesin	PR=promethazine
BR=brompheniramine	DM=dextromethorphan	HY=hydrocodone	PS=pseudoephedrine
CH=chlorpheniramine	DBR=dexbrompheniramine	LO=loratadine	PT=phenyltoloxamine
CO=codeine	DPH=diphenhydramine	PE=phenylephrine	PY=pyrilamine
CX=carbinoxamine	FE=fexofenadine	PH=pheniramine	TR=triprolidine

*5 mL/dose for 6-11 yo. 2.5 mL if 2-5yo. †1 mL/dose if 10-18 mo. ¾ mL if 7-9 mo. ½ mL if 4-6 mo. ¼ mL if 1-3 months old. ‡10 mL/dose if 6-11 yo. 5 mL if 2-5 yo. 2.5 mL if 13-23 mo. 1.25 mL if 4-12 mo. ✦Also contains acetaminophen guaifenesin (**Robitussin, Hytuss, Guiatuss, Mucinex**): 100-400 mg PO q4h. 600-1200 mg PO q12h (extended release). 100-200 mg/dose if 6-11 yo. 50-100 mg/dose if 2-5 yo. [OTC: Tabs 100, 200 mg. Caps 200 mg. Extended release tabs 600 & 1200 mg. Syrup 100 & 200 mg/5 ml. Generic: Syrup 100 mg/5 ml. Rx: Trade: Tabs 200, 1200 mg. Syrup 100 mg/5 ml.] ▶L ♀C ▶+ $

Decongestants

phenylephrine (**Sudafed PE**): 10 mg PO q4h. [OTC: Trade tabs 10 mg] ▶L ♀C ▶+ $

pseudoephedrine (**Sudafed, Sudafed 12 Hour, Efidac/24, Dimetapp Decongestant Infant Drops, PediaCare Infants' Decongestant Drops, Triaminic Oral Infant Drops, ★Pseudofrin**): Adult: 60 mg PO q4-6h. Peds: 30 mg/dose if 6-12 yo, 15 mg/dose if 2-5 yo. Extended release tabs: 120 mg PO bid or 240 mg PO daily. Dimetapp, PediaCare, & Triaminic Infant Drops: (7.5 mg/0.8 ml): Give PO q4-6h. Max 4 doses/day. 2-3: 1.6 ml. 12-23: 1.2 ml. 4-11 mo: 0.8 ml. 0-3 mo: 0.4 ml. [OTC: Generic/Trade: Tabs 30, 60 mg. Chewable tabs 15 mg. Trade only: Tabs, extended release 120, 240 mg. Trade only: Liquid 15 mg/5 ml. Generic/Trade: Liquid 30 mg/5 ml. Infant drops 7.5 mg/0.8 ml.] ▶L ♀C ▶+ $

Ear Preparations

Auralgan (benzocaine + antipyrine): 2-4 drops in ear(s) tid-qid prn. [Generic/Trade: Otic soln 10 & 15 ml.] ▶Not absorbed ♀C ▶? $

carbamide peroxide (**Debrox, Murine Ear**): 5-10 drops in ear(s) bid x 4 days. [OTC: Trade: Otic soln 6.5%, 15 or 30 ml bottle.] ▶Not absorbed ♀? ▶? $

Cipro HC Otic (ciprofloxacin + hydrocortisone): ≥1 yo to adult: 3 drops in ear(s) bid x 7 days. [Trade: Otic suspension 10 ml.] ▶Not absorbed ♀C ▶- $$$

Ciprodex Otic (ciprofloxacin + dexamethasone): ≥6 mo to adult: 4 drops in ear(s) bid x 7 days. [Trade: Otic suspension 5 & 7.5 ml.] ▶Not absorbed ♀C ▶- $$$

Cortisporin Otic (hydrocortisone + polymyxin + neomycin): 4 drops in ear(s) tid-qid up to 10 days of soln or suspension. Peds: 3 drops in ear(s) tid-qid up to 10 days. Caveats with perforated TMs or tympanostomy tubes: (1) Risk of neomycin ototoxicity, especially if use prolonged or repeated; (2) Use suspension rather than acidic soln. [Generic/Trade: Otic soln or suspension 7.5 & 10 ml.] ▶Not absorbed ♀? ▶? $$

Cortisporin TC Otic (hydrocortisone + neomycin + thonzonium + colistin): 4-5 drops in ear(s) tid-qid up to 10 days. [Trade: Otic suspension, 10 ml.] ▶Not absorbed ♀? ▶? $$$

docusate sodium (**Colace**): Cerumen removal: Instill 1 ml in affected ear. [Generic/Trade: Liquid 150 mg/15 ml.] ▶Not absorbed ♀+ ▶+ $

Domeboro Otic (acetic acid + aluminum acetate): 4-6 drops in ear(s) q2-3h. Peds: 2-3 drops in ear(s) q3-4h. [Generic/Trade Otic soln 60 ml.] ▶Not absorbed ♀? ▶? $

ofloxacin (**Floxin Otic**): >12 yo: 10 drops in ear(s) bid. 1-12 yo: 5 drops in ear(s) bid. [Trade: Otic soln 0.3% 5,10 ml. "Singles": single-dispensing containers 0.25 ml (5 drops), 2 per foil pouch.] ▶Not absorbed ♀? ▶? $$

Pediotic (hydrocortisone + polymyxin + neomycin): 3-4 drops in ear(s) tid-qid up to 10 days. [Trade: Otic suspension 7.5 ml.] ▶Not absorbed ♀C ▶- $$

Swim-Ear (isopropyl alcohol + anhydrous glycerins): 4-5 drops in ears after swimming. [OTC: Trade: Otic soln 30 ml.] ▶Not absorbed ♀? ▶? $

triethanolamine (**Cerumenex**): Fill ear canal x 15-30 mins to loosen cerumen, then flush. [Trade: Otic soln 6 & 12 ml with dropper.] ▶Not absorbed ♀C ▶- $$

VoSol Otic (acetic acid + propylene glycol): 5 drops in ear(s) tid-qid. Peds >3 yo: 3-4 drops in ear(s) tid-qid. VoSoL HC adds hydrocortisone 1%. [Generic/Trade: Otic soln 2%, 15 & 30 ml.] ▶Not absorbed ♀? ▶? $

Mouth & Lip Preparations

amlexanox (**Aphthasol, OraDisc A**): Aphthous ulcers: Apply ¼ inch paste or mucoadhesive patch to affected area qid after oral hygiene for up to 10 days. Up to 3 patches may be applied at one time. [Trade: Oral paste 5%, 5 g tube. Mucoadhesive patch 2 mg, #20.] ▶LK ♀B ▶? $

cevimeline (**Evoxac**): Dry mouth due to Sjogren's syndrome: 30 mg PO tid. [Trade: Caps 30 mg.] ▶L ♀C ▶- $$$

chlorhexidine gluconate (**Peridex, Periogard, ✦Denticare**): Rinse with 15 ml of undiluted soln for 30 seconds bid. Do not swallow. Spit after rinsing. [Generic/trade: Oral rinse 0.12% 473-480 ml bottles.] ▶Fecal excretion ♀B ▶? $

clotrimazole (**Mycelex**): Oral troches dissolved slowly in mouth 5 times/day x 14 days. [Trade: Oral troches 10 mg.] ▶L ♀C ▶? $$$

Debacterol (sulfuric acid + sulfonated phenolics): Aphthous stomatitis, mucositis: Apply to dry ulcer. Rinse with water. [Trade: 1 ml prefilled, single-use applicator.] ▶Not absorbed ♀C ▶+ $$

docosanol (**Abreva**): Herpes labialis (cold sores): At 1st sign of infection apply 5x/day until healed. [OTC: Trade: 10% cream in 2 g tube.] ▶? ♀B ▶? $$

doxycycline (**Periostat**): Periodontitis, adjunct to scaling & root planing: 20 mg PO bid. [Generic/trade: Caps 20 mg.] ▶L ♀D ▶- $$$

Gelclair (maltodextrin + propylene glycol): Aphthous ulcers, mucositis, stomatitis: Rinse mouth with 1 packet tid or prn. [Trade: 21 /box.] ▶Not absorbed ♀+ ▶+ $$$

lidocaine viscous (**Xylocaine**): Mouth or lip pain in adults only: 15-20 ml topically or swish & spit q3h. [Generic/Trade: soln 2%, 20 ml unit dose, 50, 100, 450 ml bottles.] ▶LK ♀B ▶+ $

magic mouthwash (**Benadryl + Mylanta + Carafate**): 5 ml PO swish & spit or swish & swallow tid before meals and prn. [Compounded suspension. A standard mixture is 30 ml diphenhydramine liquid (12.5 mg/5 ml) + 60 ml Mylanta or Maalox + 4 g Carafate.] ▶LK ♀B(- in 1st trimester) ▶- $$$

nystatin (**Mycostatin, ✦Nilstat**): Thrush: 5 ml PO swish & swallow qid. Infants: 2 ml/dose with 1 ml placed in each cheek. [Generic/Trade: Suspension 100,000 units/ml 60 & 480 ml bottle. Trade: Oral lozenges (Pastilles) 200,000 units.] ▶Not absorbed ♀C ▶? $$

penciclovir (**Denavir**): Herpes labialis (cold sores): apply cream q2h while awake x 4 days. Start at first sign of symptoms. [Trade: Cream 1%, 1.5 g tube.] ▶Not absorbed ♀B ▶- $

pilocarpine (**Salagen**): Dry mouth due to radiation of head & neck or Sjogren's syndrome: 5 mg PO tid-qid. [Generic/Trade Tabs 5 mg tablet 7.5 mg.] ▶L ♀C ▶- $$$

triamcinolone (**Kenalog in Orabase, ✦Oracort**): Apply paste bid-tid, ideally pc & qhs. [Generic/trade: 0.1% oral paste, 5 g tubes.] ▶L ♀C ▶? $

Nasal Preparations

azelastine (**Astelin**): Allergic/vasomotor rhinitis: 2 sprays/nostril bid. [Trade: Nasal spray, 100 sprays/bottle.] ▶L ♀C ▶? $$$

beclomethasone (**Vancenase, Vancenase AQ Double Strength, Beconase AQ**): Vancenase: 1 spray per nostril bid-qid. Beconase AQ: 1-2 sprays per nostril bid. Vancenase AQ Double Strength: 1-2 spray(s) per nostril daily. [Trade: Vancenase 42 mcg/spray, 80,200 sprays/bottle. Beconase AQ 42 mcg/spray, 200 sprays/bottle. Vancenase AQ Double Strength 84 mcg/spray, 120 sprays/bottle.] ▶L ♀C ▶? $$$

budesonide (**Rhinocort Aqua**): 1-4 sprays per nostril daily. [Trade: Nasal inhaler 120 sprays/bottle.] ▶L ♀B ▶? $$$

cromolyn (**NasalCrom, BenaMist, Children's NasalCrom**): 1 spray per nostril tid-qid. [OTC: Generic/Trade: Nasal inhaler 200 sprays/bottle. Trade: Children's Na-salCrom w/special "child-friendly" applicator. 100 sprays/bottle.] ▶LK ♀B ▶+ $

flunisolide (**Nasalide, Nasarel, ♣Rhinalar**): Start 2 sprays/nostril bid. Max 8 sprays/nostril/day. [Generic/Trade: Nasal soln 0.025%, 200 sprays/bottle. Na-salide with pump unit. Nasarel with meter pump & nasal adapter.] ▶L ♀C ▶? $$

fluticasone (**Flonase**): 2 sprays per nostril daily. [Trade: Nasal spray 0.05%, 120 sprays/bottle.] ▶L ♀C ▶? $$$

ipratropium (**Atrovent Nasal Spray**): 2 sprays per nostril bid-qid. [Generic/Trade: Nasal spray 0.03%, 345 sprays/bottle & 0.06%, 165 sprays/bottle.] ▶L ♀B ▶? $$

levocabastine (**♣Livostin Nasal Spray**): Canada only. 2 sprays in each nostril bid, increase prn to tid-qid. [Trade: nasal spray 0.5mg/ml, plastic bottles of 15ml. Each spray delivers 50 mcg.] ▶L (but minimal absorption) ♀C ▶- ?

mometasone (**Nasonex**): Adult: 2 sprays/nostril daily. Peds 2-11 yo: 1 spray/nostril daily. [Trade: Nasal spray, 120 sprays/bottle.] ▶L ♀C ▶? $$$

oxymetazoline (**Afrin, Dristan 12 Hr Nasal, Nostrilla**): 2-3 drops/sprays per nostril bid x 3 days. [OTC: Generic/Trade: Nasal spray 0.05%, 15 & 30 ml bottles. Nose drops 0.025% & 0.05%, 20 ml w/dropper.] ▶L ♀C ▶? $

phenylephrine (**Neo-Synephrine, Sinex, Nostril**): 2-3 sprays/drops per nostril q4h prn x 3 days. [OTC: Generic/Trade: Nasal drops 0.125, 0.16%. Generic/Trade: Nasal spray/drops 0.25, 0.5, 1%.] ▶L ♀C ▶? $

saline nasal spray (**SeaMist, Pretz, NaSal, Ocean, ♣HydraSense**): 1-3 sprays or drops per nostril prn. [Generic/Trade: Nasal spray 0.4, 0.5, 0.6, 0.65, 0.75%. Na-sal drops 0.4, 0.65, & 0.75%.] ▶Not metabolized ♀A ▶+ $

triamcinolone (**Nasacort AQ, Nasacort HFA, Tri-Nasal**): Nasacort HFA, Tri-Nasal: 2 sprays per nostril daily-bid. Max 4 sprays/nostril/day. Nasacort AQ: 2 sprays per nostril daily. [Trade: Nasal spray 55 mcg/spray, 100 sprays/bottle (Nasacort HFA). Nasal spray, 55 mcg/spray, 120 sprays/bottle (Nasacort AQ). Nasal spray 50 mcg/spray, 120 sprays/bottle (Tri-Nasal).] ▶L ♀C ▶- $$

Other

Cetacaine (benzocaine + tetracaine + butyl aminobenzoate): Topical anesthesia of mucous membranes: Spray: Apply for ≤1 second. Liquid or gel: Apply with cotton applicator directly to site. [Trade: Spray 56g. Liquid 56 g. Hospital gel 29 g.] ▶LK ♀C ▶? $

GASTROENTEROLOGY

Antidiarrheals

bismuth subsalicylate (**Pepto-Bismol, Kaopectate**): 2 tabs or 30 ml (262 mg/15 ml) PO q 30 min-1 h up to 8 doses/ day. Peds: 10 ml (262 mg/15 ml) or 2/3 tab if 6-9 yo, 5 ml (262 mg/15 ml) or 1/3 tab if 3-6 yo. Risk of Reye's syndrome in children. [OTC Generic/Trade: chew tab 262 mg, susp 87 mg/5 ml (Kaopectate Children's Liquid), 262 & 524 mg/15 ml. Generic only: susp 130 mg/15 ml. Trade only: cap-lets 262 mg (Pepto-Bismol).] ▶K ♀D ▶? $

Imodium Advanced (loperamide + simethicone): 2 caplets PO initially, then 1 cap-let PO after each unformed stool to a max of 4 caplets/24 h. Peds: 1 caplet PO initially, then ½ caplet PO after each unformed stool to a max of 2 caplets/day (if 6-8 yo or 48-59 lbs) or 3 caplets/day (if 9-11 yo or 60-95 lbs). [OTC: Trade: caplet 2 mg loperamide/125 mg simethicone.] ▶L ♀B ▶+ $

Lomotil (diphenoxylate + atropine): 2 tabs or 10 ml PO qid. [Generic/Trade: soln 2.5/0.025 mg diphenoxylate/atropine per 5 ml, tab 2.5/0.025 mg.] ▶L ♀C ▶– ©V $

loperamide (**Imodium, Imodium AD**, ♥**Loperacap, Diarr-eze**): 4 mg PO initially, then 2 mg PO after each unformed stool to a maximum of 16 mg/day. Peds: 2 mg PO tid if >30 kg, 2 mg bid if 20-30 kg, 1 mg tid if 13-20 kg. [Generic/Trade: cap 2 mg, tab 2 mg. OTC generic/trade: liquid 1 mg/5 ml.] ▶L ♀B ▶+ $

Motofen (difenoxin + atropine): 2 tabs PO initially, then 1 after each loose stool q3-4 h prn. Maximum of 8 tabs/24h. [Trade only: tab difenoxin 1 mg + atropine 0.025 mg.] ▶L ♀C ▶– ©IV $

opium (**opium tincture, paregoric**): 5-10 ml paregoric PO daily-qid or 0.3-0.6 ml PO opium tincture qid. [Trade: opium tincture 10% (deodorized opium tincture, 10 mg morphine equivalent per mL). Generic: paregoric (camphorated opium tincture, 2 mg morphine equiv./5 ml).] ▶L ♀B (D with long-term use) ▶? ©II (opium tincture), III (paregoric) $

Antiemetics - 5-HT3 Receptor Antagonists

dolasetron (**Anzemet**): Nausea with chemo: 1.8 mg/kg up to 100 mg IV/PO single dose. Post-op nausea: 12.5 mg IV in adults and 0.35 mg/kg IV in children as single dose. Alternative for prevention 100 mg (adults) or 1.2 mg/kg (children) PO 2 h before surgery. [Trade only: tab 50,100 mg.] ▶LK ♀B ▶? $$$

granisetron (**Kytril**): Nausea with chemo: 10 mcg/kg IV over 5 minutes, 30 minutes prior to chemo. Oral: 1 mg PO bid x 1 day only. Radiation-induced nausea and vomiting: 2 mg PO 1 hr before first irradiation fraction of each day. [Trade only: tab 1 mg, oral soln 2 mg/10 ml.] ▶L ♀B ▶? $$$

ondansetron (**Zofran**): Nausea with chemo (≥6 month old): 32 mg IV over 15 min, or 0.15 mg/kg doses 30 min prior to chemo and repeated at 4 & 8 hrs after first dose. Oral dose if ≥12 yo: 8 mg PO and repeated 8 hrs later. If 4-11 yo: 4 mg PO 30 min prior to chemo and repeated at 4 & 8 hrs. Prevention of post-op nausea: 4 mg IV over 2-5 min or 4 mg IM or 16 mg PO 1 hr before anesthesia. If 1 month-12 yo: 0.1 mg/kg IV over 2-5 min x 1 if ≤40 kg; 4 mg IV over 2-5 min x 1 if >40 kg. Prevention of N/V associated with radiotherapy: 8 mg PO tid. [Trade only: tab 4,8,24 mg, orally disintegrating tab 4, 8 mg, solution 4 mg/5 ml.] ▶L ♀B ▶? $$$

palonosetron (**Aloxi**): Nausea with chemo: 0.25 mg IV over 30 seconds, 30 minutes prior to chemo. ▶L ♀B ▶? $$$$$

Antiemetics - Other

aprepitant (**Emend**): Prevention of nausea with chemo, in combination with dexamethasone and ondansetron: 125 mg PO on day 1 (1 h prior to chemo), then 80 mg PO qam on days 2 & 3. [Trade only: cap 80, 125 mg.] ▶L ♀B ▶? $$$$$

Diclectin (doxylamine + pyridoxine): Canada only. 2 tabs PO qhs. May add 1 tab in am and 1 tab in afternoon, if needed. [Trade: delayed-release tab doxylamine 10 mg + pyridoxine 10 mg.] ▶LK ♀A ▶? $

dimenhydrinate (**Dramamine**, ♥**Gravol**): 50-100 mg PO/IM/IV q4-6h prn. [OTC: Generic/Trade: tab/cap 50 mg. Trade only: chew tab 50 mg.] ▶LK ♀B ▶– $

doxylamine (**Unisom Nighttime Sleep Aid, others**): 12.5 mg PO bid; often used in combination with pyridoxine. [OTC Trade/Generic: tab 25 mg.] ▶L ♀A ▶? $

dronabinol (**Marinol**): Nausea with chemo: 5 mg/m^2 1-3 h before chemo then 5 mg/m^2/dose q2-4h after chemo for 4-6 doses/day. Anorexia associated with AIDS: Initially 2.5 mg PO bid before lunch and dinner. [Trade only: cap 2.5,5,10 mg.] ▶L ♀C ▶– ©III $$$$$

droperidol (*Inapsine*): 0.625-2.5 mg IV or 2.5 mg IM. May cause fatal QT prolongation, even in patients with no risk factors. Monitor ECG before, ▶L ♀C ▶? $

meclizine (*Antivert, Bonine, Medivert, Meclicot, Meni-D, ♣ Bonamine*): Motion sickness: 25-50 mg PO 1 hr before travel. May repeat q24h prn. [Rx/OTC/Generic /Trade: Tabs 12.5, 25 mg. Chew Tabs 25 mg. Rx/Trade only: Tabs 30, 50 mg. Caps 25 mg.] ▶L ♀B ▶? $

metoclopramide (*Reglan, ♣ Maxeran*): 10 mg IV/IM q2-3h prn. 10-15 mg PO qid, 30 min before meals and qhs. [Generic/Trade: tabs 5,10 mg, liquid 5 mg/5 ml.] ▶K ♀B ▶? $$

phosphorated carbohydrates (*Emetrol*): 15-30 ml PO q15min prn, max 5 doses. Peds: 5-10 ml. [OTC Generic/Trade: Solution containing dextrose, fructose, and phosphoric acid.] ▶L ♀A ▶+ $

prochlorperazine (*Compazine, ♣ Stemetil*): 5-10 mg IV over at least 2 min. 5-10 mg PO/IM tid-qid. 25 mg PR q12h. Sustained release: 15 mg PO qam or 10 mg PO q12h. Peds: 0.1 mg/kg/dose PO/PR tid-qid or 0.1-0.15 mg/kg/dose IM tid-qid. [Generic/Trade: tabs 5,10,25 mg, supp 25 mg. Trade only: extended release caps (Compazine Spansules) 10,15,30 mg, supp 2.5,5 mg, liquid 5 mg/5 ml.] ▶LK ♀C ▶? $

promethazine (*Phenergan*): Adults: 12.5-25 mg PO/IM/PR q4-6h. Peds: 0.25-1 mg/ kg PO/IM/PR q4-6h. Contraindicated if <2 yo; caution in older children. IV use common but not approved. [Generic/Trade: tab 25,50 mg, syrup 6.25 mg/5 ml, supp 50 mg. Trade only: tab 12.5 mg, syrup 25 mg/5 ml, supp 12.5,25 mg.] ▶LK ♀C ▶- $

scopolamine (*Transderm-Scop, ♣ Transderm-V*): Motion sickness: Apply 1 disc (1.5 mg) behind ear 4h prior to event; replace q3 days. [Trade only: topical disc 1.5 mg/72h, box of 4.] ▶L ♀C ▶+ $

thiethylperazine (*Torecan*): 10 mg PO/IM 1-3 times/day. [Trade only: tab 10 mg.] ▶L ♀? ▶? $

trimethobenzamide (*Tigan*): 250 mg PO q6-8h, 200 mg IM/PR q6-8h. Peds: 100-200 mg/dose PO/PR q6-8h if 13.6-40.9 kg; 100 mg PR q6-8h if <13.6kg (not newborns). [Trade/generic: cap 300 mg. Generic: cap 250 mg, supp 100,200 mg.] ▶LK ♀C but + ▶? $

Antiulcer - Antacids

Alka-Seltzer (aspirin + citrate + bicarbonate): 2 regular strength tabs in 4 oz water q4h PO prn, max 8 tab (<60 yo) or 4 tabs (>60 yo) in 24h or 2 extra-strength tabs in 4 oz water q6h PO prn, max 7 tabs (<60 yo) or 4 tabs (>60 yo) in 24h. [OTC Trade: regular strength, original: ASA 325 mg + citric acid 1000 mg + sodium bicarbonate 1916 mg. Regular strength lemon lime and cherry: 325 mg + 1000 mg + 1700 mg. Extra-strength: 500 mg + 1000 mg + 1985 mg. Not all forms contain ASA (eg, Alka Seltzer Heartburn Relief).] ▶LK ♀? (- 3rd trimester) ▶? $

aluminum hydroxide (*Alternagel, Amphojel, Alu-Tab, Alu-Cap, ♣ Basaljel, Mucaine*): 5-10 ml or 1-2 tabs PO up to 6 times daily. Constipating. [OTC Generic/Trade: cap 475 mg, susp 320, 600, mg/5 ml.] ▶K ♀+ (? 1st trimester) ▶? $

calcium carbonate (*Tums, Mylanta Children's, Titralac, Rolaids Calcium Rich, Surpass*): 1000-3000 mg PO q2h prn or 1-2 pieces gum chewed prn, max 7000 mg/day. [OTC Generic/Trade: tabs 500, 650,750, 1000 mg, susp 1250 mg/5 ml, gum (Surpass) 300, 450 mg.] ▶K ♀+ (? 1st trimester) ▶? $

Citrocarbonate (bicarbonate + citrate): 1-2 teaspoonfuls in cold water PO 15 minutes to 2 hours after meals prn. [OTC Trade: sodium bicarbonate 0.78 g + sodium citrate anhydrous 1.82 g in each 1 teaspoonful dissolved in water.] ▶K ♀? ▶? $

Gaviscon (aluminum hydroxide + magnesium carbonate): 2-4 tabs or 15-30 ml (regular strength) or 10 ml (extra strength) PO qid prn. [OTC Trade: Tab: regular strength (Al hydroxide 80 mg + Mg trisilicate 20 mg), extra strength (Al hydroxide 160 mg + Mg carbonate 105 mg). Liquid: regular strength (Al hydroxide 95 mg + Mg carbonate 358 mg per 15 ml), extra strength (Al hydroxide 508 mg + Mg carbonate 475 mg per 30 ml)] ▶K♀? ▶? $

Maalox (aluminum hydroxide + magnesium hydroxide): 10-20 ml or 1-4 tab PO prn. [OTC Generic/Trade: chew tabs, susp.] ▶K♀+ (? 1st trimester) ▶? $

magaldrate (**Riopan**): 5-10 ml PO prn. [OTC Generic/Trade: susp 540 mg/5 ml. (Riopan Plus available as susp 540, 1080/5 ml, chew tab 480, 1080).] ▶K♀+ (? 1st trimester) ▶? $

Mylanta suspension (aluminum hydroxide + magnesium hydroxide + simethicone): 2-4 tab or 10-45 ml PO prn. [OTC Generic/Trade: Liquid, double strength liquid, tab, double strength tab.] ▶K♀+ (? 1st trimester) ▶? $

Rolaids (calcium carbonate + magnesium hydroxide): 2-4 tabs PO q1h prn, max 12 tabs/day (regular strength) or 10 tabs/day (extra-strength). [OTC Trade: Tab: regular strength (Ca carbonate 550 mg, Mg hydroxide 110 mg), extra-strength (Ca carbonate 675 mg, Mg hydroxide 135 mg).] ▶K♀? ▶? $

Antiulcer - H2 Antagonists

cimetidine (**Tagamet, Tagamet HB**): 300 mg IV/IM/PO q6-8h, 400 mg PO bid, or 400-800 mg PO qhs. Erosive esophagitis: 800 mg PO bid or 400 mg PO qid. Continuous IV infusion 37.5-50 mg/h (900-1200 mg/day). [Generic/Trade: tab 200,300,400,800 mg, Liquid 300 mg/5 ml. OTC, Trade only: tab 100 mg, susp 200 mg/20 ml.] ▶LK♀B ▶+ $$$

famotidine (**Pepcid, Pepcid RPD, Pepcid AC, Maximum Strength Pepcid AC**): 20 mg IV q12h. 20-40 mg PO qhs, or 20 mg PO bid. [Generic/Trade: tab 10 mg (OTC, Pepcid AC Acid Controller), chew tab 10 (OTC), 20 (Rx and OTC, Maximum Strength Pepcid Ac), 30, 40 mg. Trade only: orally disintegrating tab (Pepcid RPD) 20, 40 mg, suspension 40 mg/5 ml.] ▶LK♀B ▶? $$$$

nizatidine (**Axid, Axid AR**): 150-300 mg PO qhs, or 150 mg PO bid. [Trade only: tabs 75 mg (OTC, Axid AR), oral solution 15 mg/mL (480 mL). Generic/Trade: cap 150,300 mg.] ▶K♀B ▶? $$$

Pepcid Complete (famotidine + calcium carbonate + magnesium hydroxide): Treatment of heartburn: 1 tab PO prn. Max 2 tabs/day. [OTC: Trade only: chew tab famotidine 10 mg with calcium carbonate 800 mg & magnesium hydroxide 165 mg.] ▶LK♀B ▶? $

ranitidine (**Zantac, Zantac 25, Zantac 75, Zantac 150, Peptic Relief**): 150 mg PO bid or 300 mg PO qhs. 50 mg IV/IM q8h, or continuous infusion 6.25 mg/h (150 mg/d). [Generic/Trade: tabs 75 mg (OTC, Zantac 75), 150,300 mg, syrup 75 mg/5 ml. Trade only: effervescent tab 25, 150 mg, caps 150,300 mg, granules 150 mg.] ▶K♀B ▶? $$$

Antiulcer - Helicobacter pylori Treatment

Helidac (bismuth subsalicylate + metronidazole + tetracycline): 1 dose PO qid for 2 weeks. To be given with an H2 antagonist. [Trade only: Each dose: bismuth subsalicylate 524 (2x262 mg) chewable tab + metronidazole 250 mg tab + tetracycline 500 mg cap.] ▶LK♀D ▶- $$$$

PrevPac (lansoprazole + amoxicillin + clarithromycin, ✿HP-Pac): 1 dose PO bid x 10-14 days. [Trade only: lansoprazole 30 mg x 2 + amoxicillin 1 g (2x500 mg) x 2, clarithromycin 500 mg x 2.] ▶LK♀C ▶? $$$$$

HELICOBACTER PYLORI THERAPY

- Triple therapy PO x 7-14 days: clarithromycin 500 mg bid + amoxicillin 1 g bid (or metronidazole 500 mg bid) + a proton pump inhibitor*
- Quadruple therapy PO x 14 days: bismuth subsalicylate 525 mg (or 30 mL) tid-qid + metronidazole 500 mg tid-qid + tetracycline 500 mg tid-qid + a proton pump inhibitor* or a H₂ blocker†

*PPI's esomeprazole 40 mg qd, lansoprazole 30 mg bid, omeprazole 20 mg bid, pantoprazole 40 mg bid, rabeprazole 20 mg bid. †H₂ blockers cimetidine 400 mg bid, famotidine 20 mg bid, nizatidine 150 mg bid, ranitidine 150 mg bid. Adapted from *Medical Letter Treatment Guidelines* 2004.

Antiulcer - Proton Pump Inhibitors

esomeprazole (***Nexium***): Erosive esophagitis: 20-40 mg PO daily x 4-8 weeks. Maintenance of erosive esophagitis: 20 mg PO daily. GERD: 20 mg PO daily x 4 weeks. GERD with esophagitis: 20-40 mg PO daily x 10 days until taking PO. Prevention of NSAID-associated gastric ulcer: 20-40 mg PO daily x up to 6 months. H pylori eradication: 40 mg PO daily with amoxicillin 1000 mg PO bid & clarithromycin 500 mg PO bid x 10 days. [Trade only: delayed release cap 20, 40 mg.] ▶L ♀B ▶? $$$$

lansoprazole (***Prevacid, Prevacid NapraPac***): Duodenal ulcer or maintenance therapy after healing of duodenal ulcer, erosive esophagitis, NSAID-induced gastric ulcer: 30 mg PO daily x 8 weeks (treatment), 15 mg PO daily for up to 12 weeks (prevention). GERD: 15 mg PO daily. Gastric ulcer: 30 mg PO daily. Erosive esophagitis: 30 mg PO daily or 30 mg IV daily x 7 days or until taking PO. [Trade only: cap 15,30 mg. Susp 15,30 mg packets. Orally disintegrating tab 15, 30 mg. *Prevacid NapraPac*: 7 lansoprazole 15 mg caps packaged with 14 naproxen tabs 375 mg or 500 mg.] ▶L ♀B ▶? $$$$

omeprazole (***Prilosec, Zegerid, Rapinex,*** ✚***Losec***): Duodenal ulcer or erosive esophagitis: 20 mg PO daily x 14 days. Heartburn (OTC): 20 mg PO daily x 14 days. Gastric ulcer: 40 mg PO daily. Hypersecretory conditions: 60 mg PO daily. [Trade/generic: cap 10, 20 mg. OTC: 20 mg. Trade only: cap 40 mg, powder for suspension 20, 40 mg (Zegerid), oral suspension 20 mg (Rapinex).] ▶L ♀C ▶? $$$$

pantoprazole (***Protonix,*** ✚***Pantoloc***): Zollinger-Ellison syndrome: 80 mg IV q8-12h x 6 days until taking PO. GERD associated with a history of erosive esophagitis: 40 mg IV daily x 7-10 days until taking PO. [Trade only: tab 40 mg.] ▶L ♀B ▶? $$$

rabeprazole (***Aciphex,*** ✚***Pariet***): 20 mg PO daily. [Trade only: tab 20 mg.] ▶L ♀B ▶? $$$$

Antiulcer - Other

dicyclomine (***Bentyl, Bentylol, Antispas,*** ✚***Formulex, Protylol, Lomine***): 10-20 mg PO/IM qid up to 40 mg PO qid. [Generic/Trade: tab 20 mg, cap 10 mg, syrup 10 mg/5 ml. Generic only: cap 20 mg.] ▶LK ♀B ▶- $$

Donnatal (phenobarbital + atropine + hyoscyamine + scopolamine): 1-2 tabs/caps or 5-10 ml PO tid-qid. 1 extended release tab PO q8-12h. [Generic/Trade: Phenobarbital 16.2 mg + hyoscyamine 0.1 mg + atropine 0.02 mg + scopolamine 6.5 mcg in each tab, cap or 5 ml. Extended-release tab 48.6 + 0.3111 + 0.0582 + 0.0195 mg.] ▶LK ♀C ▶- $

"GI cocktail", "green goddess": Acute GI upset: mixture of Maalox/Mylanta 30 ml + viscous lidocaine (2%) 10 ml + Donnatal 10 ml administered PO in a single dose. ▶LK $

hyoscyamine (**Levsin, NuLev**): 0.125-0.25 mg PO/SL q4h prn. Sustained release: 0.375-0.75 mg PO q12h. [Generic/Trade: tab 0.125,0.15 mg, SL tab 0.125 mg, solution 0.125 mg/ml. Trade only: extended release tab/cap 0.375 mg, orally disintegrating tab 0.125 mg (NuLev), elixir 0.125 mg/5 ml.] ▶LK ♀C ▶- $

mepenzolate (**Cantil**): 25-50 mg PO qid, with meals and qhs. [Trade only: tab: 25 mg.] ▶LK ♀B ▶? ?

misoprostol (**Cytotec**): Prevention of NSAID-induced gastric ulcers: Start 100 mcg PO bid, then titrate as tolerated up to 200 mcg PO qid. Abortifacient. Diarrhea in 13-40%, abd pain in 7-20%. [Trade/generic: tab 100,200 mcg.] ▶LK ♀X ▶- $$$$

propantheline (**Pro-Banthine, ✚Propanthel**): 7.5-15 mg PO 30 min ac & qhs. [Generic/Trade: tab 15 mg. Trade only: tab 7.5 mg.] ▶LK ♀C ▶- $$$

simethicone (**Mylicon, Gas-X, Phazyme, ✚Ovol**): 40-160 mg PO qid prn. Infants: 20 mg PO qid prn [OTC Generic/Trade: tab 60,95 mg, chew tab 40,80,125 mg, cap 125 mg, drops 40 mg/0.6 ml.] ▶Not absorbed ♀C but + ▶? $

sucralfate (**Carafate, ✚Sulcrate**): 1 g PO 1h before meals (2h before other medications) and qhs. [Generic/Trade: tab 1 g. Trade only: susp 1 g/10 ml.] ▶Not absorbed ♀B ▶? $$$

Laxatives

bisacodyl (**Correctol, Dulcolax, Feen-a-Mint**): 10-15 mg PO prn, 10 mg PR prn, 5-10 mg PR prn if 2-11 yo. [OTC Generic/Trade: tab 5 mg, supp 10 mg] ▶L ♀+ ▶? $

cascara: 325 mg PO qhs prn or 5 ml of aromatic fluid extract PO qhs prn. [OTC Generic: tab 325 mg, liquid aromatic fluid extract.] ▶L ♀C ▶+ $

castor oil (**Purge, Fleet Flavored Castor Oil**): 15-60 ml of castor oil or 30-60 ml emulsified castor oil PO qhs, 5-15 ml/dose of castor oil PO or 7.5-30 ml emulsified castor oil PO for child. [OTC Generic/Trade: liquid 30,60,120,480 ml, emulsified suspension 45,60,90,120 ml.] ▶Not absorbed ♀- ▶? $

docusate calcium (**Kaopectate Stool Softener**): 240 mg PO daily. [OTC Generic/Trade: cap 240 mg.] ▶L ♀+ ▶? $

docusate sodium (**Colace**): 50-500 mg/day PO divided in 1-4 doses. Peds: 10-40 mg/d if <3 yo, 20-60 mg/d if 3-6 yo, 40-150 mg/d if 6-12 yo. [OTC Generic/Trade: cap 50,100, 250 mg, tab 50,100 mg, liquid 10 & 50 mg/5 ml, syrup 16.75 & 20 mg/5 ml.] ▶L ♀+ ▶? $

glycerin: one adult or infant suppository PR prn. [OTC Generic/Trade: supp infant & adult, solution (Fleet Babylax) 4 ml/applicator.] ▶Not absorbed ♀C ▶? $

lactulose (**Chronulac, Cephulac, Kristalose**): Constipation: 15-30 ml (syrup) or 10-20 g (powder for oral solution) PO daily. Hepatic encephalopathy: 30-45 ml (syrup) PO tid-qid, or 300 ml retention enema. [Generic/Trade: syrup 0 g/15 ml. Trade only (Kristalose): 10, 20 g packets for oral soln.] ▶Not absorbed ♀B ▶? $$

magnesium citrate (**Citro-Mag**): 150- 300 ml PO divided daily-bid. Children <6 yo: 2-4 ml/kg/24h. [OTC Generic: solution 300 ml/bottle.] ▶K ♀+ ▶? $

magnesium hydroxide (**Milk of Magnesia**): Laxative: 30-60 ml regular strength liquid PO. Antacid: 5-15 ml regular strength liquid or 622-1244 mg PO qid prn. [OTC Generic/Trade: liquid 400 & 800 (concentrated) mg/5 ml, chew tab 311 mg.] ▶K ♀+ ▶? $

methylcellulose (**Citrucel**): 1 heaping tablespoon in 8 oz. water PO daily-tid. [OTC Trade only: Packets, multiple use canisters.] ▶L ♀+ ▶? $

mineral oil (**Agoral, Kondremul, Fleet Mineral Oil Enema, ✚Lansoyl**): 15-45 ml PO. Peds: 5-15 ml/dose PO. Mineral oil enema: 60-150 ml PR. Peds 30-60 ml PR. [OTC Generic/Trade: plain mineral oil, mineral oil emulsion (Agoral, Kondremul).] ▶Not absorbed ♀C ▶? $

Peri-Colace (docusate + sennosides): 2-4 tabs PO once daily or in divided doses prn. [OTC Generic/Trade: tab 50/8.6 mg of docusate/sennosides.] ▶L ♀C ▶? $

polycarbophil (**FiberCon, Fiberall, Konsyl Fiber, Equalactin**): Laxative: 1 g PO qid prn. Diarrhea: 1 g PO q30 min. Max daily dose 6 g. [OTC Generic/Trade: tab 500,625 mg, chew tab 500,1000 mg.] ▶Not absorbed ♀+ ▶? $

polyethylene glycol (**MiraLax, GlycoLax**): 17 g (1 heaping tablespoon) in 4-8 oz water, juice, soda, coffee, or tea PO daily. [Trade only: powder for oral solution.] ▶Not absorbed ♀C ▶? $

polyethylene glycol with electrolytes (**GoLytely, Colyte, TriLyte, NuLytely, Half-Lytely and Bisacodyl Tablet Kit, ✦Klean-Prep, Electropeg, Peg-Lyte**): Bowel prep: 240 ml q10 min PO or 20-30 ml/min per NG until 4L is consumed. [Generic/Trade: powder for oral solution. Available as a kit of 2L bottle of polyethylene glycol with electrolytes and 4 bisacodyl tabs 5 mg (HalfLytely and Bisacodyl Tablet Kit).] ▶Not absorbed ♀C ▶? $

psyllium (**Metamucil, Fiberall, Konsyl, Hydrocil, ✦Prodium Plain**): 1 tsp in liquid, 1 packet in liquid or 1-2 wafers with liquid PO daily-tid. [OTC: Generic/Trade: powder, granules, wafers, including various flavors and various amounts of psyllium.] ▶Not absorbed ♀+ ▶? $

senna (**Senokot, SenokotXTRA, Ex-Lax, Fletcher's Castoria, ✦Glysennid**): 2 tabs or 1 tsp granules or 10-15 ml syrup PO. Max 8 tabs, 4 tsp granules, 30 ml syrup per day. Take granules with full glass of water. [OTC Generic/Trade (All dosing is based on sennosides content; 1 mg sennosides = 21.7 mg standardized senna concentrate): granules 15 mg/tsp, syrup 8.8 mg/5 ml, liquid 3 mg/ml (Fletcher's Castoria), tab 8.6, 15, 17, 25 mg, chewable tab 15 mg.] ▶L ♀C ▶+ $

Senokot-S (senna + docusate): 2 tabs PO daily. [OTC Trade: tab 8.6 mg senna concentrate/50 mg docusate.] ▶L ♀C ▶+ $

sodium phosphate (**Fleet enema, Fleet Phospho-Soda, Visicol, ✦Enemol**): 1 adult or pediatric enema PR or 20-30 ml of oral soln PO prn (max 45 ml/24 h). Visicol: Evening before colonoscopy: 3 tabs with 8 oz clear liquid q15 min until 20 tabs are consumed. Day of colonoscopy: starting 3-5 before procedure, 3 tabs with 8 oz clear liquid q15 min until 20 tabs are consumed. [OTC Trade only: peds & adult enema, oral soln. Visicol tab (trade $$$) 1.5 g.] ▶Not absorbed ♀C ▶? $

sorbitol: 30-150 ml (of 70% solution) PO or 120 ml (of 25-30% solution) PR as a single dose. Cathartic: 1-2 mL/kg PO. [Generic: sol 70%.] ▶Not absorbed ♀+ ▶? $

Other GI Agents

alosetron (**Lotronex**): Diarrhea-predominant IBS in women who have failed conventional therapy: 1 mg PO daily for 4 weeks; may increase to 1 mg PO bid. Discontinue if symptoms not controlled in 4 weeks on 1 mg PO bid. [Trade: tab 0.5, 1 mg.] ▶L ♀B ▶? $$$$

alpha-galactosidase (**Beano**): 5 drops per ½ cup gassy food, 3 tabs PO (chew, swallow, crumble) or 15 drops per typical meal. [Trade: drops 150 GalU/5 drops, tab 150 GalU.] ▶Minimal absorption ♀? ▶? $

balsalazide (**Colazal**): 2.25 g PO tid x 8-12 weeks. [Trade: cap 750 mg.] ▶Minimal absorption ♀B ▶? $$$$

budesonide (**Entocort EC**): 9 mg PO daily x 8 weeks (remission induction) or 6 mg PO daily x 3 months (maintenance). [Trade: cap 3 mg.] ▶L ♀C ▶? $$$$$

domperidone: Canada only. 10-20 mg PO 3-4 times daily, 15-30 minutes before meals. [Rx:Trade / generic: tabs 10 mg.] ▶L, gut wall ♀C ▶- $

glycopyrrolate (**Robinul, Robinul Forte**): 0.1 mg/kg PO bid-tid, max 8 mg/day. [Trade: tab 1, 2 mg.] ▶K ♀B ▶? $$$

infliximab (*Remicade*): 5 mg/kg IV infusion. May be repeated at 2 & 6 weeks, then every 8 weeks for moderately to severely active Crohn's disease or fistulizing disease. Serious, life-threatening infections, including sepsis & disseminated TB have been reported. Monitor for signs/symptoms of heart failure. Hypersensitivity reactions may occur. ▶Serum ♀B ▶? $$$$$

lactase (*Lactaid*): Swallow or chew 3 caplets (Original strength), 2 caplets (Extra strength), 1 caplet (Ultra) with first bite of dairy foods. Adjust dose based on response. [OTC Trade/generic: caplets, chew tab.] ▶Not absorbed ♀+ ▶+ $

Librax (clidinium + chlordiazepoxide): 1 cap PO tid-qid. [Generic/Trade: cap clidinium 2.5 mg + chlordiazepoxide 5 mg.] ▶K ♀D ▶- $

mesalamine (**5-aminosalicylic acid, 5-ASA, Asacol, Pentasa, Rowasa, Canasa, *Mesasal, Salofalk**): Asacol: 800-1600 mg PO tid. Pentasa: 1000 mg PO qid. Rowasa: 500 mg PR bid or 4 g enema qhs. Canasa: 500 mg PR bid-tid or 1000 mg PR qhs. [Trade only: delayed release tab 400 mg (Asacol), controlled-release cap 250 mg (Pentasa), supp 500 mg (Rowasa), rectal supp 500, 1000 mg (Canasa). Rectal susp 4 g/60 ml.] ▶Gut ♀B ▶? $$$$

neomycin (*Mycifradin*): Hepatic encephalopathy: 4-12 g/day PO divided q6-8h. Peds: 50-100 mg/kg/day PO divided q6-8h. [Generic/Trade: tab 500 mg, solution 125 mg/5 ml.] ▶Minimally absorbed ♀D ▶? $$$

octreotide (*Sandostatin, Sandostatin LAR*): Variceal bleeding: Bolus 50-100 mcg IV followed by infusion 25-50 mcg/hr. AIDS diarrhea: 100-500 mcg SC tid. Other indications with varying doses. [Trade/generic: injection vials 0.05,0.1,0.2,0.5,1 mg, long-acting injectable susp (Sandostatin LAR) 10,20,30 mg.] ▶LK ♀B ▶? $$$$$

olsalazine (*Dipentum*): Ulcerative colitis: 500 mg PO bid. [Trade only: cap 250 mg.] ▶L ♀C ▶- $$$$

orlistat (*Xenical*): Weight loss: 120 mg PO tid with meals. [Trade only: cap 120 mg.] ▶Gut ♀B ▶? $$$$

pancreatin (*Creon, Donnazyme, Ku-Zyme, *Entozyme*): 8,000-24,000 units lipase (1-2 tab/cap) PO with meals and snacks. [Tab, cap with varying amounts of pancreatin, lipase, amylase and protease.] ▶Gut ♀C ▶? $$$

pancrelipase (*Viokase, Pancrease, Pancrecarb, Cotazym, Ku-Zyme HP*): 4,000-33,000 units lipase (1-3 tab/cap) PO with meals and snacks. [Tab, cap, powder with varying amounts of lipase, amylase and protease.] ▶Gut ♀C ▶? $$$

pinaverium (**Dicetel*): Canada only. 50-100 mg PO bid. [Trade: tabs 50, 100 mg.] ▶? ♀C ▶- $$-$$$

secretin (*SecreMax, ChiRhoClin*): Test dose 0.2 mcg IV. If tolerated, 0.2-0.4 mcg/kg IV over 1 minute. ▶Serum ♀C ▶? $$$$$

sulfasalazine (*Azulfidine, Azulfidine EN-tabs, *Salazopyrin, Salazopyrin EN, S.A.S.*): 500-1000 mg PO qid. Peds: 30-60 mg/kg/day divided q4-6h. [Generic/Trade: tab 500 mg.] ▶K ♀- ▶? $$

tegaserod (*Zelnorm*): Constipation-predominant IBS in women: 6 mg PO bid before meals for 4-6 weeks. Chronic idiopathic constipation in those <65 yo: 6 mg PO bid before meals. [Trade: tab 2, 6 mg.] ▶stomach/L ♀B ▶? $$$$

trimebutine (**Modulon*): Canada only. Up to 600 mg PO in divided doses (eg, 200 mg tid). [Rx:Trade: tabs 100, 200 mg.] ▶? ♀C ▶? $$

ursodiol (*Actigall, Ursofalk, URSO*): Gallstone dissolution (Actigall): 8-10 mg/kg/day PO divided bid-tid. Prevention of gallstones associated with rapid weight loss (Actigall): 300 mg PO bid. Primary biliary cirrhosis (URSO): 13-15 mg/kg/day PO divided in 2-4 doses. [Trade/generic: cap 300 mg. Trade only: Tab 250, 500 mg (URSO).] ▶Bile ♀B ▶? $$$$

HEMATOLOGY (See cardiology section for antiplatelet drugs & thrombolytics.)

Anticoagulants - Heparin, LMW Heparins, & Fondaparinux

dalteparin (Fragmin): DVT prophylaxis, abdominal surgery: 2,500 units SC 1-2 h preop & daily postop x 5-10d. DVT prophylaxis, abdominal surgery in patients with malignancy: 5,000 units SC evening before surgery and daily postop x 5-10 days. DVT prophylaxis, hip replacement: Give SC for up to 14 days. Pre-op start: 2,500 units given 2 h preop and 4-8h postop, then 5,000 units daily starting ≥6h after second dose. Postop start: 2,500 units 4-8h postop, then 5,000 units daily starting ≥6h after first dose. Unstable angina or non-Q-wave MI: 120 units/kg up to 10,000 units SC q12h with aspirin (75-165 mg/day PO) until clinically stable. DVT prophylaxis, acute medical illness with restricted mobility: 5,000 units SC daily x 12-14 days. [Trade: Single-dose syringes 2,500 & 5,000 anti-Xa units/0.2 ml, 7500 anti-Xa/0.3 ml, 10,000 anti-Xa units/1 ml; multi-dose vial 10,000 units/ml, 9.5 ml and 25,000 units/ml, 3.8 ml.] ▶KL ♀B ▶+ $$$$

enoxaparin (Lovenox): DVT prophylaxis, hip/knee replacement: 30 mg SC q12h starting 12-24 h postop (severe renal impairment, CrCl <30 ml/min: 30 mg SC daily). Alternative for hip replacement: 40 mg SC daily starting 12h preop. Abdominal surgery: 40 mg SC daily starting 2 h preop (severe renal impairment 30 mg SC daily). Acute medical illness with restricted mobility: 40 mg SC daily (severe renal impairment 30 mg SC daily). Outpatient treatment of DVT without pulmonary embolus: 1 mg/kg SC q12h until PO anticoagulation established. Inpatient treatment of DVT with/without pulmonary embolus: 1 mg/kg SC q12h or 1.5 mg/kg SC q24h (severe renal impairment 1 mg/kg SC daily) until therapeutic oral anticoagulation established. Unstable angina or non-Q-wave MI: 1 mg/kg SC q12h with aspirin (100-325 mg PO daily) for ≥2 days and until clinically stable (severe renal impairment 1 mg/kg SC daily). [Trade: Multi-dose vial 300 mg; Syringes 30,40 mg; graduated syringes 60,80,100,120,150 mg. Concentration is 100 mg/mL except for 120,150 mg which are 150 mg/mL.] ▶KL ♀B ▶+ $$$$

fondaparinux (Arixtra): DVT prophylaxis, hip/knee replacement or hip fracture surgery, abdominal surgery: 2.5 mg SC daily starting 6-8 h postop. Usual duration is 5-9 days; extend prophylaxis up to 24 additional days (max 32 days) in hip fracture surgery. DVT / PE treatment based on weight: 5 mg (if <50 kg), 7.5 mg (if 50-100 kg), 10 mg (if >100 kg) SC daily for ≥5 days & therapeutic oral anticoagulation. [Trade: Pre-filled syringes 2.5 mg/0.5 mL, 5 mg/0.4 mL, 7.5 mg/0.6 mL, 10 mg/0.8 mL.] ▶K ♀B ▶? $$$$$

WEIGHT-BASED HEPARIN DOSING FOR DVT/PE*

Initial dose: 80 units/kg IV bolus, then 18 units/kg/h. Check PTT in 6 h.
PTT <35 secs (<1.2 x control): 80 units/kg IV bolus, then ↑ infusion rate by 4 units/kg/h.
PTT 35-45 secs (1.2-1.5 x control): 40 units/kg IV bolus, then ↑ infusion by 2 units/kg/h.
PTT 46-70 seconds (1.5-2.3 x control): No change.
PTT 71-90 seconds (2.3-3 x control): ↓ infusion rate by 2 units/kg/h.
PTT >90 seconds (>3 x control): Hold infusion for 1 h, then ↓ infusion rate by 3 units/kg/h.

* PTT = Activated partial thromboplastin time. Reagent-specific target PTT may differ; use institutional nomogram when appropriate. Adjusted dosing may be appropriate in obesity. Consider establishing a max bolus dose / max initial infusion rate or use an adjusted body weight in obesity. Monitor PTT q6h during first 24h of therapy and 6h after each heparin dosage adjustment. The frequency of PTT monitoring can be reduced to q morning when PTT is stable within therapeutic range. Check platelets between days 3-5. Can begin warfarin on 1st day of heparin; continue heparin for ≥4 to 5 days of combined therapy. Adapted from *Ann Intern Med* 1993;119:874; *Chest* 2004:126:192S, *Circulation* 2001; 103:2994.

heparin (✚*Hepalean*): Venous thrombosis/pulmonary embolism treatment: Load 80 units/kg IV, then mix 25,000 units in 250 ml D5W (100 units/ml) and infuse at 18 units/kg/h. Adjust based on coagulation testing (PTT). DVT prophylaxis: 5,000 units SC q8-12h. Peds: Load 50 units/kg IV, then infuse 25 units/kg/h. [Generic: 1000, 2500, 5000, 7500, 10,000, 20,000 units/ml in various vial and syringe sizes.] ▶Reticuloendothelial system ♀C but ▶ ▶+ $

tinzaparin (*Innohep*): DVT with/without pulmonary embolism: 175 units/kg SC daily for ≥6 days and until adequate anticoagulation with warfarin. [Trade: 20,000 anti-Xa units/ml, 2 ml multi-dose vial.] ▶K ♀B ▶+ $$$$$

Anticoagulants - Other

argatroban: Heparin-induced thrombocytopenia: Start 2 mcg/kg/min IV infusion. Get PTT at baseline and 2 h after starting infusion. Adjust dose (not >10 mcg/kg/min) until PTT is 1.5-3 times baseline (not >100 seconds). ▶L ♀B ▶- $$$$$

bivalirudin (*Angiomax*): Anticoagulation during PCI: 0.75 mg/kg IV bolus prior to intervention, then 1.75 mg/kg/hr for duration of procedure (with provisional Gp IIb/IIIa inhibition). Use with aspirin 300-325 mg PO daily. Additional bolus of 0.3 mg/kg if activated clotting time <225 sec. ▶proteolysis/K ♀B ▶? $$$$$

lepirudin (*Refludan*): Anticoagulation in heparin-induced thrombocytopenia and associated thromboembolic disease: Bolus 0.4 mg/kg up to 44 mg IV over 15-20 seconds, then infuse 0.15 mg/kg/h up to 16.5 mg/h. ▶K ♀B ▶? $$$$$

warfarin (*Coumadin, Jantoven*): Start 2-10 mg PO daily x 3-4 days, then adjust dose to PT/INR. [Generic/Trade: Tabs 1, 2, 2.5, 3, 4, 5, 6, 7.5, 10 mg] ▶L ♀X ▶+ $

THERAPEUTIC GOALS FOR ANTICOAGULATION

INR Range*	Indication
2.0-3.0	Atrial fibrillation, deep venous thrombosis, pulmonary embolism, bioprosthetic heart valve, mechanical prosthetic heart valve (aortic position, bileaflet or tilting disk with normal sinus rhythm and normal left atrium)
2.5-3.5	Mechanical prosthetic heart valve: (1) mitral position, (2) aortic position with atrial fibrillation, (3) caged ball or caged disk

*Aim for an INR in the middle of the INR range (e.g. 2.5 for range of 2-3 and 3.0 for range of 2.5-3.5). Adapted from: *Chest suppl 2004*; 126: 416S, 450S, 474S; see this manuscript for additional information and other indications.

Other Hematological Agents (See endocrine section for vitamins and minerals.)

aminocaproic acid (*Amicar*): Hemostasis: 4-5 g PO/IV over 1h, then 1 g/h prn. [Generic/Trade: Syrup or oral soln 250 mg/ml, tabs 500 mg.] ▶K ♀D ▶? $$

anagrelide (*Agrylin*): Thrombocythemia due to myeloproliferative disorders: Start 0.5 mg PO qid or 1 mg PO bid, then after 1 week adjust to lowest effective dose. Max 10 mg/d. [Generic/Trade: Caps, 0.5, 1 mg.] ▶LK ♀C ▶? $$$$$

aprotinin (*Trasylol*): To reduce blood loss during CABG: 1 ml IV test dose ≥10 min before loading dose. Regimen A: 200 ml loading dose, then 200 ml pump prime dose, then 50 ml/h. Regimen B: 100 ml loading dose, then 100 ml pump prime dose, then 25 ml/h. May cause anaphylaxis. ▶lysosomal enzymes,K ♀B ▶? $$$$$

darbepoetin (*Aranesp, NESP*): Anemia of chronic renal failure: 0.45 mcg/kg IV/SC once weekly, or q2 weeks in some patients. Cancer chemo anemia: 2.25 mcg/kg SC q week. Adjust dose based on Hb. [Trade: Single-dose vials 25, 40, 60, 100, 200, 300, 500 mcg/1 ml. Additionally 150 mcg/0.75 ml. Prefilled syringes: 60, 100, 150, 200, 300, 500 mcg.] ▶cellular sialidases, L ♀C ▶? $$$$$

desmopressin (*DDAVP, Stimate, ♥Octostim*): Hemophilia A, von Willebrand's disease: 0.3 mcg/kg IV over 15-30 min, or 150-300 mcg intranasally. [Trade: Stimate nasal spray 150 mcg/0.1 ml (1 spray), 2.5 ml bottle (25 sprays). Generic/Trade (DDAVP nasal spray): 10 mcg/0.1 ml (1 spray), 5 ml bottle (50 sprays). Note difference in concentration of nasal solutions.] ►LK ♀B ▶? $$$$$

erythropoietin (*Epogen, Procrit, epoetin, ♥Eprex*): Anemia: 1 dose IV/SC 3 times /week. Initial dose if renal failure = 50-100 units/kg, AZT = 100 units/kg, or chemo = 150 units/kg. Alternate for chemo-associated anemia: 40,000 units SC once/ week. [Trade: Single-dose 1 ml vials 2,000, 3,000, 4,000, 10,000, 40,000 units/ml. Multi-dose vials 10,000 units/ml 2 ml & 20,000 units/ml 1 ml.] ►L ♀C ▶? $$$$$

factor VIIa (*NovoSeven, ♥Niastase*): Specialized dosing. [Trade: 1200, 2400, 4800 mcg/vial.] ►L ♀C ▶? $$$$$

factor VIII (*Advate, Hemofil M, Monoclate P, Monarc-M, ReFacto, ♥Kogenate, Recombinate*): Specialized dosing. [Specific formulation usually chosen by specialist in Hemophilia Treatment Center. Advate is only current recombinant formulation of factor VIII.] ►L ♀C ▶? $$$$$

factor IX (*Benefix, Mononine, ♥Immunine VH*): Specialized dosing. [Specific formulation usually chosen by specialist in Hemophilia Treatment Center.] ►L ♀C ▶? $$$$$

filgrastim (*G-CSF, Neupogen*): Neutropenia: 5 mcg/kg SC/IV daily. [Trade: Single-dose vials 300 mcg/1 ml, 480 mcg/1.6 ml. Single-dose syringes 300 mcg/0.5 ml, 480 mcg/0.8 ml.] ►L ♀C ▶? $$$$$

oprelvekin (*Neumega*): Chemotherapy-induced thrombocytopenia in adults: 50 mcg/kg SC daily. [Trade: 5 mg single-dose vial with diluent.] ►K ♀C ▶? $$$$$

pegfilgrastim (*Neulasta*): 6 mg SC once each chemo cycle. [Trade: Single-dose syringes 6 mg/0.6 ml.] ►Plasma ♀C ▶? $$$$$

protamine: Reversal of heparin: 1 mg antagonizes ~100 units heparin. Reversal of low molecular weight heparin: 1 mg protamine per 100 anti-Xa units of dalteparin or tinzaparin. 1 mg protamine per 1 mg enoxaparin. Give IV (max 50 mg) over 10 minutes. May cause allergy/anaphylaxis. ►Plasma ♀C ▶? $

sargramostim (*GM-CSF, Leukine*): Specialized dosing for marrow transplant. ►L ♀C ▶? $$$$$

HERBAL & ALTERNATIVE THERAPIES

> **NOTE**: In the US, herbal and alternative therapy products are regulated as dietary supplements, not drugs. Premarketing evaluation and FDA approval are not required unless specific therapeutic claims are made. Since these products are not required to demonstrate efficacy, it is unclear whether many of them have health benefits. In addition, there may be considerable variability in content from lot to lot or between products. See www.tarascon.com/herbals for the evidence-based efficacy ratings used by Tarascon editorial staff.

aloe vera (*acemannan, burn plant*): Topical: Efficacy unclear for seborrheic dermatitis, psoriasis, genital herpes, skin burns. Do not apply to surgical incisions; impaired healing reported. Oral: Mild to moderate active ulcerative colitis (possibly effective): 100 ml PO bid. Efficacy unclear for type 2 diabetes. OTC laxatives containing aloe removed from US market due to possible increased risk of colon cancer. ►LK ♀oral- topical +? ▶oral- topical +? $

androstenedione (*andro*): Marketed as anabolic steroid to enhance athletic performance. May cause androgenic (primarily in women) and estrogenic (primarily in men) side effects. FDA warned manufacturers to stop marketing as dietary supplement in March 2004. ►L, peripheral conversion to estrogens & androgens ♀- ▶- $

aristolochic acid (*Aristolochia, Asarum, Bragantia*): Nephrotoxic & carcinogenic; do not use. Was promoted for weight loss. ▶?♀-▶-$

arnica (*Arnica montana, leopard's bane, wolf's bane*): Do not take by mouth. Topical promoted for treatment of skin wounds, bruises, aches, and sprains; but insufficient data to assess efficacy. Do not use on open wounds. ▶?♀-▶-$

artichoke leaf extract (*Cynara-SL, Cynara scolymus*): May reduce total cholesterol, but clinical significance is unclear. Cynara-SL is promoted as digestive aid (possibly effective for dyspepsia) at a dose of 1-2 caps PO daily (320 mg dried artichoke leaf extract/cap). ▶?♀?▶?$

astragalus (*Astragalus membranaceus, huang qi, vetch*): Used in combination with other herbs in traditional Chinese medicine, but efficacy unclear for CHD, CHF, chronic kidney disease, viral infections, URIs, and as adjunct to cancer chemotherapy. ▶?♀?▶?$

bilberry (*Vaccinium myrtillus, huckleberry, Tegens, VMA extract*): Cataracts (efficacy unclear): 160 mg PO bid of 25% anthocyanosides extract. Insufficient data to evaluate efficacy for macular degeneration. Does not appear effective for improving night vision. ▶Bile, K ♀-▶-$

bitter melon (*Momordica charantia, karela*): Possibly effective for type 2 diabetes. Dose unclear; juice may be more potent than dried fruit powder. Hypoglycemic coma reported in 2 children ingesting tea. Seeds can cause hemolytic anemia in G6PD deficiency. ▶? ♀-▶-$$

bitter orange (*Citrus aurantium, Seville orange, Acutrim Natural AM, Dexatrim Natural Ephedrine Free*): Sympathomimetic similar to ephedra; safety and efficacy not established. Do not use with MAOIs. ▶K ♀-▶-$

black cohosh (*Cimicifuga racemosa, Remifemin, Menofem*): Menopausal symptoms (possibly effective): 20 mg PO bid of Remifemin. Efficacy unclear (conflicting data) for vasomotor symptoms induced by breast cancer treatment (including tamoxifen). North American Menopause Society considers black cohosh plus lifestyle changes an option for relief of mild symptoms. ▶?♀-▶-$

butterbur (*Petesites hybridus, Petadolex, Petaforce, Tesalin, ZE 339*): Migraine prophylaxis (possibly effective): Petadolex 50-75 mg PO bid. Allergic rhinitis prophylaxis (possibly effective): Petadolex 50 mg PO bid or Tesalin 1 tab PO qid or 2 tabs tid. Efficacy unclear for asthma or allergic skin disease. [Not by prescription. Standardized pyrrolizidine-free extracts: Petadolex (7.5 mg of petasin & isopetasin/50 mg tab). Tesalin (ZE 339; 8 mg petasin/tab).] ▶?♀-▶-$

chamomile (*Matricaria recutita - German chamomile, Anthemis nobilis - Roman chamomile*): Promoted as a sedative or anxiolytic, to relieve GI distress, for skin infections or inflammation, many other indications. Efficacy unclear for any indication. ▶?♀-▶?$

chaparral (*Larrea divaricata, creosote bush*): Hepatotoxic; do not use. Promoted as cancer cure. ▶?♀-▶-$

chasteberry (*Vitex agnus castus fruit extract, Femaprin*): Premenstrual syndrome (possibly effective): 20 mg PO daily of extract ZE 440. ▶?♀-▶-$

chondroitin: Osteoarthritis (possibly effective): 200-400 mg PO bid-tid or 1200 mg PO daily. ▶K ♀?▶?$

coenzyme Q10 (*CoQ-10, ubiquinone*): Heart failure (efficacy unclear): 100 mg/day PO divided bid-tid. Parkinson's disease ($$$$): 1200 mg/day PO divided qid at meals and has slowed progression of early disease in phase II study. Efficacy unclear for improving athletic performance. Appears ineffective for diabetes. Statins may reduce CoQ10 blood levels, but no evidence that CoQ10 supplements treat or prevent statin myopathy. ▶Bile ♀-▶-$

comfrey (**Symphytum officinale**): May cause hepatic cancer; do not use, even topically. ▶? ♀– ▶– $

cranberry (**Cranactin, Vaccinium macrocarpon**): Prevention of UTI (possibly effective): 300 mL/day PO cranberry juice cocktail; 1-6 caps PO (hard gel caps with 300-400 mg concentrated cranberry juice extract) bid with water 1 h before or 2 h after meals. Insufficient data to assess efficacy for treatment of UTI. ▶? ♀? ▶? $

creatine: Promoted to enhance athletic performance. No benefit for endurance exercise; modest benefit for intense anaerobic tasks lasting <30 seconds. Usual loading dose of 20 g/day PO x 5 days, then 2-5 g/day taken bid. ▶LK ♀– ▶– $

dehydroepiandrosterone (**DHEA, Aslera, Fidelin, Prasterone**): No convincing evidence that DHEA slows aging or improves cognition in elderly. Rx product (Aslera) in development for treatment of women with lupus. To improve well-being in women with adrenal insufficiency (effective): 50 mg PO daily. ▶Peripheral conversion to estrogens and androgens ♀– ▶– $

devil's claw (**Harpagophytum procumbens, Phyto Joint, Doloteffin, Harpadol**): Osteoarthritis, acute exacerbation of chronic low back pain (possibly effective): 2400 mg extract/day (providing 50-100 mg harpagoside/day) PO divided bid-tid. [Not by prescription. Extracts standardized to harpagoside (iridoid glycoside) content.] ▶? ♀– ▶– $

dong quai (**Angelica sinensis**): Appears ineffective for postmenopausal symptoms; North American Menopause Society recommends against use. May increase bleeding risk with warfarin; avoid concurrent use. ▶? ♀– ▶– $

echinacea (**E. purpurea, E. angustifolia, E. pallida, cone flower, EchinaGuard, Echinacin Madaus**): Efficacy unclear for prevention or treatment of upper respiratory infections. ▶? ♀– ▶– $

elderberry (**Sambucus nigra, Rubini, Sambucol, Sinupret**): Efficacy unclear for influenza, sinusitis, and bronchitis. ▶? ♀– ▶– $

ephedra (**Ephedra sinica, ma huang, Metabolife 356, Biolean, Ripped Fuel, Xenadrine**): Little evidence of efficacy, other than modest short-term weight loss. In 2004 FDA banned ephedra supplements. ▶K ♀– ▶– $$

evening primrose oil (**Oenothera biennis**): Appears ineffective for premenstrual syndrome, postmenopausal symptoms, atopic dermatitis. ▶? ♀? ▶? $

fenugreek (**Trigonelle foenum-graecum**): Efficacy unclear for diabetes or hyperlipidemia. ▶? ♀– ▶? $$

feverfew (**Chrysanthemum parthenium, Migra-Lief, MigraSpray, Tanacetum parthenium L.**): Prevention of migraine (possibly effective): 50-100 mg extract PO daily; 2-3 fresh leaves PO with or after meals daily; 50-125 mg freeze-dried leaf PO daily. May take 1-2 months to begin working. Inadequate data to evaluate efficacy for acute migraine. ▶? ♀– ▶– $

garcinia (**Garcinia cambogia, Citri Lean**): Appears ineffective for weight loss. ▶? ♀– ▶– $

garlic supplements (**Allium sativum, Kwai, Kyolic**): Modest reduction in lipids in short-term studies, but long-term benefit in hyperlipidemia unclear. Small reductions in BP, but efficacy in HTN unclear. Does not appear effective for diabetes. Cytochrome P450 3A4 inducer. Significantly decreases saquinavir levels. May increase bleeding risk with warfarin with/without increase in INR. ▶LK ♀– ▶– $

ginger (**Zingiber officinale**): Prevention of motion sickness (efficacy unclear): 500-1000 mg powdered rhizome PO single dose 1 h before exposure. American College of Obstetrics and Gynecology considers ginger 250 mg PO qid a nonpharmacologic option for N/V of pregnancy. Efficacy unclear for postop N/V (conflicting study results). ▶? ♀? ▶? $

ginkgo biloba (*EGb 761, Ginkgold, Ginkoba, Quanterra Mental Sharpness*): Dementia (modestly effective): 40 mg PO tid of standardized extract containing 24% ginkgo flavone glycosides and 6% terpene lactones. Benefit may be delayed for up to 4 weeks. Does not appear to improve memory in elderly with normal cognitive function. Does not appear effective for prevention of acute altitude sickness. Limited benefit in intermittent claudication. ▶K ♀- ▶- $

ginseng - American (*Panax quinquefolius L.*): Reduction of postprandial glucose in type 2 diabetes (possibly effective): 3 g PO taken with or up to 2h before meal. ▶K ♀- ▶- $

ginseng - Asian (*Panax ginseng, Ginsana, Ginsai, G115, Korean red ginseng*): Promoted to improve vitality and well-being: 200 mg PO daily. Ginsana: 2 caps PO daily or 1 cap PO bid. Ginsana Sport: 1 cap PO daily. Preliminary evidence of efficacy for erectile dysfunction. Efficacy unclear for improving physical or psychomotor performance, diabetes, herpes infections, cognitive or immune function, postmenopausal hot flashes (American College of Obstetrics and Gynecologists and North American Menopause Society recommend against use). ▶? ♀- ▶- $

glucosamine (*Aflexa, Cosamin DS, Dona, Flextend, Promotion*): Osteoarthritis (effective for decreasing pain and joint space narrowing in knee OA): 500 mg PO tid. Dona: 1 packet (1500 mg) dissolved in glass of water PO daily. ▶? ♀+ ▶- $

goldenseal (*Hydrastis canadensis*): Often used in attempts to achieve false-negative urine test for illicit drug use (efficacy unclear). Often combined with echinacea in cold remedies; but insufficient data to assess efficacy for common cold or URIs. ▶? ♀- ▶- $

grape seed extract (*Vitus vinifera L., procyanidolic oligomers, PCO*): Small clinical trials suggest benefit in chronic venous insufficiency. No benefit in single study of seasonal allergic rhinitis. ▶? ♀? ▶? $

green tea (*Camellia sinensis*): Efficacy unclear for cancer prevention, weight loss, hypercholesterolemia. Do not use in patients receiving irinotecan. May decrease INR with warfarin due to vitamin K content. Contains caffeine. [Not by prescription. Green tea extract available in caps standardized to polyphenol content.] ▶? ♀+ in moderate amount in food, - in supplements ▶+ in moderate amount in food, - in supplements ?

guarana (*Paullinia cupana*): Marketed as an ingredient in weight-loss dietary supplements. Seeds contain caffeine. Guarana in weight loss dietary supplements has the potential to provide high doses of caffeine. ▶? ♀+ in food, - in supplements ▶+ in food, - in supplements ?

guggulipid (*Commiphora mukul extract, guggul*): Efficacy unclear for treatment of hyperlipidemia (conflicting study results). ▶? ♀- ▶- $$

hawthorn (*Crataegus laevigata, monogyna, oxyacantha, standardized extract WS 1442 - Crataegutt novo, HeartCare*): Mild heart failure (possibly effective): 80 mg PO bid to 160 mg PO tid of standardized extract (19% oligomeric procyanidins; WS 1442; HeartCare 80 mg tabs). ▶? ♀- ▶- $

horse chestnut seed extract (*Aesculus hippocastanum, HCE50, Venastat*): Chronic venous insufficiency (effective): 1 cap Venastat (16% aescin standardized extract) PO bid with water before meals. ▶? ♀- ▶- $

kava (*Piper methysticum, One-a-day Bedtime & Rest, Sleep-Tite*): Promoted as anxiolytic (possibly effective) or sedative. Do not use due to hepatotoxicity. ▶K ♀- ▶- $

kombucha tea (*Manchurian or Kargasok tea*): Recommend against use; has no proven benefit for any indication; may cause severe acidosis. Avoid. ▶? ♀- ▶- $

licorice (*Glycyrrhiza glabra, Glycyrrhiza uralensis*): Insufficient data to assess efficacy for postmenopausal vasomotor symptoms. Chronic high doses can cause pseudo-primary aldosteronism (with HTN, edema, hypokalemia). ▶Bile ♀- ▶- $

melatonin (*N-acetyl-5-methoxytryptamine*): To reduce jet lag after flights over >5 time zones (possibly effective): 0.5-5 mg PO qhs x 3-6 nights starting on day of arrival. ▶L ♀- ▶- $

methylsulfomethane (*MSM, dimethyl sulfone, crystalline DMSO2*): Insufficient data to assess efficacy of oral and topical MSM for arthritis pain. ▶? ♀- ▶? $

milk thistle (*Silybum marianum, Legalon, silymarin, Thisylin*): Hepatic cirrhosis (possibly effective): 100-200 mg PO tid of standardized extract with 70-80% silymarin. ▶LK ♀- ▶- $

nettle root (*stinging nettle, Urtica dioica radix*): Efficacy unclear for treatment of BPH. ▶? ♀- ▶- $

noni (*Morinda citrifolia*): Promoted for many medical disorders; but insufficient data to assess efficacy. Potassium content comparable to orange juice; hyperkalemia reported in chronic renal failure. ▶? ♀- ▶- $$$

probiotics (*Acidophilus, Bifidobacteria, Lactobacillus, Bacid, Culturelle, IntestiFlora, Lactinex, LiveBac, Power-Dophilus, Primadophilus, Probiotica, Saccharomyces boulardii*): Culturelle. Prevention of antibiotic-induced diarrhea (efficacy unclear): 1 cap PO bid during & for 1 week after antibiotic therapy. Give 2 h before/after antibiotic. Prevention of travelers' diarrhea (efficacy unclear): 1 cap PO bid from 2-3 days before until end of trip. Probiotica: 1 chew tab PO daily. Dose of other products may vary; check label. [Not by prescription. Culturelle contains Lactobacillus GG 10 billion cells/cap. Probiotica contains Lactobacillus reuteri 100 million cells/chew tab.] ▶? ♀+ ▶+ $

pycnogenol (*French maritime pine tree bark*): Promoted for many medical disorders; but insufficient data to assess efficacy. ▶L ♀- ▶- $

pygeum africanum (*African plum tree, Prostata, Prostatonin, Provol*): BPH (may have modest efficacy): 50-100 mg PO bid or 100 mg PO daily of standardized extract containing 14% triterpenes. Prostatonin (also contains Urtica dioica): 1 cap PO bid with meals; up to 6 weeks for full response. ▶? ♀- ▶- $

red clover isoflavone extract (*Trifolium pratense, trefoil, Promensil, Rimostil, Supplifem, Trinovin*): Postmenopausal vasomotor symptoms (conflicting evidence; does not appear effective overall, but may have modest benefit for severe sx): Promensil 1 tab PO daily-bid with meals. [Not by prescription. Isoflavone content (genistein, daidzein, biochanin, formononetin) is 40 mg/tab in Promensil and Trinovin, 57 mg/tab in Rimostil.] ▶Gut, L K ♀- ▶- $$

s-adenosylmethionine (*Flexium, SAM-e, sammy*): Depression (possibly effective): 400-1600 mg/day PO. Osteoarthritis (possibly effective): 400-1200 mg/day PO. Flexium (labeled for joint health): 200 mg PO bid or 400 mg PO daily on empty stomach. Onset of response in OA in 2-4 weeks. ▶L ♀? ▶? $$$

Saint John's wort (*Alterra, Hypericum perforatum, Kira, Movana, One-a-day Tension & Mood, LI-160, St John's wort*): Mild depression (effective): 300 mg PO tid of standardized extract (0.3% hypericin). May be ineffective for moderate major depression. May decrease efficacy of many drugs (eg, oral contraceptives) by inducing liver metabolism. May cause serotonin syndrome with SSRIs, MAOIs. ▶L ♀- ▶- $

saw palmetto (*Serenoa repens, One-a-day Prostate Health, Prostata, Quanterra*): BPH (effective): 160 mg PO bid or 320 mg PO daily of standardized liposterolic extract. Take with food. Brewed teas may not be effective. ▶? ♀- ▶- $

shark cartilage (**BeneFin, Cancenex, Cartilade**): Efficacy unclear for palliative care of advanced cancer. ▶? ♀- ▶- $$$$$

silver - colloidal (**mild & strong silver protein, silver ion**): Promoted as antimicrobial; unsafe and ineffective for any use. Silver accumulates in skin (leads to grey tint), conjunctiva, and internal organs with chronic use. [Not by prescription. May come as silver chloride, cyanide, iodide, oxide, or phosphate.] ▶? ♀- ▶- $

soy (**Genisoy, Healthy Woman, Novasoy, Phytosoya, Supplifem, Supro**): Cardiovascular risk reduction: ≥25 g/day soy protein (50 mg/day isoflavones) PO. Hypercholesterolemia: ~50 g/day soy protein PO reduces LDL cholesterol by ~13%; efficacy unclear for isoflavone supplements. Postmenopausal vasomotor symptoms (conflicting evidence; modest benefit possible): 20-60 g/day soy protein PO (40-80 mg/day isoflavones). Does not appear to improve lipids, cognition, or bone mineral density in healthy postmenopausal women. ▶Gut, L, K ♀+ for food, ? for supplements ▶+ for food, ? for supplements $

stevia (**Stevia rebaudiana**): Leaves traditionally used as sweetener. Efficacy unclear for treatment of type 2 diabetes or hypertension. ▶L ♀? ▶? $

tea tree oil (**melaleuca oil, Melaleuca alternifolia**): Not for oral use; CNS toxicity reported. Efficacy unclear for onychomycosis, tinea pedis, acne vulgaris, dandruff. ▶? ♀- ▶- $

valerian (**Valeriana officinalis, Alluna, One-a-day Bedtime & Rest, Sleep-Tite**): Insomnia (possibly effective): 400-900 mg of standardized extract PO 30 minutes before bedtime. Alluna: 2 tabs PO 1 h before bedtime. ▶? ♀- ▶- $

wild yam (**Dioscorea villosa**): Ineffective as topical "natural progestin". Was used historically to synthesize progestins, cortisone, and androgens; it is not converted to them or DHEA in the body. ▶L ♀? ▶? $

willow bark extract (**Salix alba, Salicis cortex, Assalix, salicin**): Osteoarthritis, low back pain (possibly effective): 60 to 240 mg/day salicin PO divided bid-tid. [Not by prescription. Some products standardized to 15% salicin content.] ▶K ♀- ▶- $

yohimbe (**Corynanthe yohimbe, Pausinystalia yohimbe, Potent V**): Nonprescription yohimbe promoted for impotence and as aphrodisiac, but these products rarely contain much yohimbine. FDA considers yohimbe bark in herbal remedies an unsafe herb. [Yohimbine is the primary alkaloid in the bark of the yohimbe tree. Yohimbine HCl is a prescription drug in the US; yohimbe bark is available without prescription. Yohimbe bark (not by prescription) and prescription yohimbine HCl are not interchangeable.] ▶L ♀- ▶- $

IMMUNOLOGY

Immunizations (For vaccine info see CDC website www.cdc.gov.)

BCG vaccine (**Tice BCG, ♣Pacis, Oncotice, Immucyst**): 0.2-0.3 ml percutaneously. ♀C ▶? $$$$

Comvax (haemophilus b + hepatitis B vaccine): 0.5 ml IM. ♀C ▶? $$$

diphtheria tetanus & acellular pertussis vaccine (**DTaP, Tripedia, Infanrix, Daptacel, Boostrix, ♣Tripacel, Adacel**): 0.5 ml IM. ♀C ▶- $

diphtheria-tetanus toxoid (**Td, DT, ♣D2T5**): 0.5 ml IM. [Injection DT (pediatric: 6 weeks- 6 yo). Td (adult and children: ≥7 years).] ♀C ▶? $

haemophilus b vaccine (**ActHIB, HibTITER, PedvaxHIB**): 0.5 ml IM. ♀C ▶? $

hepatitis A vaccine (**Havrix, Vaqta, ♣Avaxim, Epaxal**): Adult formulation 1 ml IM, repeat in 6-12 months. Peds: 0.5 ml IM, repeat 6-18 months later. [Single dose vial (specify pediatric or adult).] ♀C ▶+ $$$

hepatitis B vaccine (*Engerix-B, Recombivax HB*): Adults: 1 ml IM, repeat in 1 and 6 months. Separate pediatric formulations and dosing. ♀C ▶+ $$$

influenza vaccine (*Fluzone, Fluvirin, FluMist, ♥Fluviral, Vaxigrip*): 0.5 ml IM or 1 dose (0.5 mL) intranasally (FluMist). ♀C ▶+ $

Japanese encephalitis vaccine (*JE-Vax*): 1.0 ml SC x 3 doses on days 0, 7, and 30. ♀C ▶? $$$$$

measles mumps & rubella vaccine (*M-M-R II, ♥Priorix*): 0.5 ml SC. ♀C ▶+ $$

meningococcal polysaccharide vaccine (*Menomune-A/C/Y/W-135, Menactra, ♥Menjugate*): 0.5 ml SC (Menomune) or IM (Menactra). ♀C ▶? $$$

Pediarix (DTaP + hepatitis B + polio): 0.5 ml at 2, 4, 6 months IM. ♀C ▶? $$$

plague vaccine (*Plague vaccine*): Age 18-61 yo: 1 ml IM x 3 doses, then 0.2 ml IM 1-3 months after the 1st injection, then 0.2 ml IM 5-6 months later. ♀C ▶+ $

pneumococcal 23-valent vaccine (*Pneumovax, ♥Pneumo 23*): 0.5 ml IM/SC. ♀C ▶+ $

pneumococcal 7-valent conjugate vaccine (*Prevnar*): 0.5 ml IM x 3 doses 6-8 weeks apart starting at 2-6 months of age, followed by a fourth dose at 12-15 months. ♀C ▶? $$$

poliovirus vaccine (*Orimune, IPOL*): An all-IPV schedule is recommended. Inactivated (IPOL): 0.5 ml SC. ♀C ▶? $$

rabies vaccine (*RabAvert, Imovax Rabies, BioRab, Rabies Vaccine Adsorbed*): 1 ml IM in deltoid region on days 0, 3, 7, 14, 28. ♀C ▶? $$$$

smallpox vaccine (*Dryvax*): Prevention of smallpox or monkeypox: Specialized administration using a bifurcated needle SC x 1. ♀C ▶- ?

tetanus toxoid: 0.5 ml IM/SC. ♀C ▶+ $

TriHibit (haemophilus b + DTaP): 4th dose only, 15-18 mos: 0.5 ml IM. ♀C ▶- $$

Twinrix (hepatitis A inactivated + hepatitis B recombinant vaccines): Adults: 1 ml IM in deltoid, repeat in 1 & 6 months. ♀C ▶? $$$

typhoid vaccine (*Vivotif Berna, Typhim Vi, ♥Typherix*): 0.5 ml IM x 1 dose (Typhim Vi); 1 cap qod x 4 doses (Vivotif Berna). May revaccinate q2-5 yrs if high risk. [Trade only: Caps] ♀C ▶? $$$

varicella vaccine (*Varivax, ♥Varilrix*): Children 1 to 12 yo: 0.5 ml SC x 1 dose. Age ≥13: 0.5 ml SC, repeat 4-8 weeks later. ♀C ▶+ $$$

yellow fever vaccine (*YF-Vax*): 0.5 ml SC. ♀C ▶+ $$$

CHILDHOOD IMMUNIZATION SCHEDULE*						Months				Years	
Age	Birth	1	2	4	6	12	15	18	24	4-6	11-12
Hepatitis B	HB-1	HB-2			HB-3						
DTP†			DTP	DTP	DTP		DTP			DTP	Td
H influenza b			Hib	Hib	Hib	Hib					
Pneumococci			PCV	PCV	PCV	PCV					
Polio§			IPV	IPV		IPV				IPV	
MMR						MMR				MMR	
Varicella						Varicella					
Meningococcal											MCV
Influenza					Influenza‡						
Hepatitis A¶										HA (some areas)	

*2005 schedule from the CDC, ACIP, AAP, & AAFP, see CDC website (www.cdc.gov). †Acellular form preferred for all DTP doses. §Inactivated form (IPV) preferred for all doses in the US. ‡Also annually immunize older children (and contacts) with risk factors such as asthma, cardiac disease, sickle cell diseases, HIV, DM. Live-attenuated influenza (nasal form) only for healthy children ≥5 yo. ¶HA series recommended for selected high-risk areas, consult local public health authorities.

TETANUS WOUND MANAGEMENT (www.cdc.gov)	Uncertain or <3 prior tetanus immunizations	≥3 prior tetanus immunizations
Non tetanus prone wound, Ie, clean & minor	Td (DT if <7 yo)	Td if >10 years since last dose
Tetanus prone wound, eg, dirt, contamination, punctures, crush components	Td (DT if <7 yo), plus tetanus immune globulin 250 units IM at site other than Td.	Td if >5 years since last dose

Immunoglobulins

antivenin - crotalidae immune Fab ovine polyvalent (*CroFab*): Rattlesnake envenomation: Give 4-6 vials IV infusion over 60 minutes, within 6 hours of bite if possible. Administer 4-6 additional vials if no initial control of envenomation syndrome, then 2 vials q6h for up to 18 hours (3 doses) after initial control has been established. ▶? ♀C ▶? $$$$$

botulism immune globulin (*BabyBIG*): Infant botulism <1 yo: 1 mL (50 mg)/kg IV. ▶L ♀? ▶? ?

hepatitis B immune globulin (*H-BIG, BayHep B, NABI-HB*): 0.06 ml/kg IM within 24 h of needlestick, ocular, or mucosal exposure, repeat in 1 month. ▶L ♀C ▶? $$$

immune globulin - intramuscular (*Baygam*): Hepatitis A prophylaxis: 0.02-0.06 ml/ kg IM depending on length of stay. Measles (within 6 days post-exposure): 0.2-0.25 ml/kg IM. ▶L ♀C ▶? $$$$

immune globulin - intravenous (*Carimune, Gamimune, Polygam, Panglobulin, Octagam, Flebogamma, Sandoglobulin, Gammagard, Gamunex, Iveegam, Venoglobulin*): IV dosage varies by indication and product. ▶L ♀C ▶? $$$$$

lymphocyte immune globulin human (*Atgam*): Specialized dosing. ▶L ♀C ▶? $$$$$

rabies immune globulin human (*Imogam, BayRab*): 20 units/kg, as much as possible infiltrated around bite, the rest IM. ▶L ♀C ▶? $$$$$

RSV immune globulin (*RespiGam*): IV infusion for RSV. ▶Plasma ♀C ▶? $$$$$

tetanus immune globulin (*BayTet*): Prophylaxis: 250 units IM. ▶L ♀C ▶? $$$$

varicella-zoster immune globulin (*VZIG*): Specialized dosing. ▶L ♀C ▶? $$$$$

Immunosuppression

basiliximab (*Simulect*): Specialized dosing for organ transplantation. ▶Plasma ♀B ▶? $$$$$

cyclosporine (*Sandimmune, Neoral, Gengraf*): Specialized dosing for organ transplantation, rheumatoid arthritis, and psoriasis. [Generic/Trade: microemulsion Caps 25, 100 mg. Generic/Trade: Caps (Sandimmune) 25, 100 mg, solution (Sandimmune) 100 mg/ml, microemulsion solution (Neoral, Gengraf) 100 mg/ml.] ▶L ♀C ▶- $$$$$

daclizumab (*Zenapax*): Specialized dosing, organ transplantation. ▶L♀C ▶? $$$$$

mycophenolate mofetil (*Cellcept, Myfortic*): Specialized dosing, organ transplantation. [Trade only (CellCept): caps 250 mg, tabs 500 mg, oral suspension 200 mg/ml. Trade (Myfortic): tablet, extended-release: 180, 360 mg.] ▶? ♀C ▶? $$$$$

sirolimus (*Rapamune*): Specialized dosing for organ transplantation. [Trade: oral solution 1 mg/ml. Tablet 1, 2, 5 mg.] ▶L ♀C ▶- $$$$$

tacrolimus (*Prograf, FK 506*): Specialized dosing for organ transplantation. [Trade only: Caps 1,5 mg.] ▶L ♀C ▶- $$$$$

Other

tuberculin PPD (*Aplisol, Tubersol, Mantoux, PPD*): 5 TU (0.1 ml) intradermally, read 48-72h later. ▶L ♀C ▶+ $

NEUROLOGY

Alzheimer's Disease

donepezil (*Aricept*): Start 5 mg PO qhs. May increase to 10 mg PO qhs in 4-6 wks. [Trade: Tabs 5,10 mg. Orally disintegrating tabs 5,10 mg] ▶LK ♀C ▶? $$$$

galantamine (*Razadyne, Razadyne ER*): Extended release: Start 8 mg PO q am with food; increase to 16 mg q am after 4 wks. May increase to 24 q am after another 4 wks. Immediate release: Start 4 mg PO bid with food; increase to 8 mg bid after 4 wks. May increase to 12 mg bid after another 4 wks. [Trade: Razadyne tabs 4, 8, 12 mg; oral solution 4 mg/mL. Razadyne ER extended release caps 8, 16, 24 mg. Prior to April 2005 was called Reminyl.] ▶LK ♀B ▶? $$$$

memantine (*Namenda, ✦Ebixa*): Start 5 mg PO daily. Increase by 5 mg/d at weekly intervals to max 20 mg/d. Doses >5 mg/d should be divided bid. [Trade: Tabs 5, 10 mg. Oral soln 2 mg/ml.] ▶KL ♀B ▶? $$$$

rivastigmine (*Exelon*): Start 1.5 mg PO bid with food. Increase to 3 mg bid after 2 wks. Max 12 mg/d. [Trade: Caps 1.5,3,4.5,6 mg. Oral soln 2 mg/ml]▶K♀B▶? $$$$

Anticonvulsants

carbamazepine (*Tegretol, Tegretol XR, Carbatrol, Epitol*): 200-400 mg PO bid-qid. extended-release: 200 mg PO bid. Age 6-12 yo: 100 mg PO bid or 50 mg PO qid; increase by 100 mg/d at weekly intervals divided tid-qid (regular release), bid (extended-release), or qid (suspension). Age <6 yo: 10-20 mg/kg/d PO divided bid-qid. Aplastic anemia. [Trade: Tabs 200 mg (Tegretol, Epitol). Chew tabs 100 mg (Tegretol, Epitol). Susp 100 mg/5 ml (Tegretol). extended-release tabs 100, 200, 400 mg (Tegretol XR). extended-release caps 200, 300 mg. Generic: Tabs 200 mg. Chew tabs 100, 200 mg. Susp 100 mg/5 ml.] ▶LK ♀D ▶+ $

clobazam (✦*Frisium*): Canada only. Adults: Start 5-15 mg PO daily. Increase prn to max 80 mg daily. Children <2 yo : 0.5-1mg/kg PO daily. Children 2-16 yo: Start 5 mg PO daily. May increase prn to max 40 mg daily. [Generic-Trade: Tabs 10 mg.] ▶L ♀X (first trimester) D (2nd/3rd trimesters) ▶- $

clonazepam (*Klonopin, Klonopin Wafer, ✦Clonapam, Rivotril*): Start 0.5 mg PO tid. Max 20 mg/d. [Generic/Trade: Tabs 0.5,1,2 mg. Orally disintegrating tabs 0.125,0.25,0.5,1,2 mg.] ▶LK ♀D ▶- ⊙IV $$$

diazepam (*Valium, Diastat, ✦Vivol, E Pam, Diazemuls*): Active seizures: 5-10 mg IV q10-15 min to max 30 mg, or 0.2-0.5 mg/kg rectal gel PR. Muscle spasm: 2-10 mg PO tid-qid. [Generic/Trade: Tabs 2,5,10 mg. Soln 5 mg/5 ml. Trade only: Intensol concentrated soln 5 mg/ml. Rectal gel (Diastat) 2.5,5,10,15,20 mg] ▶LK ♀D ▶- ⊙IV $$

ethosuximide (*Zarontin*): Start 250 mg PO daily (or divided bid) if 3-6 yo, or 500 mg PO daily (or divided bid) if >6 yo. Max 1.5 g/d. [Generic/Trade: Caps 250 mg. Syrup 250 mg/5 ml.] ▶LK ♀C ▶- $$$$

felbamate (*Felbatol*): Start 400 mg PO tid. Max 3,600 mg/d. Peds: Start 15 mg/kg/day PO divided tid-qid. Max 45 mg/kg/d. Aplastic anemia, hepatotoxicity. [Trade: Tabs 400, 600 mg. Susp 600 mg/5 ml.] ▶KL ♀C ▶- $$$$$

fosphenytoin (*Cerebyx*): Load: 15-20 mg "phenytoin equivalents" (PE) per kg IM/IV no faster than 150 mg/min. Maintenance: 4-6 PE/kg/d. ▶L ♀D ▶+ $$$$$

gabapentin (*Neurontin*): Start 300 mg PO qhs. Increase gradually to 300-600 mg PO tid. Max 3,600 mg/d. Postherpetic neuralgia: Start 300 mg PO on day one; increase to 300 mg bid on day 2, and to 300 mg tid on day 3. Max 1,800 mg/d. Partial seizures, initial monotherapy: Titrate as with earlier indications. Usual effective dose is 900-1,800 mg/day. [Generic: Tabs 100, 300, 400 mg. Trade/generic: caps 100, 300, 400 mg. Tabs 600, 800 mg (scored). Soln 50 mg/ml.] ▶K ♀C ▶? $$$$

lamotrigine (*Lamictal, Lamictal CD*): Partial seizures or Lennox-Gastaut syndrome, adjunctive therapy with a single enzyme-inducing anticonvulsant. Age >12 yo: 50 mg PO daily x 2 wks, then 50 mg bid x 2 wks, then gradually increase to 150-250 mg PO bid. Age 2-12 yo: dosing is based on weight and concomitant meds (see package insert). Also approved for conversion to monotherapy (age ≥16 yo): see package insert. Drug interaction with valproate (see package insert for adjusted dosing guidelines). Potentially life-threatening rashes reported in 0.3% of adults and 0.8% of children; discontinue at first sign of rash. [Trade: Tabs 25, 100, 150, 200 mg. Chewable dispersible tabs (Lamictal CD) 2, 5, 25 mg.] ▸LK ♀C ▶- $$$$$

levetiracetam (*Keppra*): Start 500 mg PO bid. Increase by 1,000 mg/d q2 wks prn. Max 3,000 mg/d. [Trade: Tabs 250, 500, 750 mg. Oral solution 100 mg/ml.] ▸K ♀C ▶? $$$$$

lorazepam (*Ativan*): Status epilepticus (unapproved): 0.05-0.1 mg/kg IV over 2-5 min. ▸LK ♀D ▶- ©IV $$$

oxcarbazepine (*Trileptal*): Start 300 mg PO bid. Titrate to 1200 mg/d (adjunctive) or 1,200-2,400 mg/d (monotherapy). Peds 4-16 yo: Start 8-10 mg/kg/d divided bid. [Trade: Tabs 150, 300, 600 mg. Oral suspension 300 mg/5 ml.] ▸LK ♀C ▶- $$$$$

phenobarbital (*Luminal*): Load: 20 mg/kg IV at rate ≤60 mg/min. Maintenance: 100-300 mg/d PO divided daily-bid; peds 3-5 mg/kg/day PO divided bid-tid. Multiple drug interactions. [Generic/Trade: Tabs 15, 16, 30, 32, 60, 65, 100 mg. Elixir 20 mg/5 ml.] ▸L ♀D ▶- ©IV $

phenytoin (*Dilantin, Phenytek*): Status epilepticus: Load 10-15 mg/kg IV no faster than 50 mg/min, then 100 mg IV/PO q6-8h. Epilepsy: Oral load: 400 mg PO initially, then 300 mg in 2h and 4h. Maintenance: 5 mg/kg (or 300 mg PO) given daily (extended-release) or divided tid (standard release). [Generic/Trade: Extended-release caps 100 mg (Dilantin). Suspension 125 mg/5 ml. Trade only: Extended-release caps 30 mg (Dilantin), 200, 300 mg (Phenytek). Chew tabs 50 mg. Generic: Prompt-release caps 100 mg.] ▸L ♀D ▶+ $$

pregabalin (*Lyrica*): Dosing information unavailable at press time.

primidone (*Mysoline*): Start 100-125 mg PO qhs. Increase over 10d to 250 mg tid-qid. Metabolized to phenobarbital. [Generic/Trade: Tabs 50,250 mg.] ▸LK ♀D ▶-$$$

tiagabine (*Gabitril*): Start 4 mg PO daily. Increase by 4-8 mg/wk prn to max 32 mg/d (children ≥12 yo) or 56 mg/d (adults) divided bid-qid. [Trade: Tabs 2, 4, 12, 16 mg.] ▸L ♀C ▶? $$$$$

topiramate (*Topamax*): Partial seizures, primary generalized tonic-clonic seizures, monotherapy age >10 yrs: Start 25 mg PO bid week 1, 50 mg bid week 2, 75 mg bid week 3, 100 mg bid week 4, 150 mg bid week 5, then 200 mg bid as tolerated. Partial seizures, primary generalized tonic-clonic seizures, or Lennox Gastaut Syndrome, adjunctive therapy: Start 25-50 mg PO qhs. Increase weekly by 25-50 mg/d to usual effective dose of 200 mg PO bid. Doses >400 mg not shown to be more effective. Migraine prophylaxis: 50 mg PO bid. [Trade only: Tabs 25, 100, 200 mg. Sprinkle Caps 15, 25 mg.] ▸K ♀C ▶? $$$$$

valproic acid (*Depakene, Depakote, Depakote ER, Depacon, divalproex, ✦Epiject, Epival, Deproic*): Epilepsy: 10-15 mg/kg/d PO/IV divided bid-qid (standard release or IV) or given once daily (Depakote ER). Titrate to max 60 mg/kg/d. Parenteral (Depacon): ≤20 mg/min IV. Hepatotoxicity, drug interactions, reduce dose in elderly. [Trade only: Tabs, delayed release (Depakote, divalproex sodium) 125, 250, 500 mg. Tabs, extended release (Depakote ER) 250, 500 mg. Caps, sprinkle (Depakote) 125 mg. Generic/Trade: Syrup (Depakene, valproic acid) 250 mg/5 ml. Caps (Depakene) 250 mg.] ▸L ♀D ▶+ $$$$$

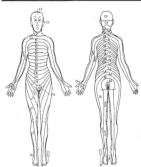

DERMATOMES

MOTOR NERVE ROOTS

Level	Motor function
C4	Spontaneous breathing
C5	Shoulder shrug / deltoid
C6	Biceps / wrist extension
C7	Triceps / wrist flexion
C8/T1	finger flexion
T1-T12	Intercostal/abd muscles
T12	cremasteric reflex
L1/L2	hip flexion
L2/L3/L4	hip adduction / quads
L5	great toe dorsiflexion
S1/S2	foot plantarflexion
S2-S4	rectal tone

LUMBOSACRAL NERVE ROOT COMPRESSION	Root	Motor	Sensory	Reflex
	L4	quadriceps	medial foot	knee-jerk
	L5	dorsiflexors	dorsum of foot	medial hamstring
	S1	plantarflexors	lateral foot	ankle-jerk

GLASGOW COMA SCALE		
Eye Opening	Verbal Activity	Motor Activity
4. Spontaneous	5. Oriented	6. Obeys commands
3. To command	4. Confused	5. Localizes pain
2. To pain	3. Inappropriate	4. Withdraws to pain
1. None	2. Incomprehensible	3. Flexion to pain
	1. None	2. Extension to pain
		1. None

zonisamide (**Zonegran**): Start 100 mg PO daily. Titrate q2 wks to 300-400 mg PO daily (or divided bid). Max 600 mg/d. Contraindicated in sulfa allergy. [Trade: Caps 25, 50, 100 mg.] ▶LK ♀C ▶? $$$$

Migraine Therapy - Triptans (5-HT1 Receptor Agonists)

NOTE: May cause vasospasm. Avoid in ischemic or vasospastic heart disease, cerebrovascular syndromes, peripheral arterial disease, uncontrolled HTN, and hemiplegic or basilar migraine. Do not use within 24 hours of ergots or other triptans. Risk of serotonin syndrome if used with SSRIs.

almotriptan (**Axert**): 6.25-12.5 mg PO. May repeat in 2h prn. Max 25 mg/d. [Trade: Tabs 6.25, 12.5 mg.] ▶LK ♀C ▶? $

eletriptan (**Relpax**): 20-40 mg PO. May repeat in >2 h prn. Max 40 mg/dose or 80 mg/d. [Trade: Tabs 20 mg, 40 mg] ▶LK ♀C ▶? $

frovatriptan (**Frova**): 2.5 mg PO. May repeat in 2h prn. Max 7.5 mg/24h. [Trade: Tabs 2.5 mg.] ▶LK ♀C ▶? $

naratriptan (**Amerge**): 1-2.5 mg PO. May repeat in 4h prn. Max 5 mg/24h. [Trade: Tabs 1, 2.5 mg.] ▶KL ♀C ▶? $$

rizatriptan (**Maxalt, Maxalt MLT**): 5-10 mg PO. May repeat in 2h prn. Max 30 mg/24h. MLT form dissolves on tongue without liquids. [Trade: Tabs 5, 10 mg. Orally disintegrating tabs (MLT) 5, 10 mg.] ▶LK ♀C ▶? $$

sumatriptan (*Imitrex*): 6 mg SC. May repeat in 1h prn. Max 12 mg/24h. Tablets: 25-100 mg PO (50 mg most common). May repeat q2h prn with 25-100 mg doses. Max 200 mg/24h. Intranasal spray: 5-20 mg q2h. Max 40 mg/24h. [Trade: Tabs 25, 50, 100 mg. Nasal spray 5, 20 mg/ spray. Injection 6 mg/0.5 ml.] ▶K ♀C ▶+ $$

zolmitriptan (*Zomig, Zomig ZMT*): 1.25-2.5 mg PO q2h. May repeat in 2h prn. Max 10 mg/24h. Orally disintegrating tabs (ZMT) 2.5 mg PO. May repeat in 2h prn. Max 10 mg/24h. Nasal spray: 5 mg (1 spray) in one nostril. May repeat in 2h. Max 10 mg/24h. [Trade: Tabs 2.5, 5 mg. ZMT 2.5, 5 mg ($$$). Nasal spray 5 mg/spray.] ▶L ♀C ▶? $$

Migraine Therapy - Other

Cafergot (ergotamine + caffeine): 2 tabs (1/100 mg each) PO at onset, then 1 tab q30 min prn. Max 6 tabs/attack or 10/wk. Suppositories (2/100 mg): 1 PR at onset; may repeat in 1h prn. Max 2/attack or 5/wk. [Trade: Supp 2/100 mg ergotamine/caffeine. Generic: Tabs 1/100 mg ergotamine/caffeine.] ▶L ♀X ▶- $

dihydroergotamine (*D.H.E. 45, Migranal*): Solution (DHE 45) 1 mg IV/IM/SC. May repeat in 1h prn. Max 2 mg (IV) or 3 mg (IM/SC) per day. Nasal spray (Migranal): 1 spray in each nostril. May repeat in 15 min prn. Max 6 sprays/24h or 8 sprays/wk. [Trade: Nasal spray 0.5 mg/spray. Self-injecting soln: 1 mg/ml.] ▶L ♀X ▶- $$

flunarizine (✚ *Sibelium*): Canada only. 10 mg PO qhs. [Generic/Trade: Caps 5 mg] ▶L ♀C ▶- $$

Midrin (isometheptene + dichloralphenazone + acetaminophen): Tension & vascular headache treatment: 1-2 caps PO q4h. Max 8 caps/d. Migraine treatment: 2 caps PO x 1, then 1 cap q1h prn to max 5 caps/12h. [Generic/Trade: Caps 65/100 /325 mg of isometheptene/dichloralphenazone/acetaminophen.] ▶L ♀? ▶? ◎IV $

Multiple sclerosis

glatiramer (*Copaxone*): Multiple sclerosis: 20 mg SC daily. ▶Serum ♀B ▶? $$$$$

interferon beta-1A (*Avonex, Rebif*): Multiple sclerosis: Avonex- 30 mcg (6 million units) IM q wk. Rebif- start 8.8 mcg SC three times weekly, and titrate over 4 wks to maintenance dose of 44 mcg three times weekly over 4 wks. Follow LFTs and CBC. [Trade: Avonex: Injection 33 mcg (6.6 million units) single dose vial. Rebif: Starter kit 20 mcg pre-filled syringe, 44 mcg prefilled syringe.] ▶L ♀C ▶? $$$$$

interferon beta-1B (*Betaseron*): Multiple sclerosis: Start 0.0625 mg SC qod; titrate over six weeks to 0.25 mg (8 million units) SC qod. [Trade: Injection 0.3 mg (9.6 million units) single dose vial.] ▶L ♀C ▶? $$$$$

Myasthenia Gravis

edrophonium (*Tensilon, Enlon, Reversol*): Myasthenia gravis eval: 2 mg IV over 15-30 seconds (test dose) while on cardiac monitor, then 8 mg IV after 45 sec. Atropine should be readily available in case of cholinergic reaction. ▶Plasma♀C▶?$

neostigmine (*Prostigmin*): 15-375 mg/d PO in divided doses, or 0.5 mg IM/SC. [Trade: Tablets 15 mg.] ▶L ♀C ▶? $$$

pyridostigmine (*Mestinon, Mestinon Timespan, Regonal*): Myasthenia gravis: 60-200 mg PO tid (standard release) or 180 mg PO daily-bid (extended release). [Trade: Tabs 60 mg. Extended release tabs 180 mg. Syrup 60 mg/5 ml.] ▶Plasma, K ♀C ▶+ $$

Parkinsonian Agents - Anticholinergics

benztropine mesylate (*Cogentin*): 0.5-2 mg IM/PO/IV daily-bid. [Generic/Trade: Tabs 0.5, 1, 2 mg.] ▶LK ♀C ▶? $$

biperiden (**Akineton**): 2 mg PO tid-qid. [Trade: Tabs 2 mg] ▶LK ♀C ▶? $$

trihexyphenidyl (**Artane**): Start 1 mg PO daily. Increase gradually to 6-10 mg/d, divided tid. Max 15 mg/d. [Generic/Trade: Tabs 2,5 mg. Elixir 2 mg/5 ml.] ▶LK♀C▶? $

Parkinsonian Agents - COMT Inhibitors

entacapone (**Comtan**): Start 200 mg PO with each dose of carbidopa/levodopa. Max 8 tabs/d (1600 mg). [Trade: Tabs 200 mg.] ▶L ♀C ▶? $$$$

tolcapone (**Tasmar**): Start 100 mg PO tid. Max 600 mg/d. Must be taken concurrently with carbidopa/levodopa. Hepatotoxicity; monitor LFTs. [Trade: Tabs 100, 200 mg.] ▶LK ♀C ▶? $$$$

Parkinsonian Agents - Dopaminergic Agents & Combinations

amantadine (**Symmetrel**, ✦**Endantadine**): 100 mg PO bid. Max 300-400 mg/d. [Trade only: Tabs 100 mg. Generic: Caps 100 mg. Generic/Trade: Syrup 50 mg/ 5 ml.] ▶K ♀C ▶- $

apomorphine (**Apokyn**): Start 0.2 ml SC prn. May increase in 0.1 ml increments every few days. Monitor for orthostatic hypotension after initial dose and with dose escalation. Max 0.6 ml/dose or 2 ml/d. Potent emetic - start trimethobenzamide 300 mg PO tid 3d prior to use, and continue for ≥2 months. [Trade only: Cartridges (for injector pen, 10 mg/ml) 3 ml. Ampules (10 mg/ml) 2 ml.] ▶L ♀C ▶? $$$$$

bromocriptine (**Parlodel**): Start 1.25 mg PO bid. Usual effective dose 10-40 mg/d. Max 100 mg/d. [Generic/Trade: Tabs 2.5 mg. Caps 5 mg.] ▶L ♀B ▶- $$$$$

carbidopa (**Lodosyn**): Adjunct to carbidopa/levodopa. Give 12.5-25 mg PO prn with each dose of carbidopa/levodopa. [Trade: Tabs 25 mg.] ▶LK ♀C ▶? $$$$

carbidopa-levodopa (**Atamet, Sinemet, Sinemet CR, Parcopa**): Start 1 tab (25/100 mg) PO tid. Increase q1-4 d as needed. Sustained release: Start 1 tab (50/200 mg) PO bid; increase q 3d as needed. [Generic/Trade: Tabs (carbidopa/levodopa) 10/100, 25/100, 25/250. Tabs, sustained release (Sinemet CR, carbidopa-levodopa ER) 25/100, 50/200 mg. Tabs: orally disintegrating tablet (Parcopa) 10/100, 25/100, 25/250.] ▶L ♀C ▶- $$$$

pergolide (**Permax**): Start 0.05 mg PO daily. Gradually increase to 1 mg PO tid. Max 5 mg/d. [Generic/Trade: Tabs 0.05, 0.25, 1 mg.] ▶K ♀B ▶? $$$$$

pramipexole (**Mirapex**): Start 0.125 mg PO tid. Gradually increase to 0.5-1.5 mg PO tid. [Trade: Tabs 0.125, 0.25, 0.5, 1, 1.5 mg.] ▶K ♀C ▶? $$$$$

ropinirole (**Requip**): Parkinsonism: Start 0.25 mg PO tid, then gradually increase to 1 mg PO tid. Max 24 mg/d. Restless legs syndrome: Start 0.25 mg PO 1-3 hr before sleep for 2 days, then increase to 0.5 mg/d days 3-7. Increase by 0.5 mg/d at weekly intervals as tolerated to max dose of 4 mg/d. [Trade: Tabs 0.25, 0.5, 1, 2, 4, 5 mg.] ▶L ♀C ▶? $$$$

selegiline (**Eldepryl, Atapryl, Carbex, Selpak**): 5 mg PO q am and q noon. [Generic/Trade: Caps 5 mg. Tabs 5 mg.] ▶LK ♀C ▶? $$$$

Stalevo (carbidopa + levodopa + entacapone): Parkinson's disease (conversion from carbidopa-levodopa +/- entacapone): Start Stalevo tab with same amount of carbidopa-levodopa, titrate to desired response. May need to reduce levodopa dose if not already taking entacapone. [Trade: Tabs (carbidopa/levodopa/entacapone): 12.5/50/200 mg, 25/100/200 mg, 37.5/150/200 mg.] ▶L ♀C ▶- $$$$$

Other Agents

alteplase (**tpa, t-PA, Activase**, ✦**Activase rt-PA**): Thrombolysis for acute ischemic stroke with symptoms ≤3h: 0.9 mg/kg (max 90 mg); give 10% of total dose as an IV bolus, and the remainder IV over 60 min. Multiple exclusions. ▶L ♀C ▶? $$$$$

dexamethasone (**Decadron, ✦Dexasone**): Cerebral edema: Load 10-20 mg IV/IM, then give 4 mg IV/IM q6h or 1-3 mg PO tid. Bacterial meningitis: 0.15 mg/kg IV/IM q6h. [Generic/Trade: Tabs 0.25, 0.5, 0.75, 1.0, 1.5, 2, 4, 6 mg. Elixir/ solution 0.5 mg/5 ml. Trade only: Solution concentrate 0.5 mg/ 0.5 ml (Intensol).] ▶L ♀C ▶- $$$

mannitol (**Osmitrol, Resectisol**): Intracranial HTN: 0.25-2 g/kg IV over 30-60 min. ▶K ♀C ▶? $$

meclizine (**Antivert, Bonine, Medivert, Meclicot, Meni-D, ✦Bonamine**): Motion sickness: 25-50 mg PO 1 hr prior to travel, then 25-50 mg PO q24h. Vertigo: 25 mg PO q6h prn. [Rx/OTC/Generic/Trade: Tabs 12.5, 25 mg. Chew tabs 25 mg. Rx/Trade only: Tabs 30, 50 mg. Caps 25 mg.] ▶L ♀B ▶? $

nimodipine (**Nimotop**): Subarachnoid hemorrhage: 60 mg PO q4h x 21 d. [Trade: Caps 30 mg.] ▶L ♀C ▶- $$$$$

oxybate (**Xyrem, GHB, gamma hydroxybutyrate**): Cataplexy associated with narcolepsy: 2.25 g PO qhs. Repeat in 2.5-4h. May increase by 1.5 g/d at >2 wk intervals to max 9 g/d. [Trade: Soln 180 ml (500 mg/ml).] ▶L ♀B ▶? ©III $$$$$

riluzole (**Rilutek**): ALS: 50 mg PO q12h. Monitor LFTs. [Trade: Tabs 50 mg.] ▶LK ♀C ▶- $$$$$

OB/GYN

Contraceptives – Other (Oral contraceptives on table on next page)

levonorgestrel (**Plan B**): Emergency contraception: 1 tab PO ASAP but within 72h of intercourse. 2nd tab 12h later. [Trade: Kit contains 2 tabs 0.75 mg.] ▶L ♀X ▶- $

NuvaRing (ethinyl estradiol + etonogestrel): Contraception: 1 ring intravaginally x 3 weeks each month. [Trade: Flexible intravaginal ring, 15 mcg ethinyl estradiol/0.120 mg etonogestrel/day. 1 and 3 rings/box.] ▶L ♀X ▶- $$

Ortho Evra (norelgestromin + ethinyl estradiol, ✦Evra): Contraception: 1 patch q week x 3 weeks, then 1 week patch-free. [Trade: Transdermal patch: 150 mcg norelgestromin + 20 mcg ethinyl estradiol/day. 1 and 3 patches/box.] ▶L ♀X ▶- $$

Estrogens (See also Hormone Replacement Combinations)

esterified estrogens (**Menest**): HRT: 0.3 to 1.25 mg PO daily. [Trade: Tabs 0.3, 0.625, 1.25, 2.5 mg.] ▶L ♀X ▶- $

estradiol (**Estrace, Estradiol, Gynodiol**): HRT: 1-2 mg PO daily. [Generic/Trade: Tabs, micronized 0.5,1,2 mg, scored. Trade only: 1.5 mg (Gynodiol).] ▶L ♀X ▶- $$

estradiol acetate (**Femtrace**): HRT: 0.45-1.8 mg PO daily. [Trade: Tabs, 0.45, 0.9, 1.8 mg.] ▶L ♀X ▶- $$

estradiol acetate vaginal ring (**Femring**): Menopausal atrophic vaginitis & vasomotor symptoms: Insert & replace after 90 days. [Trade: 0.05 mg/day and 0.1 mg/day.] ▶L ♀X ▶- $$

estradiol cypionate (**Depo-Estradiol**): HRT: 1-5 mg IM q 3-4 weeks. ▶L ♀X ▶- $

estradiol gel (**Estrogel**): HRT: Thinly apply contents of one complete pump depression (1.25 g) to one entire arm. [Trade: Gel 0.06% in non-aerosol, metered-dose pump with 64 1.25 g doses.] ▶L ♀X ▶- $$

estradiol topical emulsion (**Estrasorb**): HRT: Rub contents of one pouch each to left and right legs (spread over thighs & calves) qam. Daily dose = two 1.74 g pouches. [Trade: Topical emulsion, 56 pouches/carton.] ▶L ♀X ▶- $$

estradiol transdermal system (**Alora, Climara, Esclim, Estraderm, FemPatch, Menostar, Vivelle, Vivelle Dot, ✦Estradot, Oesclim**): HRT: Apply one patch weekly (Climara, FemPatch, Estradiol, Menostar) or twice per week (Esclim, Estra derm, Vivelle, Vivelle Dot, Alora). [Trade: Transdermal patches doses in mg/day:

ORAL CONTRACEPTIVES* ►L ♀X Monophasic	Estrogen (mcg)	Progestin (mg)
Norinyl 1+50, Ortho-Novum 1/50, Necon 1/50	50 mestranol	1 norethindrone
Ovcon-50	50 ethinyl estradiol	1 norethindrone
Demulen 1/50, Zovia 1/50E		1 ethynodiol
Ovral, Ogestrel		0.5 norgestrel
Norinyl 1+35, Ortho-Novum 1/35, Necon 1/35, Nortrel 1/35	35 ethinyl estradiol	1 norethindrone
Brevicon, Modicon, Necon 0.5/35, Nortrel 0.5/35		0.5 norethindrone
Ovcon-35		0.4 norethindrone
Previfem		0.18 norgestimate
Ortho-Cyclen, MonoNessa, Sprintec-28		0.25 norgestimate
Demulen 1/35, Zovia 1/35E, Kelnor 1/35		1 ethynodiol
Loestrin 21 1.5/30, Loestrin Fe 1.5/30, Junel 1.5/30, Junel 1.5/30 Fe, Microgestin Fe 1.5/30	30 ethinyl estradiol	1.5 norethindrone
Cryselle, Lo/Ovral, Low-Ogestrel		0.3 norgestrel
Apri, Desogen, Ortho-Cept, Reclipsen		0.15 desogestrel
Levlen, Levora, Nordette, Portia, Seasonale		0.15 levonorgestrel
Yasmin		3 drospirenone
Loestrin 21 1/20, Loestrin Fe 1/20, Junel 1/20, Junel Fe 1/20, Microgestin 1/20	20 ethinyl estradiol	1 norethindrone
Alesse, Aviane, Lessina, Levlite, Lutera		0.1 levonorgestrel
Progestin-only		
Micronor, Nor-Q.D., Camila, Errin, Jolivette, Nora-BE	none	0.35 norethindrone
Ovrette		0.075 norgestrel
Biphasic (estrogen & progestin contents vary)		
Kariva, Mircette	20/10 eth estrad	0.15/0 desogestrel
Ortho Novum 10/11, Necon 10/11	35 eth estradiol	0.5/1 norethindrone
Triphasic (estrogen & progestin contents vary)		
Cyclessa, Velivet	25 ethinyl estradiol	0.100/0.125/0.150 desogestrel
Ortho-Novum 7/7/7, Necon 7/7/7, Nortrel 7/7/7	35 ethinyl estradiol	0.5/0.75/1 norethindr
Tri-Norinyl		0.5/1/0.5 norethindr
Enpresse, Tri-Levlen, Triphasil, Trivora-28	30/40/30 ethinyl estradiol	0.5/0.75/0.125 levonorgestrel
Ortho Tri-Cyclen, Trinessa, Tri-Sprintec, Tri-Previfem	35 eth estradiol	0.18/0.215/0.25 norgestimate
Ortho Tri-Cyclen Lo	25 eth estradiol	
Estrostep Fe	20/30/35 estr	1 norethindrone

*All: Not recommended in smokers. Increase risk of thromboembolism, stroke, MI, hepatic neoplasia & gallbladder disease. Nausea, breast tenderness, & breakthrough bleeding are common transient side effects. Effectiveness reduced by hepatic enzyme-inducing drugs such as certain anticonvulsants and barbiturates, rifampin, rifabutin, griseofulvin, & protease inhibitors. Coadministration with St. John's wort may decrease efficacy. Vomiting or diarrhea may also increase the risk of contraceptive failure. Consider an additional form of birth control in above circumstances. See product insert for instructions on missing doses. Most available in 21 and 28 day packs. **Progestin only**: Must be taken at the same time every day. Because much of the literature regarding OC adverse effects pertains mainly to estrogen/progestin combinations, the extent to which progestin-only contraceptives cause these effects is unclear. No significant interaction has been found with broad-spectrum antibiotics. The effect of St. John's wort is unclear. No placebo days, start new pack immediately after finishing current one. Available in 28 day packs. Readers may find the following website useful: www.managingcontraception.com.

Climara (q week) 0.025,0.0375, 0.05, 0.06, 0.075, 0.1. FemPatch (q week) 0.025. Esclim (twice/week) 0.025, 0.0375, 0.05, 0.075, 0.1. Vivelle, Vivelle Dot (twice/week) 0.025, 0.0375, 0.05, 0.075, 0.1. Estraderm (twice/week) 0.05, & 0.1. Alora (twice/week) 0.025, 0.05, 0.075, 0.1. Generic: Estradiol transdermal patches: (q week) 0.025, 0.05, 0.075, 0.1.] ▶L ♀X ▶- $-$$

estradiol vaginal ring (*Estring*): Menopausal atrophic vaginitis: Insert & replace after 90 days. [Trade: 2 mg ring single pack.] ▶L ♀X ▶- $$

estradiol vaginal tab (*Vagifem*): Menopausal atrophic vaginitis: one tablet vaginally daily x 2 weeks, then one tablet vaginally 2x/week. [Trade: Vaginal tab: 25 mcg in disposable single-use applicators, 8 & 18/pack.] ▶L ♀X ▶- $-$$

estradiol valerate (*Delestrogen*): HRT: 10-20 mg IM q4 weeks. ▶L ♀X ▶- $

estrogen cream (*Premarin, Estrace*): Menopausal atrophic vaginitis: Premarin: 0.5-2 g daily. Estrace: 2-4 g daily x 2 weeks, then reduce. [Trade: Vaginal cream. Premarin: 0.625 mg conjugated estrogens/g in 42.5 g with w/o calibrated applicator. Estrace: 0.1 mg estradiol/g in 42.5 g w/calibrated applicator.] ▶L ♀X ▶? $$$

estrogens conjugated (*Premarin, C.E.S., Congest*): HRT: 0.3 to 1.25 mg PO daily. Abnormal uterine bleeding: 25 mg IV/IM. Repeat in 6-12h if needed. [Trade: Tabs 0.3, 0.45, 0.625, 0.9, 1.25 mg.] ▶L ♀X ▶- $$

estrogens synthetic conjugated A (*Cenestin*): HRT: 0.3 to 1.25 mg PO daily. [Trade: Tabs 0.3, 0.45, 0.625, 0.9, 1.25 mg.] ▶L ♀X ▶- $$

estrogens synthetic conjugated B (*Enjuvia*): HRT: 0.3 to 1.25 mg PO daily. [Trade: Tabs 0.3, 0.45, 0.625, 1.25 mg.] ▶L ♀X ▶- $$

estropipate (*Ogen, Ortho-Est*): HRT: 0.75 to 6 mg PO daily. [Generic/Trade: Tabs 0.75, 1.5, 3, & 6 mg of estropipate.] ▶L ♀X ▶- $$

GnRH Agents

cetrorelix acetate (*Cetrotide*): Infertility: 0.25 mg SC daily during the early to mid follicular phase or 3 mg SC x 1 usually on stimulation day 7. [Trade: Injection 0.25 mg in 1 & 7-dose kits. 3 mg in 1 dose kit.] ▶Plasma ♀X ▶- $$$$$

ganirelix (*Follistim-Antagon Kit, ✦Orgalutran*): Infertility: 250 mcg SC daily during the early to mid follicular phase. Continue until hCG administration. [Trade: Injection 250 mcg/0.5 ml in pre-filled, disposable syringes with 3 vials follitropin beta.] ▶Plasma ♀X ▶? $$$$$

goserelin (*Zoladex*): Endometriosis: 3.6 mg implant SC q28 days or 10.8 mg implant q12 weeks x 6 months. ▶LK ♀X ▶- $$$$$

leuprolide (*Lupron, Lupron Depot*): Endometriosis or fibroid-associated anemia, Depot: 3.75 mg IM q4 month or 11.25 mg IM q3 months, for total therapy of 6 months (endometriosis) or 3 months (fibroids). Concurrent iron for fibroid-associated anemia. ▶L ♀X ▶- $$$$$

nafarelin (*Synarel*): Endometriosis: 200-400 mcg intranasal bid x 6 months. [Trade: Nasal soln 2 mg/ml in 8 ml bottle (200 mcg per spray) about 80 sprays/bottle.] ▶L ♀X ▶- $$$$$

EMERGENCY CONTRACEPTION within 72 hours of unprotected sex: Take first dose ASAP, then identical dose 12h later. Each dose is either 2 pills of *Ovral* or *Ogestrel*, 4 pills of *Cryselle, Levlen, Levora, Lo/Ovral, Nordette, Tri-Levlen**, *Triphasil**, *Trivora**, or *Low Ogestrel*, or 5 pills of *Alesse, Aviane, Lessina,* or *Levlite*. If vomiting occurs within 1 hour of taking either dose of medication, consider whether or not to repeat that dose with an antiemetic 1h prior. *Plan B* kit contains 2 levonorgestrel 0.75mg tabs. Each dose is 1 pill. The progestin-only method causes less nausea & may be more effective. More info at: www.not-2-late.com.

*Use 0.125 mg levonorgestrel/30 mcg ethinyl estradiol tabs.

Hormone Replacement Combinations (See also estrogens.)

Activella (estradiol + norethindrone): HRT: 1 tab PO daily. [Trade: Tab 1 mg estradiol/0.5 mg norethindrone acetate in calendar dial pack dispenser.] ▶L ♀X ▶- $$

Climara Pro (estradiol + levonorgestrel): HRT: 1 patch weekly. [Trade: Transdermal 0.045/0.015 estradiol/levonorgestrel in mg/day, 4 patches/box.] ▶L ♀X ▶- $$

CombiPatch (estradiol + norethindrone, ✿Estalis): HRT: 1 patch twice weekly. [Trade: Transdermal patch 0.05 estradiol/ 0.14 norethindrone & 0.05 estradiol/ 0.25 norethindrone in mg/day, 8 patches/box.] ▶L ♀X ▶- $$

Estratest (esterified estrogens + methyltestosterone): HRT: 1 tab PO daily. [Trade: Tabs 1.25 mg esterified estrogens/2.5 mg methyltestosterone.] ▶L ♀X ▶- $$

Estratest H.S. (esterified estrogens + methyltestosterone): HRT: 1 tab PO daily. [Trade: Tabs 0.625 mg esterified estrogens/1.25 mg methyltestost.] ▶L ♀X ▶- $$

FemHRT (ethinyl estradiol + norethindrone): HRT: 1 tab PO daily. [Trade: Tabs 5/1 and 2.5/0.5 mcg ethinyl estradiol/mg norethindrone, 28/blister card.] ▶L ♀X ▶- $$

Prefest (estradiol + norgestimate): HRT: 1 pink tab PO daily x 3 days followed by 1 white tab PO daily x 3 days, sequentially throughout the month. [Trade: Tabs in 30-day blister packs 1 mg estradiol (15 pink) & 1 mg estadiol/0.09 mg norgestimate (15 white).] ▶L ♀X ▶- $$

Premphase (estrogens conjugated + medroxyprogesterone): HRT: 1 tab PO daily. [Trade: Tabs in 28-day EZ-Dial dispensers: 0.625 mg conjugated estrogens (14) & 0.625 mg/5 mg conjugated estrogens/medroxyprogesterone (14).] ▶L ♀X ▶- $$

Prempro (estrogens conjugated + medroxyprogesterone, ✿PremPlus): HRT: 1 tab PO daily. [Trade: Tabs in 28-day EZ-Dial dispensers: 0.625 mg/5 mg, 0.625 mg/2.5 mg, 0.45 mg/1.5 mg, or 0.3 mg/1.5 mg conjugated estrogens/medroxyprogesterone.] ▶L ♀X ▶- $$

Syntest D.S. (esterified estrogens + methyltestosterone): HRT: 1 tab PO daily. [Trade: Tabs 1.25 mg esterified estrogens/2.5 mg methyltestost.] ▶L ♀X ▶- $$

Syntest H.S. (esterified estrogens + methyltestosterone): HRT: 1 tab PO daily. [Trade: Tabs 0.625 mg esterified estrogens/1.25 mg methyltestost.] ▶L ♀X ▶- $$

Labor Induction / Cervical Ripening

dinoprostone (*PGE2, Prepidil, Cervidil*, ✿Prostin E2): Cervical ripening: One syringe of gel placed directly into the cervical os for cervical ripening or one insert in the posterior fornix of the vagina. [Trade: Gel (Prepidil) 0.5 mg/3 g syringe. Vaginal insert (Cervidil) 10 mg.] ▶Lung ♀C ▶? $$$$

misoprostol (*PGE1, Cytotec*): Cervical ripening: 25 mcg intravaginally q3-6h (or 50 mcg q6h). [Generic/Trade: Oral tabs 100 & 200 mcg.] ▶LK ♀X ▶- $

oxytocin (*Pitocin*): Labor induction: 10 units in 1000 ml NS (10 milliunits/ml), start at 6-12 ml/h (1-2 milliunits/min). Uterine contractions/postpartum bleeding: 10 units IM or 10-40 units in 1000 ml NS IV, infuse 20-40 milliunits/minute. ▶LK ♀? ▶- $

Ovulation Stimulants

clomiphene (*Clomid, Serophene*): Specialized dosing for ovulation induction. [Generic/Trade: Tabs 50 mg, scored.] ▶L ♀D ▶? $$

Progestins

hydroxyprogesterone caproate: Amenorrhea, dysfunctional uterine bleeding, metrorrhagia: 375 mg IM. Production of secretory endometrium & desquamation: 125-250 mg IM on 10th day of the cycle, repeat q7days until suppression no longer desired. ▶L ♀X ▶? $

DRUGS GENERALLY ACCEPTED AS SAFE IN PREGNANCY (selected)

<u>Analgesics:</u> acetaminophen, codeine*, meperidine*, methadone*. <u>Antimicrobials:</u> penicillins, cephalosporins, erythromycins (not estolate), azithromycin, nystatin, clotrimazole, metronidazole**, nitrofurantoin***, Nix. <u>Antivirals:</u> acyclovir, valacyclovir, famciclovir. <u>CV:</u> labetalol, methyldopa, hydralazine. <u>Derm:</u> erythromycin, clindamycin, benzoyl peroxide. <u>Endo:</u> insulin, liothyronine, levothyroxine. <u>ENT:</u> chlorpheniramine, diphenhydramine, dimenhydrinate, dextromethorphan, guaifenesin, nasal steroids, nasal cromolyn. <u>GI:</u> trimethobenzamide, antacids*, simethicone, cimetidine, famotidine, ranitidine, nizatidine, psyllium, metoclopramide, bisacodyl, docusate, doxylamine, meclizine. <u>Psych:</u> fluoxetine****, desipramine, doxepin. <u>Pulmonary:</u> short-acting inhaled beta-2 agonists, cromolyn, nedocromil, beclomethasone, budesonide, theophylline, prednisone**. <u>Other –</u> heparin.
*Except if used long-term and in high does at term   **Except 1st trimester.
***Contraindicated at term and during labor and delivery.   ****Except 3rd trimester.

medroxyprogesterone (***Provera, Amen***): HRT: 10 mg PO daily for last 10-12 days of month, or 2.5-5 mg PO daily. Secondary amenorrhea, abnormal uterine bleeding: 5-10 mg PO daily x 5-10 days. Endometrial hyperplasia: 10-30 mg PO daily. [Generic/Trade: Tabs 2.5, 5, & 10 mg, scored.] ▶L ♀X ▶+ $

medroxyprogesterone - injectable (***Depo-Provera, depo-subQ provera 104***): Contraception/Endometriosis: 150 mg IM in deltoid or gluteus maximus or 104 mg SC in anterior thigh or abdomen q13 weeks. ▶L ♀X ▶+ $$

megestrol (***Megace, Megace ES***): Endometrial hyperplasia: 40-160 mg PO daily x 3-4 mo. AIDS anorexia: 800 mg (20 ml) susp PO daily or 625 mg (5 ml) ES daily. [Generic/Trade: Tabs 20 & 40 mg. Suspension 40 mg/ml in 237 ml. Trade: Megace ES suspension 125 mg/ml (150 ml).] ▶L ♀D ▶? $$$$$

norethindrone (***Aygestin***): Amenorrhea, abnormal uterine bleeding: 2.5-10 mg PO daily x 5-10 days during the second half of the menstrual cycle. Endometriosis: 5 mg PO daily x 2 weeks. Increase by 2.5 mg q 2 weeks to 15 mg. [Generic/trade: Tabs 5 mg, scored.] ▶L ♀D ▶? $

progesterone gel (***Crinone, Prochieve***): Secondary amenorrhea: 45 mg (4%) intravaginally qod up to 6 doses. If no response, use 90 mg (8%) qod up to 6 doses. Infertility: special dosing. [Trade: 4%, 8% single-use, prefilled applicators.] ▶Plasma ♀- ▶? $$$

progesterone micronized (***Prometrium***): HRT: 200 mg PO qhs 10-12 days/month or 100 mg qhs daily. Secondary amenorrhea: 400 mg PO qhs x 10 days. Contraindicated in peanut allergy. [Trade: Caps 100 & 200 mg.] ▶L ♀B ▶+ $

Selective Estrogen Receptor Modulators

raloxifene (***Evista***): Osteoporosis prevention/treatment: 60 mg PO daily. [Trade: Tabs 60 mg.] ▶L ♀X ▶- $$$

tamoxifen (***Nolvadex, Tamone, ✦Tamofen***): Breast cancer prevention: 20 mg PO daily x 5 years. Breast cancer: 10-20 mg PO bid. [Generic/Trade: Tabs 10 & 20 mg.] ▶L ♀D ▶- $$$

APGAR SCORE		0	1	2
	Heart rate	0. Absent	1. <100	2. >100
	Respirations	0. Absent	1. Slow/irreg	2. Good/crying
	Muscle tone	0. Limp	1. Some flexion	2. Active motion
	Reflex irritability	0. No response	1. Grimace	2. Cough/sneeze
	Color	0. Blue	1. Blue extremities	2. Pink

Tocolytics

indomethacin (**Indocin, Indocid**): Preterm labor: initial 50-100 mg PO/PR followed by 25 mg PO/PR q6-12h up to 48 hrs. [Generic/Trade: Immediate release caps 25 & 50 mg. Trade: Oral suspension 25 mg/5 ml. Suppositories 50 mg.] ▶L ♀? ▶- $

magnesium sulfate: Eclampsia: 4-6 g IV over 30min, then 1-2 g/h. Drip: 5 g in 250 ml D5W (20 mg/ml), 2 g/h = 100 ml/h. Preterm labor: 6 g IV over 20 minutes, then 2-3 g/h titrated to decrease contractions. Monitor respirations & reflexes. If needed, may reverse hypocalcemic effects with calcium gluconate 1g IV. ▶K ♀A ▶+ $$

nifedipine (**Procardia, Adalat, Procardia XL, Adalat CC, ✿Adalat XL**): Preterm labor: loading dose: 10 mg PO q20-30 min if contractions persist, up to 40 mg within the first hour. Maintenance dose: 10-20 mg PO q4-6h or 60-160 mg extended release PO daily. [Generic/Trade: immediate release caps 10 & 20 mg. Extended release tabs 30, 60, 90 mg.] ▶L ♀C ▶? $$$

terbutaline (**Brethine, Bricanyl**): Preterm labor: 0.25 mg SC q30 min up to 1 mg/4 hours. Infusion: 2.5-10 mcg/min IV, gradually increased to effective max doses of 17.5-30 mcg/minute. Tachycardia common. [Generic/Trade: Tabs 2.5, 5 mg (Brethine scored)] ▶L ♀B ▶+ $$$$$

Uterotonics

carboprost (**Hemabate, 15-methyl-prostaglandin F2 alpha**): Refractory postpartum uterine bleeding: 250 mcg deep IM. ▶LK ♀C ▶? $$$

methylergonovine (**Methergine**): Refractory postpartum uterine bleeding: 0.2 mg IM/PO tid-qid prn. [Trade: Tabs 0.2 mg.] ▶LK ♀C ▶? $

Vaginitis Preparations (See also STD/vaginitis table in antimicrobial section)

boric acid: Resistant vulvovaginal candidiasis: 1 vag supp qhs x 2 weeks. [No commercial preparation; must be compounded by pharmacist. Vaginal suppositories 600 mg in gelatin capsules.] ▶Not absorbed ♀? ▶- $

butoconazole (**Gynazole, Mycelex-3**): Vulvovaginal candidiasis: Mycelex 3: 1 applicatorful qhs x 3-6 days. Gynazole-1: 1 applicatorful intravaginally qhs x 1. [OTC: Trade (Mycelex 3): 2% vaginal cream in 5 g pre-filled applicators (3s) & 20 g tube with applicators. Rx: Cream (Gynazole-1): 2% vaginal cream in 5 g pre-filled applicator.] ▶LK ♀C ▶? $(OTC)

clindamycin (**Cleocin, Clindesse, ✿Dalacin**): Bacterial vaginosis: Cleocin: 1 applicatorful cream qhs x 7d or one vaginal supp qhs x 3d. Clindesse: 1 applicatorful cream x 1. [Generic/Trade: 2% vaginal cream in 40 g tube with 7 disposable applicators (Cleocin). Vag supp (Cleocin Ovules) 100 mg (3) w/applicator. 2% vaginal cream in a single-dose prefilled applicator (Clindesse).] ▶L ♀- ▶+ $$

clotrimazole (**Mycelex 7, Gyne-Lotrimin, ✿Canesten, Clotrimaderm**): Vulvovaginal candidiasis: 1 applicatorful 1% cream qhs x 7 days. 1 applicatorful 2% cream qhs x 3 days. 1 vag supp 100 mg qhs x 7 days. 1 vag tab 200 mg qhs x 3 days. [OTC: Generic/Trade: 1% vaginal cream with applicator (some pre-filled). 2% vaginal cream with applicator. Vaginal suppositories 100 mg (7) & 200 mg (3) with applicators. 1% topical cream in some combination packs.] ▶LK ♀B ▶? $

metronidazole (**MetroGel-Vaginal, Flagyl**): Bacterial vaginosis: 1 applicatorful qhs or bid x 5 days. [Generic/Trade: 0.75% gel in 70 g tube with applicator.] ▶LK ♀B ▶? $$$

miconazole (**Monistat, Femizol-M, M-Zole, Micozole, Monazole**): Vulvovaginal candidiasis: 1 applicatorful qhs x 3 (4%) or 7 (2%) days. 100 mg vag supp qhs x 7 days. 400 mg vag supp qhs x 3 days. 1200 mg vag supp x 1. [OTC: Generic/

Trade: 2% vaginal cream in 45 g with 1 applicator or 7 disposable applicators. Vaginal suppositories 100 mg (7) OTC: Trade: 400 mg (3) & 1200 mg (1) with applicator. Generic/Trade: 4% vaginal cream in 25 g tubes or 3 prefilled applicators. Some in combo packs with 2% miconazole cream for external use.] ▸LK ♀+ ▶? $

nystatin (*Mycostatin*, ♥*Nilstat, Nyaderm*): Vulvovaginal candidiasis: 1 vag tab qhs x 14 days. [Generic/Trade: Vaginal Tabs 100,000 units in 15s & 30s with or without applicator(s).] ▸Not metabolized ♀A ▶? $$

terconazole (*Terazol*): Vulvovaginal candidiasis: 1 applicatorful of 0.4% cream qhs x 7 days, or 1 applicatorful of 0.8% cream qhs x 3 days, or 80 mg vag supp qhs x 3 days. [All forms supplied with applicators: Generic/trade: Vag cream 0.4% in 45 g tube, 0.8% in 20 g tube. Vag supp 80 mg (3).] ▸LK ♀C ▶- $$

tioconazole (*Monistat 1-Day, Vagistat-1*): Vulvovaginal candidiasis: 1 applicatorful of 6.5% ointment intravaginally qhs single-dose. [OTC: Trade: Vaginal ointment: 6.5% (300 mg) in 4.6 g prefilled single-dose applicator.] ▸Not absorbed ♀C ▶- $

Other OB/GYN Agents

clonidine (*Catapres, Catapres-TTS*, ♥*Dixirit*): Menopausal flushing: 0.1-0.4 mg/day PO divided bid-tid. Transdermal system applied weekly: 0.1 mg/day. [Generic/Trade: Tabs, non-scored 0.1, 0.2, 0.3 mg. Trade only: transdermal weekly patch 0.1 mg/day (TTS-1), 0.2 mg/day (TTS-2), 0.3 mg/day (TTS-3).] ▸LK ♀C ▶? $

danazol (*Danocrine*, ♥*Cyclomen*): Endometriosis: Start 400 mg PO bid, then titrate downward to maintain amenorrhea x 3-6 months. Fibrocystic breast disease: 100-200 mg PO bid x 4-6 months. [Generic/Trade: Caps 50, 100, 200 mg.] ▸L ♀X ▶- $$$

mifepristone (*Mifeprex, RU-486*): 600 mg PO x 1 followed by 400 mcg misoprostol on day 3, if abortion not confirmed. [Trade: Tabs 200 mg.] ▸L ♀X ▶? $$$$$

Premesis-Rx (B6 + folic acid + B12 + calcium carbonate): Pregnancy-induced nausea: 1 tab PO daily. [Trade: Tabs 75 mg vitamin B6 (pyridoxine), sustained-release, 12 mcg vitamin B12 (cyanocobalamin), 1 mg folic acid, and 200 mg calcium carbonate.] ▸L ♀A ▶+ $

RHO immune globulin (*RhoGAM, BayRho-D, WinRho SDF, MICRhoGAM, BayRho-D Mini Dose*): 300 mcg vial IM to mother at 28 weeks gestation followed by a 2nd dose ≤72 hours of delivery (if mother Rh- and baby is or might be Rh+). Microdose (50 mcg, MICRhoGAM) OK if spontaneous abortion <12 weeks gestation. ▸L ♀C ▶? $$$$

ONCOLOGY

Alkylating agents: altretamine (*Hexalen*), busulfan (*Myleran, Busulfex*), carmustine (*BCNU, BiCNU, Gliadel*), chlorambucil (*Leukeran*), cyclophosphamide (*Cytoxan, Neosar*), dacarbazine (*DTIC-Dome*), ifosfamide (*Ifex*), lomustine (*CeeNu, CCNU*), mechlorethamine (*Mustargen*), melphalan (*Alkeran*), procarbazine (*Matulane*), streptozocin (*Zanosar*), temozolomide (*Temodar*, ♥*Temodal*), thiotepa (*Thioplex*). **Antibiotics**: bleomycin (*Blenoxane*), dactinomycin (*Cosmegen*), daunorubicin (*DaunoXome, Cerubidine*), doxorubicin liposomal (*Doxil*, ♥*Caelyx, Myocet*), doxorubicin non-liposomal (*Adriamycin, Rubex*), epirubicin (*Ellence*, ♥*Pharmorubicin*), idarubicin (*Idamycin*), mitomycin (*Mutamycin, Mitomycin-C*), mitoxantrone (*Novantrone*), valrubicin (*Valstar*, ♥*Valtaxin*). **Antimetabolites**: azacitidine (*Vidaza*), capecitabine (*Xeloda*), cladribine (*Leustatin, chlorodeoxyadenosine*), clofarabine (*Clolar*), cytarabine (*Cytosar-U, Tarabine, Depo-Cyt, AraC*), floxuridine (*FUDR*), fludarabine (*Fludara*), fluorouracil (*Adrucil, 5-FU*), gemcitabine (*Gemzar*), hydroxyurea (*Hydrea, Droxia*), mercaptopurine (*6-MP, Purinethol*), methotrexate (*Rheumatrex, Trexall*), pemetrexed (*Alimta*), pentostatin (*Nipent*), thioguanine (*Tabloid*, ♥*Lanvis*). **Cytoprotective Agents**: amifostine (*Ethyol*), dexrazoxane (*Zinecard*), mesna (*Mesnex*, ♥*Uromitexan*), palifermin (*Kepivance*). **Hormones**: abarelix (*Plenaxis*), anastrozole (*Arimidex*), bicalutamide (*Casodex*), cyproterone, ♥*Androcur, Androcur Depot*, estramustine (*Emcyt*), exemestane (*Aromasin*), flutamide (*Eulexin*, ♥*Euflex*), fulvestrant (*Faslodex*), goserelin (*Zoladex*), histrelin (*Vantas*), letrozole (*Femara*), leuprolide (*Eligard, Lupron, Oaklide, Viadur*), nilutamide (*Nilandron*, ♥*Anandron*), testolactone (*Teslac*), toremifene (*Fareston*), triptorelin (*Trelstar Depot*). **Immunomodulators**: aldesleukin (*Proleukin, interleukin-2*), alemtuzumab (*Campath*), BCG (*Bacillus of Calmette & Guerin, Pacis, TheraCys, TICE BCG*, ♥*Oncotice, Immucyst, Pacis*), bevacizumab (*Avastin*), cetuximab (*Erbitux*), denileukin (*Ontak*), erlotinib (*Tarceva*), gemtuzumab (*Mylotarg*), ibritumomab (*Zevalin*), imatinib (*Gleevec*), interferon alfa-2a (*Roferon-A*), interferon alfa-2b (*Intron A*), interferon alfa-n3 (*Alferon N*), rituximab (*Rituxan*), tositumomab (*Bexxar*), trastuzumab (*Herceptin*). **Mitotic Inhibitors**: docetaxel (*Taxotere*), etoposide (*VP-16, Etopophos, Toposar, VePesid*), paclitaxel (*Taxol, Abraxane, Onxol*), teniposide (*Vumon, VM-26*), vinblastine (*Velban, VLB*), vincristine (*Oncovin, Vincasar, VCR*), vinorelbine (*Navelbine*). **Platinum-Containing Agents**: carboplatin (*Paraplatin*), cisplatin (*Platinol-AQ*), oxaliplatin (*Eloxatin*). **Radiopharmaceuticals**: samarium 153 (*Quadramet*), strontium-89 (*Metastron*). **Miscellaneous**: arsenic trioxide (*Trisenox*), asparaginase (*Elspar*, ♥*Kidrolase*), bexarotene (*Targretin*), bortezomib (*Velcade*), gefitinib (*Iressa*), irinotecan (*Camptosar*), leucovorin (*Wellcovorin, folinic acid*), levamisole (*Ergamisol*), mitotane (*Lysodren*), pegaspargase (*Oncaspar*), porfimer (*Photofrin*), topotecan (*Hycamtin*), tretinoin (*Vesanoid*).

OPHTHALMOLOGY

Antiallergy - Decongestants & Combinations

naphazoline (*Albalon, AK-Con, Vasocon, Naphcon, Allerest, Clear Eyes*): 1 gtt qid prn for up to 4 days. [OTC Generic/Trade: solution 0.012, 0.02, 0.03% (15, 30 mL). Rx generic/Trade: 0.1% (15 mL).] ▶? ♀C ▶? $

Naphcon-A (naphazoline + pheniramine, *Visine-A*): 1 gtt qid prn for up to 4 days. [OTC Trade only: solution 0.025% + 0.3% (15 mL).] ▶L ♀C ▶? $

Vascon-A (naphazoline + antazoline): 1 gtt qid prn for up to 4 days. [OTC Trade only: solution 0.1% + 0.5% (15 mL).] ▶L ♀C ▶? $

Antiallergy - Dual Antihistamine & Mast Cell Stabilizer

azelastine (*Optivar*): 1 gtt bid. [Trade only: solution 0.05% (3, 6 mL).] ▶L ♀C ▶? $$

epinastine (*Elestat*): 1 gtt bid. [Trade only: soln 0.05% (5,10 mL).] ▶K ♀C ▶? $$$

ketotifen (*Zaditor*): 1 gtt in each eye q8-12h. [Trade only: solution 0.025% (5 mL).] ▶Minimal absorption ♀C ▶? $$

olopatadine (*Patanol*): 1-2 gtts of 0.1% solution in each eye bid at an interval of 6-8h (Patanol) or 1 gtt of 0.2% solution in each eye daily (Patanol ES). [Trade: solution 0.1% (5 mL, Patanol), 0.2% (2.5 mL, Patanol ES).] ▶K ♀C ▶? $$$

Antiallergy - Pure Antihistamines

emedastine (*Emadine*): 1 gtt up to qid. [Trade: soln 0.05% (5 mL).] ▶L ♀B ▶? $$

levocabastine (*Livostin*): 1 gtt qid. [Trade only: suspension 0.05% (5,10 mL).] ▶Minimal absorption ♀C ▶? $$$

Antiallergy - Pure Mast Cell Stabilizers

cromolyn sodium (*Crolom, Opticrom*): 1-2 gtts in each eye 4-6 times per day. [Generic/Trade: solution 4% (10 mL).] ▶LK ♀B ▶? $$$

lodoxamide (*Alomide*): 1-2 gtts in each eye qid. [Trade only: solution 0.1% (10 mL).] ▶K ♀B ▶? $$$

nedocromil (*Alocril*): 1-2 gtts in each eye bid. [Trade: soln 2% (5 mL).] ▶L ♀B ▶? $$

pemirolast (*Alamast*): 1-2 gtts in each eye qid. [Trade only: solution 0.1% (10 mL).] ▶? ♀C ▶? $$$

Antibacterials - Aminoglycosides

gentamicin (*Garamycin, Genoptic, Gentak, ♣Alcomicin, Diogent*): 1-2 gtts q2-4h; ½ inch ribbon of oint bid-tid. [Generic/Trade: solution 0.3% (5 ,15 mL), ointment 0.3% (3.5 g tube).] ▶K ♀C ▶? $

tobramycin (*Tobrex*): 1-2 gtts q1-4h or ½ inch ribbon of ointment q3-4h or bid-tid. [Generic/Trade: soln 0.3% (5 mL). Trade only: oint 0.3% (3.5 g tube).] ▶K ♀B ▶- $

Antibacterials - Fluoroquinolones

ciprofloxacin (*Ciloxan*): 1-2 gtt q1-6h or ½ inch ribbon ointment bid-tid. [Trade/generic: soln 0.3% 2.5,5,10 mL. Trade only: oint 0.3% (3.5 g tube).] ▶LK ♀C ▶? $$

gatifloxacin (*Zymar*): 1-2 gtts q2h while awake up to 8 times/day on days 1 & 2, then 1-2 gtts q4h up to 4 times/day on days 3-7. [Trade only: solution 0.3%.] ▶K ♀C ▶? $$

levofloxacin (*Iquix, Quixin*): Quixin: 1-2 gtts q2h while awake up to 8 times/day on days 1 & 2, then 1-2 gtts q4h up to 4 times/day on days 3-7. Iquix: 1-2 gtts q30 min to 2h while awake and q4-6h overnight on days 1-3, then 1-2 gtts q1-4h while awake on days 4 to completion of therapy. [Trade only: solution 0.5% (Quixin, 5 mL), 1.5% (Iquix, 5 mL).] ▶KL ♀C ▶? $$

moxifloxacin (*Vigamox*): 1 gtt tid x 7 days. [Trade only: soln 0.5%.] ▶LK ♀C ▶? $$

ofloxacin (*Ocuflox*): 1-2 gtts q1-6h x 7-10 days. [Trade/generic solution 0.3% (5 mL, 10 mL).] ▶LK ♀C ▶? $$

Antibacterials - Other

bacitracin (*AK Tracin*): Apply ¼-½ inch ribbon of ointment q3-4h or bid-qid. [Generic/Trade: ointment 500 units/g (3.5g tube)] ▶Minimal absorption ♀C ▶? $

erythromycin (*Ilotycin, AK-Mycin*): ½ inch ribbon of ointment q3-4h or 2-8 times/day. [Generic: ointment 0.5% (1, 3.5 g tube).] ▶L ♀B ▶+ $

Neosporin ointment (neomycin + bacitracin + polymyxin B): ½ inch ribbon of ointment q3-4h x 7-10 days or ½ inch ribbon 2-3 times/day for mild-moderate infection. [Generic/Trade: ointment. (3.5 g tube).] ▶K ♀C ▶? $

Neosporin solution (neomycin + polymyxin + gramicidin): 1-2 gtts q1-6h x 7-10 days. [Trade/Trade: solution (10 mL).] ▶K ♀C ▶? $$

Polysporin (polymyxin B + bacitracin): ½ inch ribbon of ointment q3-4h x 7-10 days or ½ inch ribbon bid-tid for mild-moderate infection. [Generic/Trade: ointment (3.5 g tube).] ▶K ♀C ▶? $

Polytrim (polymyxin B + trimethoprim): 1-2 gtts q3-6h x 7-10d, max 6 gtts/day. [Generic/Trade: solution (10 mL).] ▶LK ♀C ▶? $$

sulfacetamide (*Sulamyd, Bleph-10, Sulf-10, Isopto Cetamide, AK-Sulf*): 1-2 gtts q2-6h x 7-10d or ½ inch ribbon of ointment q3-8h x 7-10d. [Generic only: solution 10%, 30% (15 mL). Generic/Trade: ointment 10% (3.5g tube). Trade only: solution 10% (2.5,5,15 mL), 10, 15, 30% (15 mL).] ▶K ♀C ▶- $

Antiviral Agents

trifluridine (*Viroptic*): Herpes: 1 gtt q2-4h x 7-14d, max 9 gtts/day, 21 days. [Trade only: solution 1% (7.5 mL).] ▶Minimal absorption ♀C ▶- $$$

vidarabine (*Vira-A*): ½ inch ribbon of ointment up to 5 times daily x 5-7 days. After re-epithelialization, ½ inch ribbon bid x 5-7 days. [Trade only: ointment 3% (3.5 g tube).] ▶Cornea ♀C ▶? $$$

Corticosteroid & Antibacterial Combinations

> NOTE: Recommend that only ophthalmologists or optometrists prescribe due to infection, cataract, corneal/scleral perforation, and glaucoma risk. Monitor intraocular pressure.

Blephamide (prednisolone + sodium sulfacetamide): 1-2 gtts q1-8h or ½ inch ribbon of ointment daily-qid. [Generic/Trade: solution/suspension (5,10 mL), Trade only: ointment (3.5 g tube).] ▶KL ♀C ▶? $

Cortisporin (neomycin + polymyxin + hydrocortisone): 1-2 gtts or ½ inch ribbon of ointment q3-4h or more frequently prn. [Generic/Trade: suspension (7.5 mL), ointment (3.5 g tube).] ▶LK ♀C ▶? $

FML-S Liquifilm (prednisolone + sodium sulfacetamide): 1-2 gtts q1-8h or ½ inch ribbon of ointment daily-qid. [Trade only: suspension (5,10 mL).] ▶KL ♀C ▶? $

Maxitrol (dexamethasone + neomycin + polymyxin): 1-2 gtts q1-8h or ½ -1 inch ribbon of ointment daily-qid. [Trade/Generic: suspension (5 mL), ointment (3.5 g tube).] ▶KL ♀C ▶? $

Pred G (prednisolone + gentamicin): 1-2 gtts q1-8h daily-qid or ½ inch ribbon of ointment bid-qid. [Trade: susp (2,5,10 mL), ointment (3.5 g tube).] ▶KL ♀C ▶? $$

TobraDex (tobramycin + dexamethasone): 1-2 gtts q2-6h or ½ inch ribbon of ointment bid-qid. [Trade: suspension (2.5,5,10 mL), oint (3.5 g tube).] ▶L ♀C ▶? $$

Vasocidin (prednisolone + sodium sulfacetamide): 1-2 gtts q1-8h or ½ inch ribbon of ointment daily-qid. [Generic/Trade: solution (5,10 mL)] ▶KL ♀C ▶? $

Zylet (loteprednol + tobramycin): 1-2 gtts q1-2h x 1-2 days then 1-2 gtts q4-6h. [Trade: suspension 0.5% loteprednol + 0.3% tobramycin 2.5,5,10 mL] ▶LK ♀C ▶?

Corticosteroids

> NOTE: Recommend that only ophthalmologists or optometrists prescribe due to infection, cataract, corneal/scleral perforation, and glaucoma risk. Monitor intraocular pressure.

fluorometholone (*FML, FML Forte, Flarex, Fluor-Op*): 1-2 gtts q1-12h or ½ inch ribbon of ointment q4-24h. [Generic/Trade: suspension 0.1% (5,10,15 mL). Trade only: suspension 0.25% (5,10,15 mL), ointment 0.1% (3.5 g tube)] ▶L ♀C ▶? $$$

loteprednol (*Alrex, Lotemax*): 1-2 gtts qid. [Trade only: suspension 0.2% (Alrex 5,10 mL), 0.5% (Lotemax 2.5, 5,10,15 mL).] ▶L ♀C ▶? $$

prednisolone (*AK-Pred, FML Forte, Pred Mild, Inflamase, Inflamase Forte, Econopred, Econopred Plus, ✦AK Tate, Diopred*): Solution: 1-2 gtts up to q1h during day and q2h at night, when response observed, then 1 gtt q4h, then 1 gtt tid-qid. Suspension: 1-2 gtts bid-qid. [Generic/Trade: suspension 1% (5,10,15 mL), solution 0.125 (5 mL), 1% (5,10,15 mL). Trade only: suspension 0.12% (5,10 mL), solution 0.125% (5,10 mL).] ▶L ♀C ▶? $

rimexolone (*Vexol*): 1-2 gtts q1-6h. [Trade only: susp 1% (5,10 mL).] ▶L ♀C ▶? $$

Glaucoma Agents - Beta Blockers (Use caution in cardiac conditions and asthma.)

betaxolol (*Betoptic, Betoptic S*): 1-2 gtts bid. [Trade only: suspension 0.25% (2.5,5,10,15 mL). Generic only: solution 0.5% (5,10,15 mL).] ▶LK ♀C ▶? $$

carteolol (*Ocupress*): 1 gtt bid. [Generic/Trade: soln 1% 5,10,15 mL] ▶KL ♀C ▶? $

levobetaxolol (*Betaxon*): 1 gtt bid. [Trade only: solution 0.5%.] ▶KL ♀C ▶? ?

levobunolol (***Betagan***): 1- 2 gtts daily-bid. [Generic/Trade: solution 0.25% (5,10 mL) 0.5% (5,10,15 mL - Trade only 2 mL).] ▶? ♀C ▶- $

metipranolol (***Optipranolol***): 1 gtt bid. [Generic/Trade: solution 0.3% (5,10 mL).] ▶? ♀C ▶? $

timolol (***Betimol, Timopic, Timoptic XE, Istalol, Tomoptic Ocudose***): 1 gtt bid. Timoptic XE, Istalol: 1 gtt daily. [Generic/Trade: solution 0.25, 0.5% (5,10,15 mL), preservative free 0.2 mL. Generic/Trade: gel forming solution 0.25, 0.5% (2.5*, 5 mL). Trade: soln 0.5% (Istalol) 10 mL). Note: * 0.25%Timoptic XE.] ▶LK ♀C ▶+ $

Glaucoma Agents - Carbonic Anhydrase Inhibitors

NOTE: Sulfonamide derivatives; verify absence of sulfa allergy before prescribing.

acetazolamide (***Diamox, Diamox Sequels***): Glaucoma: 250 mg PO up to qid (immediate release) or 500 mg PO up to bid (ext'd release). Max 1 g/day. [Generic/ Trade: Tabs 125, 250 mg. Trade only: ext'd release caps 500 mg.] ▶LK ♀C ▶+ $$

brinzolamide (***Azopt***): 1 gtt tid. [Trade: susp 1% (5,10,15 mL).] ▶LK ♀C ▶? $$

dorzolamide (***Trusopt***): 1 gtt tid. [Trade only: solution 2% (5,10 mL).] ▶KL ♀C ▶- $$

methazolamide (***Neptazane***): 25-50 mg PO daily-tid. [Generic only: Tabs 25, 50 mg.] ▶LK ♀C ▶? $

Glaucoma Agents - Miotics

pilocarpine (***Pilocar, Pilopine HS, Isopto Carpine, Ocusert, Ocu Carpine, ✦Diocarpine, Akarpine***): 1-2 gtts tid-qid up to 6 times/day or ½ inch ribbon of gel qhs. [Generic/Trade: solution 0.5, 1, 2, 3, 4, 6% (15mL). Trade only: 5%, 8% (15 mL), gel 4% (4 g tube).] ▶Plasma ♀C ▶? $

Glaucoma Agents - Prostaglandin Analogs

bimatoprost (***Lumigan***): 1 gtt qhs. [Trade only: solution 0.03% (2.5, 5, 7.5 mL).] ▶LK ♀C ▶? $$$

latanoprost (***Xalatan***): 1 gtt qhs. [Trade only: soln 0.005% 2.5 mL] ▶LK ♀C ▶? $$$

travoprost (***Travatan***): 1 gtt qhs. [Trade only: soln 0.004% (2.5,5 mL).] ▶L ♀C ▶? $$

unoprostone (***Rescula***): 1 gtt bid. [Trade: soln 0.15% 5 mL] ▶Plasma, K ♀C ▶? $$

Glaucoma Agents - Sympathomimetics

brimonidine (***Alphagan, Alphagan P, ✦Alphaga***): 1 gtt tid. [Trade only: solution 0.15% (Alphagan P: 5,10,15 mL). Generic: 0.2%.] ▶L ♀B ▶? $$

Glaucoma Agents - Other

Cosopt (dorzolamide + timolol): 1 gtt bid. [Trade only: solution dorzolamide 2% + timolol 0.5% (5,10 mL).] ▶LK ♀D ▶- $$

Mydriatics & Cycloplegics

atropine (***Isopto Atropine***): 1-2 gtts before procedure or daily-qid, 1/8-1/4 inch ointment before procedure or daily-tid. Cycloplegia may last up to 5-10d and mydriasis may last up to 7-14d. [Generic/Trade: solution 1% (5,15 mL) Generic only: ointment 1% (3.5 g tube).] ▶? ♀C ▶? $

cyclopentolate (***AK-Pentolate, Cyclogyl, Pentolair***): 1-2 gtts x 1-2 doses before procedure. Cycloplegia may last 6-24h; mydriasis may last 1 day. [Generic/Trade: solution 1% (2,15 mL). Trade only: 0.5% (15 mL), 2% (2,5,15 mL).] ▶? ♀C ▶? $

homatropine (***Isopto Homatropine***): 1-2 gtts before procedure or bid-tid. Cycloplegia & mydriasis lasts 1-3 days. [Trade only: solution 2% (5 mL), 5% (15 mL). Generic/Trade: solution 5% (5 mL).] ▶? ♀C ▶? $

phenylephrine (*Neo-Synephrine, Mydfrin, Relief*): 1-2 gtts before procedure or tid-qid. No cycloplegia; mydriasis may last up to 5 hours. [Generic/Trade: solution 2.5,10% (3*, 5, 15 mL) Note: * 2.5% Mydfrin.] ▶Plasma, L ♀C ▶? $

tropicamide (*Mydriacyl*): 1-2 gtts before procedure. Mydriasis may last 6 hours. [Generic/Trade: solution 0.5% (15 mL), 1% (2, 3, 15 mL)] ▶? ♀? ▶? $

Nonsteroidal Anti-Inflammatories

bromfenac (*Xibrom*): 1 gtt bid x 2 weeks. [Trade: solution 0.09% (5 mL).] ▶Minimal absorption ♀C, D (3rd trimester) ▶? ?

diclofenac (*Voltaren*, ✚*Voltaren Ophtha*): 1 gtt up to qid. [Trade: solution 0.1% (2.5, 5 mL).] ▶L ♀B, D (3rd trimester) ▶? $

ketorolac (*Acular, Acular LS*): 1 gtt qid. [Trade only: solution (Acular LS) 0.4% (5 ml), (Acular) 0.5% (3,5,10 mL), preservative free (Acular) 0.5% unit dose (0.4 ml).] ▶L ♀C ▶? $$$

Other Ophthalmologic Agents

artificial tears (*Tears Naturale, Hypotears, Refresh Tears, Lacrilube, GenTeal*): 1-2 gtts tid-qid prn. [OTC solution (15, 30 mL among others).] ▶Minimal absorption ♀A ▶+ $

cyclosporine (*Restasis*): 1 gtt in each eye q12h. [Trade: emulsion 0.05% (0.4 mL single-use vials).] ▶Minimal absorption ♀C ▶? $$$$

dapiprazole (*Rev-Eyes*): 2 gtt in each eye, repeat in 5 mins. [Trade only: powder for solution 0.5% (5 mL).] ▶Minimal absorption ♀B ▶? $

petrolatum (*Lacrilube, Dry Eyes, Refresh PM*, ✚*Duolube*): Apply ¼-½ inch ointment to inside of lower lid prn. [OTC oint 3.5g tube.] ▶Minimal absorption ♀A ▶+ $

proparacaine (*Ophthaine, Ophthetic*, ✚*Alcaine*): Do not prescribe for unsupervised/prolonged use. Corneal toxicity and ocular infections may occur with repeated use. 1-2 gtts before procedure. [Generic/Trade: solution 0.5% (15 mL).] ▶L ♀C ▶? $

tetracaine (*Pontocaine*): Do not prescribe for unsupervised or prolonged use. Corneal toxicity and ocular infections may occur with repeated use. 1-2 gtts or ½-1 inch ribbon of ointment before procedure. [Generic/Trade: solution 0.5% (15 mL).] ▶Plasma ♀C ▶? $

PSYCHIATRY

Antidepressants - Heterocyclic Compounds

amitriptyline (*Elavil*): Start 25-100 mg PO qhs, gradually increase to usual effective dose of 50-300 mg/d. Primarily serotonin. Demethylated to nortriptyline. [Generic: Tabs 10, 25, 50, 75, 100, 150 mg. Elavil brand no longer available.] ▶L ♀D ▶- $$

clomipramine (*Anafranil*): Start 25 mg PO qhs, gradually increase to usual effective dose of 150-250 mg/d, max 250 mg/d. Primarily serotonin. Seizures. [Generic/Trade: Caps 25, 50, 75 mg.] ▶L ♀C ▶+ $$$

desipramine (*Norpramin*): Start 25-100 mg PO daily or in divided doses. Gradually increase to usual effective dose of 100-200 mg/d, max 300 mg/d. Primarily norepinephrine. [Generic/Trade: Tabs 10, 25, 50, 75, 100, 150 mg.] ▶L ♀C ▶+ $$

doxepin (*Sinequan*): Start 75 mg PO qhs. Usual effective dose 75-150 mg/d, max 300 mg/d. Primarily norepinephrine. [Generic/Trade: Caps 10, 25, 50, 75, 100, 150 mg. oral concentrate 10 mg/mL.] ▶L ♀C ▶? $$

imipramine (*Tofranil, Tofranil PM*): Start 75-100 mg PO qhs or in divided doses, gradually increase to max 300 mg/d. Mixed serotonin and norepinephrine. Demethylated to desipramine. [Generic/Trade: Tabs 10, 25, 50 mg. Trade only: Caps 75, 100, 125, 150 mg. (as pamoate salt)] ▶L ♀D ▶- $$$

nortriptyline (**Aventyl, Pamelor**): Start 25 mg PO daily-qid. Usual effective dose 75-100 mg/d, max 150 mg/d. Primarily norepinephrine reuptake inhibitor. [Generic/Trade: Caps 10, 25, 50, 75 mg. Oral Solution 10 mg/5 mL.] ▶L ♀D ▶+ $$

protriptyline (**Vivactil**): 15-40 mg PO divided tid-qid. [Trade: Tabs 5, 10 mg.] ▶L ♀C ▶+ $$$

Antidepressants - Monoamine Oxidase Inhibitors (MAOIs)

> **NOTE:** May interfere with many medications; avoid qhs dosing. Must be on tyramine-free diet, stay on diet for 2 weeks after stopping. Risk of hypertensive crisis and serotonin syndrome with many medications, including OTC. Evaluate thoroughly for drug interactions. Allow at least 2 weeks wash-out when changing between MAOIs and SSRIs (6 weeks after fluoxetine), TCAs, and other antidepressants.

isocarboxazid (**Marplan**): Start 10 mg PO bid, increase by 10 mg q2-4 days. Usual effective dose is 20- 40 mg/d. [Trade: Tabs 10 mg.] ▶L ♀C ▶? $$$

phenelzine (**Nardil**): Start 15 mg PO tid. Usual effective dose is 60-90 mg/d in divided doses. [Trade: Tabs 15 mg.] ▶L ♀C ▶? $$

tranylcypromine (**Parnate**): Start 10 mg PO qam, increase by 10 mg/d at 1-3 week intervals to usual effective dose of 10-40 mg/d divided bid. [Trade: Tabs 10 mg.] ▶L ♀C ▶- $$

Antidepressants - Selective Serotonin Reuptake Inhibitors (SSRIs)

citalopram (**Celexa**): Depression: Start 20 mg PO daily, usual effective dose 20-40 mg/d, max 60 mg/d. [Trade/generic: Tabs 10,20,40 mg. Oral solution 10 mg/5 mL.] ▶LK ♀C but - in 3rd trimester ▶- $$$

escitalopram (**Lexapro**): Depression, generalized anxiety disorder: Start 10 mg PO daily, max 20 mg/day. [Trade: Tabs 5, 10, 20 mg, with the 10 & 20 mg scored. Oral Solution 1 mg/mL.] ▶LK ♀C but - in 3rd trimester ▶- $$$

fluoxetine (**Prozac, Prozac Weekly, Sarafem**): Depression & OCD: Start 20 mg PO q am, usual effective dose 20-40 mg/day, max 80 mg/day. Depression, maintenance: 20-40 mg/day OR 90 mg PO once weekly delayed release (start 7 days after last dose of 20 mg/day). Bulimia: 60 mg PO daily; may need to titrate up to 60 mg/day over several days. Panic disorder: Start 10 mg PO q am; titrate to 20 mg/day after one week; max dose 60 mg/day. Premenstrual Dysphoric Disorder (PMDD): Sarafem: 20 mg PO daily continuously, or 20 mg PO daily for 14 days prior to menses, max 80 mg/day. Doses >20 mg/d can be divided am & noon. [Trade/generic: tabs 10 mg, caps 10, 20, 40 mg, oral solution 20 mg/5 mL. Trade: caps (Sarafem) 10, 20 mg, caps delayed release (Prozac Weekly) 90 mg. Generic: tabs 20, 40 mg.] ▶L ♀C but - in 3rd trimester ▶- $$$

fluvoxamine (♣**Luvox**): OCD: Start 50 mg PO qhs, usual effective dose 100-300 mg/day divided bid, max 300 mg/day. OCD in ≥8 yo: Start 25 mg PO qhs, usual effective dose 50-200 mg/day divided bid, max 200 mg/day. Avoid with cisapride, diazepam, pimozide, and MAOIs; caution with benzodiazepines, TCAs, theophylline, warfarin. [Generic: Tabs 25,50,100 mg.] ▶L ♀C but - in 3rd trimester ▶- $$$$

paroxetine (**Paxil, Paxil CR, Pexeva**): Depression: Start 20 mg PO daily, usual effective dose 20-50 mg/day, max 50 mg/day. Controlled release: Start 25 mg PO qam, max 62.5 mg/day. OCD: Start 10-20 mg PO qam, usual effective dose 10-60 mg/day, max 60 mg/day. Social anxiety disorder: Start 10-20 mg PO qam, usual effective dose 10-60 mg/day, max 60 mg/day. Controlled-release: Start 12.5 mg PO qam, max 37.5 mg/day. Generalized anxiety disorder: Start 20 mg PO qam, max 50 mg/day. Panic disorder: Start 10 mg PO qam, increase by 10 mg/day at intervals ≥1 week to usual effective dose of 10-60 mg/day. Max 60 mg/day. Controlled-release: Start 12.5 mg PO qam, max 75 mg/d. Post-traumatic stress disorder: Start 20 mg PO qam, usual effective dose 20-40 mg/day, max 50 mg per day. Premenstrual dysphoric disorder: Controlled-release: Continuous dosing: Start 12.5 mg PO qam, may increase dose after 1 wk to max 25 mg qam. Intermittent dosing: Start 12.5 mg PO qam 2 wks prior to menses, max 25 mg/d. [Trade/Generic: Tabs 10,20,30,40 mg. Trade: Extended-release tabs 12.5,25,37.5 mg. Oral suspension 10 mg/5 mL.] ▶LK ♀D, - in 3rd trimester ▶? $$$

sertraline (**Zoloft**): Depression/OCD: Start 50 mg PO daily, usual effective dose 50-200 mg/d, max 200 mg/d. Panic disorder/ Posttraumatic stress disorder/Social anxiety disorder: Start 25 mg PO daily, max 200 mg/d. Premenstrual dysphoric disorder: Start 50 mg PO daily (continuous) or 14 days prior to menses (intermittent), max 150 mg daily continuous or 100 mg daily intermittent. If used intermittently, start 50 mg PO daily x 3 days then increase to 100 mg. [Trade: Tabs 25, 50, 100 mg. Oral concentrate 20 mg/mL.] ▶LK ♀C but - in 3rd trimester ▶+ $$$

Antidepressants - Other

bupropion (**Wellbutrin, Wellbutrin SR, Wellbutrin XL**): Depression: Start 100 mg PO bid, after 4-7 days can increase to 100 mg tid. Usual effective dose 300-450 mg/day. Max 150 mg/dose and 450 mg/day. Sustained release: Start 150 mg PO q am, after 4-7 days may increase to 150 mg bid, max 400 mg/d. Last dose no later than 5 pm. Extended release: Start 150 mg PO q am, after 4 days may increase to 300 mg q am, max 450 mg q am. [Generic/Trade: Tabs 75,100 mg. Sustained release tabs 100, 150, 200 mg. Extended-release tabs 150, 300 mg (Wellbutrin XL).] ▶LK ♀B ▶- $$$$

duloxetine (**Cymbalta**): Depression: 20 mg PO bid, max 60 mg/d either daily or divided bid. Diabetic peripheral neuropathic pain: 60 mg PO daily. [Trade: Caps 20, 30, 60 mg.] ▶L ♀C ▶? $$$$

mirtazapine (**Remeron, Remeron SolTab**): Start 15 mg PO qhs. Usual effective dose 15-45 mg/day. Agranulocytosis 0.1%. [Trade/generic: Tabs 15, 30, 45 mg. Tabs, orally disintegrating (SolTab) 15, 30, 45 mg. Generic: Tabs 7.5 mg.] ▶LK ♀C ▶? $$$

moclobemide (✱**Manerix**): Canada only. 300-600 mg/day PO divided twice daily after meals. [Trade: Tabs 150,300 mg. Generic tabs 100,150,300 mg] ▶L ♀C ▶- $$

nefazodone: Start 100 mg PO bid, usual effective dose 150-300 mg/day, max 600 mg/day. Hepatotoxicity. Avoid with cisapride, MAOIs, or triazolam. [Generic: Tabs 50, 100, 150, 200, 250 mg.] ▶L ♀C ▶? $$$

trazodone (**Desyrel**): Insomnia: 50-150 mg PO qhs. Depression: Start 50-150 mg/day PO in divided doses. Usual effective dose is 400-600 mg/day in divided doses. [Generic/Trade: Tabs 50, 100, 150, 300 mg.] ▶L ♀C ▶- $$$$

venlafaxine (**Effexor, Effexor XR**): Depression/ anxiety: Start 37.5-75 mg PO daily (Effexor XR), max 225 mg/d; 75 mg (Effexor) PO divided bid-tid, max 375 mg/d. Usual effective dose 150-225 mg/d. Social anxiety disorder: Start 37.5-75 mg PO daily (Effexor XR), max 225 mg/d. [Trade: Caps, extended release 37.5, 75, 150 mg. Tabs (Effexor) 25, 37.5, 50, 75, 100 mg.] ▶LK ♀C but - in 3rd trimester ▶? $$$$

Antimanic (Bipolar) Agents

carbamazepine (**Tegretol, Tegretol XR, Carbatrol, Epitol, Equetro**): Mania (American Psychiatric Association guidelines): Start 200-600 mg/d divided tid-qid (bid for extended release), increase by 200 mg/d q4-2 days. Mean effective dose 1,000 mg/d. Max 1,600 mg/d. Aplastic anemia. [Trade: Tabs 100, 200 mg (Tegretol, Epitol). Chew tabs 100 mg (Tegretol, Epitol). Susp 100 mg/5 mL (Tegretol).

Extended release tabs 100, 200, 400 mg (Tegretol XR). Extended release caps 100, 200, 300 mg (Equetro, Carbatrol). Generic: Tabs 200 mg. Chew tabs 100 mg. Susp 100 mg/5mL.] ▶LK ♀D ▶+ $

lamotrigine (*Lamictal, Lamictal CD*): Adults with bipolar disorder (maintenance): Start 25 mg PO daily, 50 mg PO daily if on enzyme-inducing drugs, or 25 mg PO qod if on valproate; titrate to 200 mg/d, or 400 mg/d divided bid if on enzyme-inducing drugs, or 100 mg/d if on valproate. Potentially life-threatening rashes in 0.3% of adults and 0.8% of children; discontinue at first sign of rash. Drug interaction with valproic acid; see product information for adjusted dosing guidelines. [Trade: Tabs 25, 100, 150, 200 mg. Chew Tabs 5, 25 mg.] ▶LK ♀C ▶- $$$$

lithium (*Eskalith, Eskalith CR, Lithobid, ✦Lithane, Carbolith, Duralith*): Acute mania: Start 300-600 mg PO tid-bid, usual effective dose 900-1800 mg/d. 300 mg = 8 mEq/mmol. Steady state in 5d. Trough levels for acute mania 1.0-1.5 mEq/L, maintenance 0.6-1.2 mEq/L. Dose increase of 300 mg/day raises level by approx 0.2 mEq/L. Monitor renal, thyroid function. Diuretics, ACE inhibitors, and angiotensin receptor blockers may increase levels. Avoid dehydration, salt restriction and many NSAIDS (ASA & sulindac OK). [Generic/Trade: caps 150, 300, 600 mg, tabs 300 mg. Ext'd release tabs 300, 450 mg. Syrup 300 mg/5 mL.] ▶K ♀D ▶- $$

topiramate (*Topamax*): Bipolar disorder (unapproved): Start 25-50 mg/day PO, titrate prn to max 400 mg/day. [Trade only: tabs 25, 100, 200 mg. sprinkle caps 15, 25 mg.] ▶K ♀C ▶? $$$$$

valproic acid (*Depakene, Depakote, Depakote ER, divalproex, ✦Epiject, Epival, Deproic*): Mania: 250 mg PO tid. Hepatotoxicity, drug interactions, reduce dose in elderly. [Generic/Trade: Caps (Depakene) 250 mg. Syrup (Depakene) 250 mg/5 mL. Trade: sprinkle Caps (Depakote) 125 mg. Tabs, enteric coated (Depakote) 125,250,500 mg. Tabs, ext'd release (Depakote ER) 250,500 mg] ▶L♀D▶- $$$$$

Antipsychotics - Atypical - Serotonin Dopamine Receptor Antagonists

clozapine (*Clozaril, FazaClo ODT*): Start 12.5 mg PO daily-bid. Usual effective dose 300-450 mg/day divided bid. Max 900 mg/day. Agranulocytosis 1-2%; check WBC counts q week x 6 months, then q2 weeks. [Generic/Trade: Tabs 25, 50, 100 mg. Trade: Orally disintegrating tab (Fazaclo ODT) 25, 100 mg (scored).] ▶L ♀B ▶- $$$$$

olanzapine (*Zyprexa, Zyprexa Zydis*): Agitation in acute bipolar mania or schizophrenia: Start 10 mg IM, may repeat in ≥2h to max 30 mg/day (reduce dose to 2.5-5 mg in the elderly or debilitated). Psychotic disorders, oral therapy: Start 5-10 mg PO daily; usual effective dose 10-15 mg/d. Bipolar disorder, monotherapy, acute manic or mixed episodes and maintenance: Start 10-15 mg PO daily. Adjust dose at intervals ≥24 h in 5 mg/day increments to usual effective dose of 5-20 mg/d. Max 20 mg/day. Bipolar mania, adjunctive: Start 10 mg PO daily; usual effective dose 5-20 mg/d. Max 20 mg/d. [Trade: Tabs 2.5,5,7.5,10,15 mg. Orally disintegrating tabs (Zyprexa Zydis) 5,10,15,20 mg.] ▶L ♀C ▶- $$$$$

quetiapine (*Seroquel*): Psychotic disorders: Start 25 mg PO bid, increase by 25-50 mg bid-tid on day 2-3, to target dose of 300-400 mg/day divided bid-tid. Usual effective dose is 150-750 mg/day. Maximum dose is 800 mg/day. Acute bipolar mania: Start 50 mg PO bid on day 1, then increase by 100 mg/day over next 3 days to reach the following maximal rate: 100 mg bid, 150 mg bid, and then 200 mg bid. If tolerated and necessary, may then increase to 300 mg bid on day 5 and 400 mg bid thereafter. Eye exam for cataracts recommended q 6 months. [Trade: Tabs 25, 100, 200, 300 mg.] ▶LK ♀C ▶- $$$$$

risperidone (**Risperdal, Risperdal Consta**): Psychotic disorders: Start 1 mg PO bid (0.5 mg/dose in the elderly), slowly increase to usual effective dose of 4-8 mg/day divided daily-bid. Max 16 mg/day. Long-acting injection (Consta): Start 25 mg IM q 2 weeks while continuing oral dose x 3 weeks. May increase q 4 weeks to max 50 mg q 2 weeks. Bipolar mania: Start 2-3 mg PO daily, may adjust by 1 mg/day at 24-hr intervals to max 6 mg/day. [Trade: Tabs 0.25,0.5,1,2,3,4 mg. Orally disintegrating tablets (M-TAB) 0.5,1,2,3,4 mg. Oral soln 1 mg/ml.] ▶LK ♀C ▶- $$$$$

ziprasidone (**Geodon**): Schizophrenia: Start 20 mg PO bid with food, adjust at >2 day intervals to max 80 mg PO bid. Acute agitation: 10-20 mg IM, max 40 mg per day. Bipolar mania: Start 40 mg PO bid with food, adjust to 60-80 mg on day 2. Usual range 40-80 mg/day. [Trade: Caps 20,40,60,80 mg.] ▶L ♀C ▶- $$$$$

Antipsychotics - D2 Antagonists - High Potency (1-5 mg = 100 mg CPZ)

fluphenazine (**Prolixin, ♥Modecate, Modeten**): 1.25-10 mg/d IM divided q6-8h. Start 0.5-10 mg/d PO divided q6-h. Usual effective dose 1-20 mg/d. Depot (fluphenazine decanoate/enanthate): 12.5-25 mg IM/SC q3 weeks = 10-20 mg/d PO fluphenazine. [Generic/Trade: Tabs 1, 2.5, 5, 10 mg. Elixir 2.5 x 5 ml. Oral concentrate 5 mg/ml.] ▶LK ♀C ▶? $$$

haloperidol (**Haldol**): 2-5 mg IM. Start 0.5- 5 mg PO bid-tid, usual effective dose 6-20 mg/d. Therapeutic range 2-15 ng/ml. Depot haloperidol (haloperidol decanoate): 100-200 mg IM q4 weeks = 10 mg/day oral haloperidol. [Generic/Trade: Tabs 0.5, 1, 2, 5, 10, 20 mg. Oral concentrate 2 mg/ml.] ▶LK ♀C ▶? $

perphenazine (**Trilafon**): Start 4-8 mg PO tid or 8-16 mg PO bid-qid (hospitalized patients), max 64 mg/d PO. Can give 5-10 mg IM q6h, max 30 mg/day IM. [Generic/Trade: Tabs 2, 4, 8, 16 mg. Oral concentrate 16 mg/5 ml.] ▶LK ♀C ▶? $$$$

pimozide (**Orap**): Tourette's: Start 1-2 mg/d PO in divided doses, increase q2 days to usual effective dose of 1-10 mg/d. [Trade only: Tabs 1, 2 mg.] ▶L ♀C ▶- $$$

thiothixene (**Navane**): Start 2 mg PO tid. Usual effective dose is 20-30 mg/d, maximum 60 mg/d PO. [Generic/Trade: Caps 2, 5, 10. Oral concentrate 5 mg/ml. Trade only: Caps 20 mg. Generic only: Caps 1 mg.] ▶LK ♀C ▶? $$

trifluoperazine (**Stelazine**): Start 2-5 mg PO bid. Usual effective dose is 15- 20 mg/d. Can give 1-2 mg IM q4-6h prn, maximum 10 mg/d IM. [Generic/Trade: Tabs 1, 2, 5, 10 mg. Trade only: oral concentrate 10 mg/ml.] ▶LK ♀C ▶- $$$

Antipsychotics - D2 Antagonists - Mid Potency (10 mg = 100 mg CPZ)

loxapine (**Loxitane, ♥Loxapac**): Start 10 mg PO bid, usual effective dose 60-100 mg/d. Max 250 mg/d. [Generic/Trade: Caps 5, 10, 25, 50 mg.] ▶LK ♀C ▶- $$$$

molindone (**Moban**): Start 50-75 mg/day PO divided tid-qid, usual effective dose 50-100 mg/day. Max 225 mg/day. [Trade: Tabs 5,10,25,50 mg.] ▶LK ♀C ▶? $$$$$

Antipsychotics - D2 Antagonists - Low Potency (50-100 mg = 100 mg CPZ)

chlorpromazine (**Thorazine, ♥Largactil**): Start 10-50 mg PO/IM bid-tid, usual dose 300-800 mg/d. [Generic/Trade: Tabs 10, 25, 50, 100, 200 mg. oral concentrate 30 mg/ml, 100 mg/ml. Trade only: sustained release Caps 30, 75, 150 mg. syrup 10 mg/5 ml. suppositories 25, 100 mg.] ▶LK ♀C ▶? $$$

thioridazine (**Mellaril, ♥Rideril**): Start 50-100 mg PO tid, usual dose 200-800 mg/day. Not first-line therapy. Causes QTc prolongation, torsade de pointes, sudden death. Contraindicated with SSRIs, propranolol, pindolol. Monitor baseline ECG and potassium. Pigmentary retinopathy with doses>800 mg/d. [Generic: Tabs 10,15,25,50,100,150,200 mg. Oral concentrate 30,100 mg/ml.] ▶LK ♀C ▶? $

Antipsychotics - Dopamine-2/serotonin-1 partial agonist & ser-2 antagonist

aripiprazole (*Abilify*): Schizophrenia: Start 10-15 mg PO daily; max 30 mg/day. Bipolar disorder: Start 30 mg PO daily; reduce dose to 15 mg if higher dose poorly tolerated. [Trade: Tabs 5,10,15,20,30 mg. Oral soln 1 mg/ml.] ▶L ♀C ▶? $$$$$

Anxiolytics / Hypnotics - Benzodiazepines - Long Half-Life (25-100 hours)

bromazepam (♥*Lectopam*): Canada only. 6-18 mg/d PO in divided doses. [Trade/generic: Tabs 1.5, 3, 6 mg.] ▶L ♀D ▶- $

chlordiazepoxide (*Librium*): Anxiety: 5-25 mg PO or 25-50 mg IM/IV tid-qid. Acute alcohol withdrawal: 50-100 mg PO/IM/IV, repeat q3-4h prn up to 300 mg/d. Half-life 5-30 h. [Generic/Trade: Caps 5, 10, 25 mg.] ▶LK ♀D ▶- ©IV $$

clonazepam (*Klonopin, Klonopin Wafer, ♥Rivotril, Clonapam*): Start 0.25-0.5 mg PO daily, max 4 mg/day. Half-life 18- 50 h. [Generic/Trade: Tabs 0.5, 1, 2 mg. Orally disintegrating tabs 0.125, 0.25, 0.5, 1, 2 mg.] ▶LK ♀D ▶? ©IV $$

clorazepate (*Tranxene, Genxene*): Start 7.5-15 mg PO qhs or bid-tid, usual effective dose is 15-60 mg/day. Acute alcohol withdrawal: 60-90 mg/day on first day divided bid-tid, reduce dose to 7.5-15 mg/day over 5 days. [Generic/Trade: Tabs 3.75, 7.5, 15 mg. Trade: ext'd release tabs 11.25, 22.5 mg.] ▶LK ♀D ▶- ©IV $$

diazepam (*Valium, ♥Vivol, E Pam, Diazemuls*): Anxiety: 2-10 mg PO bid-qid. Half-life 20-80h. Alcohol withdrawal: 10 mg PO tid-qid x 24 hr then 5 mg PO tid-qid prn. [Generic/Trade: Tabs 2,5,10 mg. Oral solution 5 mg/5 ml. Oral concentrate (Intensol) 5 mg/ml.] ▶LK ♀D ▶- ©IV $

flurazepam (*Dalmane*): 15-30 mg PO qhs. Half-life 70-90h. [Generic/Trade: Caps 15, 30 mg.] ▶LK ♀X ▶- ©IV $$

Anxiolytics / Hypnotics - Benzodiazepines - Medium Half-Life (10-15 hours)

estazolam (*ProSom*): 1-2 mg PO qhs. [Generic/Trade: Tabs 1, 2 mg.] ▶LK ♀X ▶- ©IV $$

lorazepam (*Ativan*): 0.5-2 mg IV/IM/PO q6-8h, max 10 mg/d. Half-life 10-20h. [Generic/Trade tabs 0.5,1,2 mg. Trade oral concentrate 2 mg/ml.] ▶LK ♀D ▶- ©IV $$$

temazepam (*Restoril*): 7.5-30 mg PO qhs. Half-life 8-25h. [Generic/Trade: Caps 7.5, 15, 30 mg. Trade only: Caps 22.5 mg.] ▶LK ♀X ▶- ©IV $$

Anxiolytics / Hypnotics - Benzodiazepines - Short Half-Life (<12 hours)

alprazolam (*Xanax, Xanax XR, Niravam*): 0.25-0.5 mg PO bid-tid. Half-life 12h. Multiple drug interactions. [Trade: Orally disintegrating tab (Niravam) 0.25, 0.5, 1, 2 mg. Generic/Trade: Tabs 0.25, 0.5, 1, 2 mg. Generic only: Oral concentrate 1 mg/mL. Extended release tabs: 0.5, 1, 2, 3 mg.] ▶LK ♀D ▶- ©IV $

oxazepam (*Serax*): 10-30 mg PO tid-qid. Half-life 8h. [Generic/Trade: Caps 10, 15, 30 mg. Trade only: Tabs 15 mg.] ▶LK ♀D ▶- ©IV $$$

triazolam (*Halcion*): 0.125-0.5 mg PO qhs. 0.125 mg/day in elderly. Half-life 2-3h. [Generic/Trade: Tabs 0.125, 0.25 mg.] ▶LK ♀X ▶- ©IV $

Anxiolytics / Hypnotics - Other

buspirone (*BuSpar, Vanspar*): Anxiety: Start 15 mg "dividose" daily (7.5 mg PO bid), usual effective dose 30 mg/day. Max 60 mg/day. [Generic/Trade: tabs 5, 7.5, 10, 15 mg. Trade only: Dividose tab 15, 30 mg (scored to be easily bisected or trisected).] ▶K ♀B ▶- $$$

chloral hydrate (*Aquachloral Supprettes, Somnote*): 25-50 mg/kg/day up to 1000 mg PO/PR. Many physicians use higher than recommended doses in children (eg, 75 mg/kg). [Generic/Trade: Caps 500 mg. syrup 500 mg/ 5 mL. Trade only: rectal suppositories: 325, 500, 650 mg.] ▶LK ♀C ▶+ ©IV $

diphenhydramine (*Allermax, Benadryl, Banophen, Diphen, Diphenhist, Siladryl, Sominex, ♥Allerdryl, Allernix, Nytol*): Insomnia: 25-50 mg PO qhs. Peds ≥12 yo: 50 mg PO qhs. [OTC/Generic/Trade: Tabs/Caps 25, 50 mg. Soln 6.25 mg/5 ml, 12.5 mg/5 ml. Elixir 12.5 mg/ml. OTC/Trade only: chew Tabs 12.5 mg. OTC/Rx/Generic/Trade: Caps 25, 50 mg. Oral solution 12.5 mg/5 ml.] ▶LK ♀B ▶- $

eszopiclone (*Lunesta*): 2 mg PO qhs prn. Max 3 mg. Elderly: 1 mg PO qhs prn, max 2 mg. [Trade: Tabs 1, 2, 3 mg.] ▶L ♀C ▶?

ramelteon (*Rozerem*): Insomnia: 8 mg PO qhs. [Trade: tabs 8 mg.] ▶L ♀C ▶? $$$

zaleplon (*Sonata, ♥Starnoc*): 5-10 mg PO qhs prn, max 20 mg. Do not use for benzodiazepine or alcohol withdrawal. [Trade: Caps 5, 10 mg.] ▶L ♀C ▶- ©IV $$$

zolpidem (*Ambien*): 5-10 mg PO qhs. Do not use for benzodiazepine or alcohol withdrawal. [Trade: Tabs 5, 10 mg.] ▶L ♀B ▶+ ©IV $$$

zopiclone (*♥Imovane*): Canada only. Adults: 5-7.5 mg PO qhs. Reduce dose in elderly. [Trade: tabs 5, 7.5 mg. Generic: tabs 7.5 mg.] ▶L ♀D ▶- $

Combination Drugs

Symbyax (olanzapine + fluoxetine): Bipolar depression: Start 6/25 mg PO qhs. Max 18/75 mg/day. [Trade: Caps (olanzapine/fluoxetine) 6/25, 6/50, 12/25, 12/50 mg.] ▶LK ♀C ▶- $$$$$

Drug Dependence Therapy

acamprosate (*Campral*): Maintenance of abstinence from alcohol: 666 mg (2 tabs) PO tid. Start after alcohol withdrawal and when patient is abstinent. [Trade: delayed-release tabs 333 mg.] ▶K ♀C ▶? $$$$

buprenorphine (*Subutex*): Treatment of opioid dependence: Induction 8 mg SL on day 1, 16 mg SL on day 2. Maintenance: 16 mg SL daily. Can individualize to range of 4-24 mg SL daily. [Trade: SL tabs 2, 8 mg] ▶L ♀C ▶- ©III $$$$$

bupropion (*Zyban*): Start 150 mg PO qam x 3d, then increase to 150 mg PO bid x 7-12 wks. Max dose 150 mg PO bid. Last dose no later than 5 pm. Contraindicated with seizures, bulimia, anorexia. Seizures in 0.4% at 300-450 mg/d. [Trade: Extended-release tabs 150 mg.] ▶LK ♀B ▶- $$$$

clonidine (*Catapres, Catapres-TTS*): Opioid/nicotine withdrawal, alcohol withdrawal adjunct (not FDA approved): 0.1- 0.3 mg PO tid-qid. Transdermal Therapeutic System (TTS) is designed for seven day use so that a TTS-1 delivers 0.1 mg/day x 7 days. May supplement first dose of TTS with oral x 2-3 days while therapeutic level is achieved. [Generic/Trade: Tabs, non-scored 0.1, 0.2, 0.3 mg. Trade only: transdermal weekly patch 0.1 mg/day (TTS-1), 0.2 mg/day (TTS-2), 0.3 mg/day (TTS-3).] ▶LK ♀C ▶? $

disulfiram (*Antabuse*): Sobriety: 125-500 mg PO daily. Patient must abstain from any alcohol for ≥12 h before using. Metronidazole and alcohol in any form (cough syrups, tonics, etc.) contraindicated. [Trade only: Tabs 250 mg.] ▶L ♀C ▶? $$

methadone (*Dolophine, Methadose, ♥Metadol*): Opioid dependence: 20-100 mg PO daily. Treatment >3 wks is maintenance and only permitted in approved treatment programs. [Generic/Trade: Tabs 5, 10, 40 mg. oral solution 5 & 10 mg/5 ml. oral concentrate 10 mg/ml.] ▶L ♀B ▶+ ©II $$

naltrexone (*ReVia, Depade*): Alcohol/opioid dependence: 25-50 mg PO daily. Avoid if recent ingestion of opioids (past 7-10 days). Hepatotoxicity with higher than approved doses. [Generic/Trade: Tabs 50 mg.] ▶LK ♀C ▶? $$$$$

nicotine gum (*Nicorette, Nicorette DS*): Smoking cessation: Gradually taper 1 piece q1-2h x 6 weeks, 1 piece q2-4h x 3 weeks, then 1 piece q4-8h x 3 weeks, max 30 pieces/day of 2 mg or 24 pieces/day of 4 mg. Use Nicorette DS 4 mg/piece in high cigarette use (>24 cigarettes/day). [OTC/Generic/Trade: gum 2, 4 mg.] ▶LK ♀X ▶- $$$$$

nicotine inhalation system (***Nicotrol Inhaler***, ♣***Nicorette inhaler***): 6-16 cartridges/day x 12 weeks (Range: Oral inhaler 10 mg/cartridge (4 mg nicotine delivered), 42 cartridges/box.) ▶LK ♀D ▶- $$$$$

nicotine lozenge (***Commit***): Smoking cessation: In those who smoke <30 min from waking use 4 mg lozenge; others use 2 mg. Take 1-2 lozenges q1-2 h x 6 weeks, then q2-4h in weeks 7-9, then q4-8h in weeks 10-12. Length of therapy 12 weeks. [OTC/Trade: lozenge 2,4 mg in 72,168-count packages] ▶LK ♀D ▶- $$$$$

nicotine nasal spray (***Nicotrol NS***): Smoking cessation: 1-2 doses each hour, with each dose = 2 sprays, one in each nostril (1 spray = 0.5 mg nicotine). Minimum recommended: 8 doses/day, max 40 doses/day. [Trade: nasal solution 10 mg/ml (0.5 mg/inhalation); 10 ml bottles.] ▶LK ♀D ▶- $$$$$

nicotine patches (***Habitrol, Nicoderm, Nicotrol***, ♣***Prostep***): Smoking cessation: Start one patch (14-22 mg) daily, taper after 6 wks. Ensure patient has stopped smoking. [OTC/Rx/Generic/Trade: patches 11, 22 mg/ 24 hours. 7, 14, 21 mg/ 24 h (Habitrol & NicoDerm). OTC/Trade: 15 mg/ 16 h (Nicotrol). ▶LK ♀D ▶- $$$$

Suboxone (buprenorphine + naloxone): Treatment of opioid dependence: Maintenance: 16 mg SL daily. Can individualize to range of 4-24 mg SL daily. [Trade: SL tabs 2/0.5 and 8/2 mg buprenorphine / naloxone] ▶L ♀C ▶- ©III $$$$$

Stimulants / ADHD / Anorexiants

Adderall (dextroamphetamine + amphetamine, Adderall XR): ADHD, standard-release tabs: Start 2.5 mg (3-5 yo) or 5 mg (≥6 yo) PO daily-bid, increase by 2.5-5 mg every week, max 40 mg/d. ADHD, extended-release caps (Adderall XR): If 6-12 yo, then start 5-10 mg PO daily to a max of 30 mg/d. If 13-17 yo, then start 10 mg PO daily to a max of 20 mg/d. If adult, then 20 mg PO daily. Narcolepsy, standard-release: Start 5-10 mg PO q am, increase by 5-10 mg q week, max 60 mg/d. Avoid evening doses. Monitor growth and use drug holidays when appropriate. [Trade/Generic: Tabs 5, 7.5, 10, 12.5, 15, 20, 30 mg. Caps, extended release (Adderall XR) 5,10, 15, 20, 25, 30 mg.] ▶L ♀C ▶- ©II $$$

atomoxetine (***Strattera***): ADHD: Children/adolescents >70 kg and adults: Start 40 mg PO daily, then increase after >3 days to target of 80 mg/d divided daily-bid. Max 100 mg/d. [Trade: caps 10, 18, 25, 40, 60, 80, 100 mg.] ▶K ♀C ▶? $$$$

caffeine (***NoDoz, Vivarin, Caffedrine, Stay Awake, Quick-Pep***): 100-200 mg PO q3-4h prn. [OTC/Generic/Trade: Tabs/Caps 200 mg. OTC/Trade: Extended-release tabs 200 mg. Lozenges 75 mg.] ▶L ♀B ▶? $

dexmethylphenidate (***Focalin***): ADHD, extended release, not already on stimulants: 5 mg (children) or 10 mg (adults) PO q am. Immediate release, not already on stimulants: 2.5 mg PO bid. Max 20mg/day for both. If taking racemic methylphenidate use conversion of 2.5 mg for each 5 mg of methylphenidate, max 20 mg/d. [Trade: Immediate release tabs 2.5, 5, 10 mg. Extended release caps 5, 10, 20 mg.] ▶L ♀C ▶? ©II $$

dextroamphetamine (***Dexedrine, Dextrostat***): Narcolepsy/ ADHD: 2.5-10 mg PO q am or bid-tid or 10-15 mg PO daily (sustained release), max 60 mg/d. Avoid evening doses. Monitor growth and use drug holidays when appropriate. [Trade/Generic: Tabs 5, 10 mg. Extended Release caps 5, 10, 15 mg.] ▶L ♀C ▶- ©II $$$

methylphenidate (***Ritalin, Ritalin LA, Ritalin SR, Methylin, Methylin ER, Metadate ER, Metadate CD, Concerta***): ADHD/Narcolepsy: 5-10 mg PO bid-tid or 20 mg PO qam (sustained and extended release), max 60 mg/d. Or 18-36 mg PO q am (Concerta), max 72 mg/day. Avoid evening doses. Monitor growth and use drug holidays when appropriate. [Trade: tabs 5, 10, 20 mg (Ritalin, Methylin, Metadate). Extended release tabs 10, 20 mg (Methylin ER, Metadate ER). Extended release tabs 18, 27, 36, 54 mg (Concerta). Extended release caps 10, 20, 30 mg (Metadate CD) May be sprinkled on food. Sustained-release tabs 20 mg (Ritalin SR). Extended release caps 10, 20, 30, 40 mg (Ritalin LA). Chewable tabs 2.5, 5, 10 mg (Methylin). Oral soln 5 mg/5ml, 10 mg/5 ml (Methylin). Generic: tabs 5, 10, 20 mg, extended release tabs 10, 20 mg, sustained-release tabs 20 mg.] ▶LK ♀C ▶? ©II $$$

modafinil (*Provigil, ♥Alertec*): Narcolepsy and sleep apnea/hypopnea: 200 mg PO qam. Shift work sleep disorder: 200 mg PO one hour before shift. [Trade: Tabs 100, 200 mg.] ▶LK ♀C ▶- ©IV $$$$

phentermine (*Adipex-P, Ionamin, Pro-Fast*): 8 mg PO tid or 15-37.5 mg/day q am or 10-14 h before retiring. For short-term use. [Generic/Trade: Caps 15, 18.75, 30, 37.5 mg. Tabs 8, 30, 37.5 mg. Trade only: extended release Caps 15, 30 mg (Ionamin).] ▶KL ♀C ▶- ©IV $$

sibutramine (*Meridia*): Start 10 mg PO q am, max 15 mg/d. Monitor pulse and BP. [Trade: Caps 5, 10, 15 mg.] ▶KL ♀C ▶- ©IV $$$$

BODY MASS INDEX*	Heights are in feet and inches; weights are in pounds					
BMI	*Classification*	4'10"	5'0"	5'4"	5'8"	6'0"	6'4"
<19	Underweight	<91	<97	<110	<125	<140	<156
19-24	Healthy Weight	91-119	97-127	110-144	125-163	140-183	156-204
25-29	Overweight	120-143	128-152	145-173	164-196	184-220	205-245
30-40	Obese	144-191	153-204	174-233	197-262	221-293	246-328
>40	Very Obese	>191	>204	>233	>262	>293	>328

*BMI = kg/m^2 = (weight in pounds)(703)/(height in inches)^2. Anorectants appropriate if BMI ≥30 (with comorbidities ≥27); surgery an option if BMI >40 (with comorbidities 35-40).

www.nhlbi.nih.gov

Other Agents

benztropine (*Cogentin*): EPS: 1-4 mg PO/IM/IV daily-bid. [Generic: Tabs 0.5, 1, 2 mg.] ▶LK ♀C ▶? $

clonidine (*Catapres, Catapres-TTS*): ADHD (unapproved peds): Start 0.05 mg PO qhs, titrate to 0.05-0.3 mg/d in 3-4 divided doses. Tourette's syndrome (unapproved peds and adult): 3-5 mcg/kg/d PO divided bid-qid. [Generic/Trade: Tabs 0.1, 0.2, 0.3 mg. Trade only: transdermal weekly patch 0.1 mg/day (TTS-1), 0.2 mg/day (TTS-2), 0.3 mg/day (TTS-3).] ▶LK ♀C ▶? $

diphenhydramine (*Benadryl, Banophen, Allermax, Diphen, Diphenhist, Siladryl, Sominex, ♥Allerdryl, Allernix*): EPS: 25-50 mg PO tid-qid or 10-50 mg IV/IM tid-qid. [OTC/Generic/Trade: Tabs 25, 50 mg. OTC/Trade only: chew Tabs 12.5 mg. OTC/Rx/Generic/Trade: Caps 25,50 mg, oral soln 12.5 mg/5 ml] ▶LK ♀B ▶- $

PULMONARY

Beta Agonists

albuterol (*Ventolin, Ventolin HFA, Proventil, Proventil HFA, Volmax, VoSpire ER, Ventodisk, ♥Airomir, Ventodisk, Asmavent, salbutamol*): MDI 2 puffs q4-6h prn. 0.5 ml of 0.5% soln (2.5 mg) nebulized tid-qid. One 3 ml unit dose (0.083%) nebulized tid-qid. Caps for inhalation 200-400 mcg q4-6h. 2-4 mg PO tid-qid or extended release 4-8 mg PO q12h up to 16 mg PO q12h. Children 2-5

PREDICTED PEAK EXPIRATORY FLOW (liters/min) Am Rev Resp Dis 1963; 88:644

Age	Women (height in inches)					Men (height in inches)					Child (height	
(yrs)	55"	60"	65"	70"	75"	60"	65"	70"	75"	80"	in inches)	
20	390	423	460	496	529	554	602	649	693	740	44"	160
30	380	413	448	483	516	532	577	622	664	710	46"	187
40	370	402	436	470	502	509	552	596	636	680	48"	214
50	360	391	424	457	488	486	527	569	607	649	50"	240
60	350	380	412	445	475	463	502	542	578	618	52"	267
70	340	369	400	432	461	440	477	515	550	587	54"	293

yo: 0.1-0.2 mg/kg/dose PO tid up to 4 mg tid; 6-12 yo: 2-4 mg or extended release 4 mg PO q12h. Prevention of exercise-induced bronchospasm: MDI: 2 puffs 15-30 minutes before exercise. [Generic/Trade: MDI 90 mcg/actuation, 200/canister. "HFA" inhalers use hydrofluoroalkane propellant instead of CFCs but are otherwise equivalent. Soln for inhalation 0.5% (5 mg/ml) in 20 ml with dropper. Nebules for inhalation 3 ml unit dose 0.083%. Extended release tabs 4 & 8 mg. Trade only:1.25 mg & 0.63 mg/3 ml unit dose. Tabs 2 & 4 mg. Syrup 2 mg/5 ml. Caps for inhalation 200 mcg microfine in packs of 24s & 96s w/ Rotahaler.] ▶L ♀C ▶? $

fenoterol (♥*Berotec*): Canada only. 1-2 puffs prn tid-qid. Nebulizer: up to 2.5 mg q6 hours. [Trade: MDI 100 mcg/actuation. Soln for inhalation: Unit dose 2 ml vials of 0.625 mg/ml and 0.25 mg/ml (no preservatives), and 20 ml bottles of 1 mg/ml (with preservatives that may cause bronchoconstriction in some).] ▶L ♀C ▶? $

formoterol (*Foradil*, ♥*Oxeze*): 1 puff bid. Not for acute bronchospasm. [Trade: DPI 12 mcg, 60 blisters/pack.] ▶L ♀C ▶? $$$

levalbuterol (*Xopenex, Xopenex HFA*): MDI 2 puffs q4-6h prn. 0.63-1.25 mg nebulized q6-8h. 6-11 yo: 0.31 mg nebulized tid. [Trade: MDI 45 mcg/actuation, 200 per canister. "HFA" inhalers use hydrofluoroalkane propellant. Soln for inhalation 0.31, 0.63, 1.25 mg in 3 ml unit-dose vials.] ▶L ♀C ▶? $$$$

metaproterenol (*Alupent, Metaprel, Pro-Meta*, ♥*orciprenaline*): MDI 2-3 puffs q3-4h: 0.2-0.3 ml 5% soln nebulized q4h. 20 mg PO tid-qid >9 yo, 10 mg PO tid-qid if 6-9 yo, 1.3-2.6 mg/kg/day divided tid-qid if 2-5 yo. [Trade: MDI 0.65 mg/actuation in 100 & 200/canister. Generic/Trade: Soln for inhalation 0.4, 0.6% in unit-dose vials; 5% in 10 & 30 ml with dropper. Syrup 10 mg/5 ml. Generic: Tabs 10 & 20 mg.] ▶L ♀C ▶? $$$

pirbuterol (*Maxair*): MDI: 1-2 puffs q4-6h. [Trade: MDI 0.2 mg/actuation, 400/canister.] ▶L ♀C ▶? $$$

salmeterol (*Serevent Diskus*): 1 puff bid. Not for acute bronchospasm. Use only in combo with corticosteroids. [Trade: DPI Diskus: 50 mcg 60 blisters.] ▶L♀C ▶? $$$

terbutaline (*Brethine, Bricanyl*): 2.5-5 mg PO q6h while awake in >12 yo. 0.25 mg SC. [Generic/trade: Tabs 2.5 & 5 mg (Brethine scored).] ▶L ♀B ▶- $$

WHAT COLOR IS WHAT INHALER? (Body then cap - Generics may differ)

Advair	purple	Flovent	orange/ peach	QVAR 40mcg	beige/grey
Aerobid	grey/purple	Foradil	grey/beige	QVAR 80mcg	mauve/grey
Aerobid-M	grey/green	Intal	white/blue	Serevent	green
Alupent	clear/blue	Maxair	blue/white	Diskus	
Asmanex	white/white	Maxair	white/white	Tilade	white/white
Atrovent	clear/green	Autohaler		Ventolin	light blue/navy
Azmacort	white/white	Proventil	yellow/ orange	Xopenex HFA	blue/red
Combivent	clear/orange	Pulmicort	white/brown		

Combinations

Advair (fluticasone + salmeterol): Asthma: 1 puff bid (all strengths). COPD with chronic bronchitis: 1 puff bid (250/50 only). [Trade: DPI: 100/50, 250/50, 500/50 mcg fluticasone propionate/mcg salmeterol per actuation. 60 doses per DPI.] ▶L ♀C ▶? $$$-$$$$

Combivent (albuterol + ipratropium): 2 puffs qid, max 12 puffs/day. Contraindicated with soy & peanut allergy. [Trade: MDI: 90 mcg albuterol/18 mcg ipratropium per actuation, 200/canister.] ▶L ♀C ▶? $$

DuoNeb (albuterol + ipratropium, ♥*Combivent inhalation solution*): One unit dose qid. [Trade: 2.5 mg albuterol/0.5 mg ipratropium per 3 ml vial, premixed. 30 & 60 vials/carton.] ▶L ♀C ▶? $$$$

Symbicort (budesonide + formoterol): Canada only. 1-2 puffs bid. [Trade: DPI: 100/6 and 200/6 mcg budesonide/mcg formoterol per actuation.] ▶L ♀C ▶? $$

Inhaled Steroids (See Endocrine-Corticosteroids when oral steroids necessary.)

beclomethasone (***QVAR***): 1-4 puffs bid (40 mcg). 1-2 puffs bid (80 mcg). [Trade: MDI (non-CFC): 40 & 80 mcg/actuation, 100 actuations/canister.] ▶L ♀C ▶? $$$

budesonide (***Pulmicort Turbuhaler, Pulmicort Respules***): 1-2 puffs daily-bid. [Trade: DPI: 200 mcg powder/actuation, 200/canister. Respules: 0.25 mg/2 ml & 0.5 mg/2 ml unit dose.] ▶L ♀B ▶? $$$

flunisolide (***Aerobid, Aerobid-M***): 2-4 puffs bid. [Trade: MDI: 250 mcg/actuation, 100/canister. AeroBid-M: menthol flavor.] ▶L ♀C ▶? $$$

fluticasone (***Flovent HFA***): MDI: 2-4 puffs bid. [Trade: MDI: 44, 110, 220 mcg/actuation in 120/canister.] ▶L ♀C ▶? $$$

mometasone (***Asmanex Twisthaler***): 2 puffs q pm or 1 puff bid. If prior oral corticosteroid therapy: 2 puffs bid. [Trade: DPI: 220 mcg/actuation, 60 & 120/canister.] ▶L ♀C ▶? $$$

triamcinolone (***Azmacort***): 2 puffs tid-qid or 4 puffs bid; max dose 16 puffs/day. [Trade: MDI: 100 mcg/actuation, 240/canister. Built-in spacer.] ▶L ♀D ▶? $$$

INHALED STEROIDS: ESTIMATED COMPARATIVE DAILY DOSES*

Drug	Form	ADULT			CHILD (≤12 yo)		
		Low	Medium	High	Low	Medium	High
beclomethasone MDI	40 mcg/puff	2-6	6-12	>12	2-4	4-8	>8
	80 mcg/puff	1-3	3-6	>6	1-2	2-4	>4
budesonide DPI	200 mcg/dose	1-3	3-6	>6	1-2	2-4	>4
	Soln for nebs	-	-	-	0.5 mg	1 mg	2 mg
flunisolide MDI	250 mcg/puff	2-4	4-8	>8	2-3	4-5	>5
fluticasone MDI	44 mcg/puff	2-6	6-15	>15	2-4	4-10	>10
	110 mcg/puff	1-2	3-6	>6	1	1-4	>4
	220 mcg/puff	1	2-3	>3	n/a	1-2	>2
fluticasone DPI	50 mcg/dose	2-6	6-12	>12	2-4	4-8	>8
	100 mcg/dose	1-3	3-6	>6	1-2	2-4	>4
	250 mcg/dose	1	2-3	>2	n/a	1	>1
triamcinolone MDI	100 mcg/puff	4-10	10-20	>20	4-8	8-12	>12

*MDI=metered dose inhaler. DPI=dry powder inhaler. All doses in puffs (MDI) or inhalations (DPI).
Reference: http://www.nhlbi.nih.gov/guidelines/asthma/execsumm.pdf

Leukotriene Inhibitors

montelukast (***Singulair***): Adults: 10 mg PO daily. Children 6-14 yo: 5 mg PO daily. 2-5 yo: 4 mg PO daily. 12-23 months (asthma): 4 mg (oral granules) PO daily. 6-23 months (allergic rhinitis): 4 mg (oral granules) PO daily. [Trade: Tabs 4, 5 mg (chew cherry flavor) & 10 mg. Oral granules 4 mg packet, 30/box.] ▶L ♀B ▶? $$$

zafirlukast (**Accolate**): 20 mg PO bid. Peds 5-11 yo, 10 mg PO bid. Take 1h ac or 2h pc. Potentiates warfarin & theophylline. [Trade: Tabs 10, 20 mg.] ▶L ♀B ▶- $$$

zileuton (**Zyflo**): 600 mg PO qid. Hepatotoxicity, potentiates warfarin, theophylline, & propranolol. [Trade: Tabs 600 mg.] ▶L ♀C ▶? $$$$

Other Pulmonary Medications

acetylcysteine (**Mucomyst, Mucosil-10, Mucosil-20**, ✚**Parvolex**): Mucolytic: 3-5 ml of 20% or 6-10 ml of 10% soln nebulized tid-qid. [Generic/Trade: soln 10 & 20% in 4,10, & 30 ml vials.] ▶L ♀B ▶? $$$

aminophylline (✚**Phyllocontin**): Asthma: loading dose: 6 mg/kg IV over 20-30 min. Maintenance 0.5-0.7 mg/kg/h IV. [Generic: Tabs 100 & 200 mg. Oral liquid 105 mg/5 ml. Trade: Tabs controlled release (12hr) 225 mg, scored.] ▶L ♀C ▶? $

cromolyn sodium (**Intal, Gastrocrom, Nalcrom**): Asthma: 2-4 puffs qid or 20 mg nebs qid. Prevention of exercise-induced bronchospasm: 2 puffs 10-15 min prior to exercise. Mastocytosis: Oral concentrate 200 mg PO qid for adults, 100 mg qid in children 2-12 yo. Nasal: 1 spray/nostril. [Trade: MDI 800 mcg/actuation, 112 & 200/canister. Oral concentrate 5 ml/100 mg in 8 amps/foil pouch. Generic/Trade: Soln for nebs: 20 mg/2 ml.] ▶LK ♀B ▶? $$$

dexamethasone (**Decadron**, ✚**Maxidex**): BPD preterm infants: 0.5 mg/kg PO/IV divided q12h x 3 days, then taper. Croup: 0.6 mg/kg PO or IM x 1. Acute asthma: >2 yo: 0.6 mg/kg to max 16 mg PO daily x 2 days. [Generic/Trade: Tabs 0.25, 0.5, 0.75, 1, 1.5, 2, 4, & 6 mg, various scored. Elixir: 0.5 mg/5 ml. Oral soln: 0.5 mg/5 ml & 0.5 mg/0.5 ml.] ▶L ♀C ▶- $

dornase alfa (**Pulmozyme**): Cystic fibrosis: 2.5 mg nebulized daily-bid. [Trade: soln for inhalation: 1 mg/ml in 2.5 ml vials.] ▶L ♀B ▶? $$$$$

epinephrine racemic (**AsthmaNefrin, MicroNefrin, Nephron, S-2**, ✚**Vaponefrin**): Severe croup: 0.05 ml/kg/dose diluted to 3 ml w/NS. Max dose 0.5 ml. [Trade: soln for inhalation: 2.25% epinephrine in 15 & 30 ml.] ▶Plasma ♀C ▶- $

ipratropium (**Atrovent, Atrovent HFA**): 2 puffs qid, or one 500 mcg vial neb tid-qid. Atrovent MDI contraindicated with soy/peanut allergy. [Trade: Atrovent MDI: 18 mcg/actuation, 200/canister. Atrovent HFA MDI: 17 mcg/actuation, 200/canister. Generic/Trade neb soln 0.02% (500 mcg/vial) in unit dose vials.] ▶Lung ♀B ▶? $$$

ketotifen (**Zaditen**): Canada only. 6 mo to 3 yo: 0.05 mg/kg PO bid. Children >3 yo: 1 mg PO bid. [Generic/Trade: Tabs 1 mg. Syrup 1mg/5 ml.] ▶L ♀C ▶- $$$

nedocromil (**Tilade**): 2 puffs qid. Reduce as tolerated [Trade: MDI: 1.75 mg/actuation, 112/canister.] ▶L ♀B ▶? $$

theophylline (**Elixophyllin, Uniphyl, Theo-24, T-Phyl**, ✚**Theo-Dur, Theolair**): 5-13 mg/kg/day PO in divided doses. Max dose 900 mg/day. Peds dosing variable. [Trade: Elixophyllin Liquid 80 mg/15 ml. Daily sust'd release tabs: Uniphyl 400. Caps: Theo-24: 100,200,300,400 mg. Bid sust'd release tabs T-Phyl 200 mg. Generic Theophylline ER tabs 100,200,300,600, caps: 125,200,300 mg] ▶L ♀C ▶+ $

tiotropium (**Spiriva**): COPD maintenance: Handihaler: 18 mcg inhaled daily. [Trade: Capsule for oral inhalation, 18mcg. To be used with "Handihaler" device only. Packages of 6 or 30 capsules with Handihaler device.] ▶K ♀C ▶- $$$

TOXICOLOGY

acetylcysteine (**Mucomyst, Acetadote**, ✚**Parvolex**): Acetaminophen toxicity: Mucomyst – loading dose 140 mg/kg PO or NG, then 70 mg/kg q4h x 17 doses. May be mixed in water or soft drink diluted to a 5% soln. Acetadote (IV) – loading dose

ANTIDOTES

Toxin	Antidote/Treatment	Toxin	Antidote/Treatment
acetaminophen	N-acetylcysteine	ethylene glycol	fomepizole
antidepressants*	bicarbonate	heparin	protamine
arsenic, mercury	dimercaprol (BAL)	iron	deferoxamine
benzodiazepine	flumazenil	lead	EDTA, succimer
beta blockers	glucagon	methanol	fomepizole
calcium channel	calcium chloride,	methemoglobin	methylene blue
blockers	glucagon	narcotics	naloxone
cyanide	Lilly cyanide kit	organophosphates	atropine+pralidoxime
digoxin	dig immune Fab	warfarin	vitamin K, FFP

*cyclic

150 mg/kg in 200 ml of D5W infused over 15 min; maintenance dose 50 mg/kg in 500 ml of D5W infused over 4 hours followed by 100 mg/kg in 1000 ml of D5W infused over 16 hours. [Generic/Trade: solution 10%, 20%. Trade: IV (Acetadote)] ▶L ♀B ▶? $$$$

atropine (*AtroPen*): Injector pens for insecticide or nerve agent poisoning. [Trade only: Prefilled auto-injector pen: 0.25 (yellow), 0.5 (blue), 1 (dark red), 2 mg (green).] ▶LK ♀C ▶- ?

charcoal (activated charcoal, *Actidose-Aqua, CharcoAid, EZ-Char, ♣Charco-date*): 25-100 g (1-2 g/kg or 10 times the amount of poison ingested) PO or NG ASAP. May repeat q1-4h prn at doses equivalent to 12.5 g/hr. When sorbitol is coadministered, use only with the first dose if repeated doses are to be given. [OTC/Generic/Trade: Powder 15,30,40,120,240 g. Solution 12.5 g/60 ml, 15 g/75 ml, 15g/120 ml, 25 g/120 ml, 30 g/120 ml, 50 g/240 ml. Susp 15g/120 ml, 25g/120ml, 30g/150 ml, 50g/240 ml. Granules 15g/120 ml] ▶Not absorbed ♀+ ▶+ $

deferoxamine (*Desferal*): Chronic iron overload: 500-1000 mg IM daily and 2 g IV infusion (≤15 mg/kg/hr) with each unit of blood or 1-2 g SC daily 20-40 mg/kg/day) over 8-24 h via continuous infusion pump. Acute iron toxicity: IV infusion up to 15 mg/kg/hr (consult poison center). ▶K ♀C ▶? $$$$$

dimercaprol (*BAL in oil*): Specialized dosing for arsenic, mercury, gold, lead toxicity; consult poison center. ▶KL ♀C ▶? $$$$$

edetate (*EDTA, Endrate, Meritate*): Specialized dosing for lead toxicity; consult poison center. ▶K ♀C ▶- $$$

ethanol (*alcohol*): Specialized dosing for methanol, ethylene glycol toxicity if fomepizole is unavailable or delayed. ▶L ♀D ▶+ $

flumazenil (*Romazicon, ♣Anexate*): Benzodiazepine sedation reversal: 0.2 mg IV over 15 sec, then 0.2 mg q1 min prn up to 1 mg total dose. Overdose reversal: 0.2 mg IV over 30 sec, then 0.3-0.5 mg q30 sec prn up to 3 mg total dose. Contraindicated in mixed drug OD or chronic benzodiazepine use. ▶LK ♀C ▶? $$$

fomepizole (*Antizol*): Specialized dosing in ethylene glycol or methanol toxicity. ▶L ♀C ▶? $$$$$

ipecac syrup: Emesis: 30 ml PO for adults, 15 ml if 1-12 yo. [Generic/OTC: syrup.] ▶Gut ♀C ▶? $

methylene blue (*Urolene blue*): Methemoglobinemia: 1-2 mg/kg IV over 5 min. ▶K ♀C ▶? $$

penicillamine (*Cuprimine, Depen*): Specialized dosing for copper toxicity. [Trade: Caps 125, 250 mg; Tabs 250 mg.] ▶K ♀D ▶- $$$$

pralidoxime (*Protopam, 2-PAM*): Organophosphate poisoning; consult poison center: 1-2 g IV infusion over 15-30 min or slow IV injection ≥5 min (max rate 200 mg/min). May repeat dose after 1 h if muscle weakness persists. Peds: 20-50 mg/kg/dose IV over 15-30 min. ▶K ♀C ▶? $$$

succimer (*Chemet*): Lead toxicity in children ≥1 yo: Start 10 mg/kg PO or 350 mg/m^2 q8h x 5 days, then reduce the frequency to q12h x 2 weeks. [Trade: Caps 100 mg.] ▶K ♀C ▶? $$$$$

UROLOGY

Benign Prostatic Hyperplasia

alfuzosin (*UroXatral*, ✽*Xatral*): BPH: 10 mg PO daily after a meal. [Trade: extended-release tab 10 mg.] ▶KL ♀B ▶- $$$

doxazosin (*Cardura, Cardura XL*): Immediate release: Start 1 mg PO qhs, max 8 mg/day. Extended release: 4 mg PO qam with breakfast, max 8 mg/day. [Generic/Trade: Immediate release tabs 1, 2, 4, 8 mg. Trade: XL tabs 4,8 mg.] ▶L ♀C ▶? $

dutasteride (*Avodart*): BPH: 0.5 mg PO daily. [Trade: Cap 0.5 mg.] ▶L ♀X ▶- $$$

finasteride (*Proscar*): 5 mg PO daily alone or in combo with doxazosin to reduce the risk of symptomatic progression of BPH. [Trade: Tab 5 mg.] ▶L ♀X ▶- $$$

tamsulosin (*Flomax*): 0.4 mg PO daily, 30 min after a meal. Maximum 0.8 mg/day. [Trade: Cap 0.4 mg.] ▶LK ♀B ▶- $$$

terazosin (*Hytrin*): Start 1 mg PO qhs, usual effective dose 10 mg/day, max 20 mg/day. [Generic/Trade: Caps 1, 2, 5, 10 mg.] ▶LK ♀C ▶? $

Bladder Agents - Anticholinergics & Combinations

darifenacin (*Enablex*): Overactive bladder with symptoms of urinary urgency, frequency and urge incontinence: 7.5 mg PO daily. May increase to max dose 15 mg PO daily in 2 weeks. Max dose 7.5mg PO daily with moderate liver impairment or when coadministered with potent CYP3A4 inhibitors (ketoconazole, itraconazole, ritonavir, nelfinavir, clarithromycin & nefazodone). [Trade: Extended-release tabs 7.5,15 mg.] ▶LK ♀C ▶- ?

flavoxate (*Urispas*): 100-200 mg PO tid-qid. [Trade: Tab 100 mg.] ▶K ♀B ▶? $$$$

hyoscyamine (*Anaspaz, A-spaz, Cystospaz, ED Spaz, Hyosol, Hyospaz, Levbid, Levsin, Levsinex, Medispaz, NuLev, Spacol, Spasdel, Symax*): 0.125-0.25 mg PO/SL q4h or prn. Extended release: 0.375-0.75 mg PO q12h. Max 1.5 mg/day. [Generic/Trade: Tab 0.125. Sublingual Tab 0.125 mg. Extended release Tab 0.375 mg. Extended release Cap 0.375 mg. Elixir 0.125 mg/ 5 ml. Drops 0.125 mg/1 ml. Trade: Tab 0.15 mg (Hyospaz, Cystospaz). Tab, orally disintegrating 0.125 (NuLev).] ▶LK ♀C ▶- $

oxybutynin (*Ditropan, Ditropan XL, Oxytrol*, ✽*Oxybutyn*): Bladder instability: Ditropan: 2.5-5 mg PO bid-tid, max 5 mg PO qid. Ditropan XL: 5-10 mg PO daily, increase 5 mg/day q week to 30 mg/day. Oxytrol: 1 patch twice weekly on abdomen, hips or buttocks. [Generic/Trade: Tab 5 mg. Syrup 5mg/5 ml. Trade: Extended release tablets (Ditropan XL) 5, 10, 15 mg. Transdermal (Oxytrol) 3.9 mg/day.] ▶LK ♀B ▶? $

Prosed/DS (methenamine + phenyl salicylate + methylene blue + benzoic acid + atropine + hyoscyamine): 1 tab PO qid with liberal fluids. May turn urine/contact lenses blue. [Trade: Tab (methenamine 81.6 mg/phenyl salicylate 36.2 mg/methylene blue 10.8 mg/benzoic acid 9.0 mg/atropine sulfate 0.06 mg/hyoscyamine sulfate 0.06 mg). Prosed EC = enteric coated form.] ▶KL ♀C ▶? $$$

solifenacin (*VESIcare*): Overactive bladder with symptoms of urinary urgency, frequency or urge incontinence: 5 mg PO daily. Max dose: 10 mg daily (5 mg daily if CrCl<30 mL/min, moderate hepatic impairment, or ketoconazole or other potent CYP3A4 inhibitors). [Trade: Tabs 5,10 mg] ▶LK ♀C ▶- $$$$

tolterodine (**Detrol, Detrol LA, ✚Unidet**): Overactive bladder: 1-2 mg PO bid (Detrol) or 2-4 mg PO daily (Detrol LA). [Trade: Tabs 1, 2 mg. Caps, extended release 2, 4 mg.] ▶L ♀C ▶- $$$

trospium (**Sanctura**): Overactive bladder with urge incontinence: 20 mg PO bid. If CrCl <30 ml/min: 20 mg PO qhs. If ≥75 yo may taper down to 20 mg daily. [Trade: Tab 20 mg] ▶LK ♀C ▶? ?

Urised (methenamine + phenyl salicylate + atropine + hyoscyamine + benzoic acid + methylene blue, Usept): Dysuria: 2 tabs PO qid. May turn urine/contact lenses blue, don't use with sulfa. [Trade: Tab (methenamine 40.8 mg/phenyl salicylate 18.1 mg/atropine 0.03 mg/hyoscyamine 0.03 mg/4.5 mg benzoic acid/5.4 mg methylene blue).] ▶K ♀C ▶? $$$$

UTA (methenamine + sodium phosphate + phenyl salicylate + methylene blue + hyoscyamine): 1 cap PO qid with liberal fluids. [Trade: Cap (methenamine 120 mg/sodium phosphate 40.8 mg/phenyl salicylate 36 mg/methylene blue 10 mg/hyoscyamine 0.12 mg).] ▶LK ♀C ▶? $$$

Bladder Agents - Other

bethanechol (**Urecholine, Duvoid, ✚Myotonachol**): Urinary retention: 10-50 mg PO tid-qid. [Generic/Trade: Tabs 5, 10, 25, 50 mg.] ▶L ♀C ▶? $

desmopressin (**DDAVP, ✚Minirin**): Enuresis: 10-40 mcg intranasally qhs or 0.2-0.6 mg PO qhs. Not for children <6 yo. [Generic/Trade: Tabs 0.1, 0.2 mg; Nasal solution 0.1 mg/ml (10 mcg/ spray).] ▶LK ♀B ▶? $$$$

imipramine (**Tofranil, Tofranil-PM**): Enuresis: 25-75 mg PO qhs. [Generic/Trade: Tabs 10, 25, 50 mg. Trade only: Caps (Tofranil-PM) 75, 100, 125, 150 mg.] ▶L ♀B ▶? $

methylene blue (**Methblue 65, Urolene blue**): Dysuria: 65-130 mg PO tid after meals with liberal water. May turn urine/contact lenses blue. [Trade: Tab 65 mg.] ▶Gut/K ♀C ▶? $

pentosan (**Elmiron**): Interstitial cystitis: 100 mg PO tid. [Trade: Caps 100 mg.] ▶LK ♀B ▶? $$$$

phenazopyridine (**Pyridium, Azo-Standard, Urogesic, Prodium, Pyridiate, Urodol, Baridium, UTI Relief, ✚Phenazo**): Dysuria: 200 mg PO tid x 2 days. May turn urine/contact lenses orange. [OTC Generic/Trade: Tabs 95, 97.2 mg. Rx Generic/Trade: Tabs 100, 200 mg.] ▶K ♀B ▶? $

Erectile Dysfunction

alprostadil (**Muse, Caverject, Caverject Impulse, Edex, ✚Prostin VR**): 1 intraurethral pellet (Muse) or intracavernosal injection (Caverject, Edex) at lowest dose that will produce erection. Onset of effect is 5-20 minutes. [Trade: Syringe system (Edex) 10, 20, 40 mcg. (Caverject) 5, 10, 20 mcg. (Caverject Impulse) 10, 20 mcg. Pellet (Muse) 125, 250, 500, 1000 mcg. Intracorporeal injection of locally-compounded combination agents (many variations): "Bi-mix" can be 30 mg/ml papaverine + 0.5 to 1 mg/ml phentolamine, or 30 mg/ml papaverine + 20 mcg/ml alprostadil in 5, 10 or 20 ml vials. "Tri-mix" can be 30 mg/ml papaverine + 1 mg/ml phentolamine + 10 mcg/ml alprostadil in 5, 10 or 20 ml vials.] ▶L ♀- ▶- $$$$

sildenafil (**Viagra, Revatio**): Erectile dysfunction: Start 50 mg PO 0.5-4 h prior to intercourse. Max 1 dose/day. Usual effective range 25-100 mg. Start at 25 mg if >65 yo or liver/renal impairment. Pulmonary hypertension: 20 mg PO tid. Contraindicated with nitrates. [Trade: Viagra: Tabs 25, 50, 100 mg. Unscored tab but can be cut in half. Revatio: Tabs 20 mg.] ▶LK ♀B ▶- $$$

tadalafil (*Cialis*): Start 10 mg PO ≥30-45 min prior to sexual activity. May increase to 20 mg or decrease to 5 mg prn. Max 1 dose/day. Start 5 mg (max 1 dose/day) if CrCl 31-50 ml/min. Max 5 mg/day if CrCl <30 ml/min on dialysis. Max 10 mg/day if mild to moderate hepatic impairment; avoid in severe hepatic impairment. Max 10 mg once in 72 hours if concurrent potent CYP3A4 inhibitors. Contraindicated with nitrates & alpha-blockers (except tamsulosin 0.4 mg daily). Not FDA approved for women. [Trade: Tabs 5,10,20 mg.] ▶L ♀B ▶- $$$

vardenafil (*Levitra*): Start 10 mg PO 1 h before sexual activity. Usual effective dose range 5-20 mg. Max 1 dose/day. Use lower dose (5 mg) if ≥65 yo or moderate hepatic impairment (max 10 mg). Contraindicated with nitrates and alpha-blockers. Not FDA-approved for women. [Trade: Tabs 2.5, 5, 10, 20 mg] ▶LK ♀B ▶- $$$

yohimbine (*Yocon, Yohimex*): Erectile dysfunction (not FDA approved): 5.4 mg PO tid. [Generic/Trade: Tab 5.4 mg.] ▶L ♀- ▶- $

Nephrolithiasis

acetohydroxamic acid (*Lithostat*): Chronic UTI adjunctive therapy: 250 mg PO tid-qid. [Trade: Tab 250 mg.] ▶K ♀X ▶? $$$

citrate (*Polycitra-K, Urocit-K, Bicitra, Oracit, Polycitra, Polycitra-LC*): Urinary alkalinization: 1 packet in water/juice PO tid-qid. [Trade: Polycitra-K packet (K citrate): 3300 mg. Urocit-K wax (K citrate): Tabs 5, 10 mEq. Oracit oral solution: 5 ml = Na citrate 490 mg. Generic: Polycitra-K oral solution (5 ml = K citrate 1100 mg), Bicitra oral solution (5 ml = Na citrate 500 mg), Polycitra-LC oral solution (5 ml = K citrate 550 mg/Na citrate 500 mg), Polycitra oral syrup (5 ml = K citrate 550 mg/Na citrate 550 mg).] ▶K ♀C ▶? $$$

Index

908	26t	Abenol	18b	Ophth	107t	acetic acid	72bb	activated char-		Dermatol	52t
15-methyl-pros-		Abilify	113t	acetohydroxamic		coal	120m	adrenalin	49m
taglandin	102m	Abraxane	104m	acid	123m	Activella	100t	Adriamycin	103b
292 tablet	17t	Abreva		Actonel	59m	Abocal	104t		
2-PAM	120b	Dermatol	55t	Acetoxyl	51b	ACTOPLUS met		Adult emergency	
3TC	25m	ENT	73m	acetylcysteine			61t	drugs	141
5-aminosalicylic		acamprosate		Contrast	51m	Actos	61m	Advair	118t
acid	81t		114m	Pulmonary	126t	Actron	13m	Advate	46m
5-ASA	81t	acarbose	60m	Toxicology	119b	Acular	108t	Advicor	40b
5-FU		Accolate	119t	Acidophilus	88m	Acutrim Natural		Advil	13m
Dermatol	52b	Accu-Check	62t	Aciphex	78m		89b	Aerius	69b
Oncology	104t	Accupril	36b	acitretin	54b	Acutrim		Aerobid	118m
692 tablet	104t	Accuretic	43t	Acne	51	AM	24t	Aerobid-M	118m
6-MP	104t	Accutane	52t	ActHIB	89b	acyclovir		Aesculus hippo-	
		ACE inhibitors	35	Acticin	54m	Antimicr	24t	castanum	87b
A		acebutolol	43t	Actidose-Aqua		Dermatol	55t	Aflexa	87m
A/T/S	52t	acemannan	84b		120m	Adacel	89b	African plum tree	
A1C home test-		Aceon	36b	Actigall	81b	Adalat			88m
ing	62m	Acetadote	119b	Actinic Keratosis		Cardiovas	46m	Afrin	72t
A-200	54m	acetaminophen			52	OB/GYN	102t	Aggrastat	44b
abacavir	25m	Analgesics		Actiq	14m	adapalene	51b	Aggrenox	44b
abarelix	104t	11mb, 12t, 16b,		Activase		adefovir	26b	Agoral	79b
Abbokinase	50m	17tmb, 18mb,		Cardiovas	49b	Adenocard	46m	Agrylin	45b
Abbreviations	4		19t	Neurology	96b	adenosine	38m	Airomir	116b
ABC	25t	Neurology	95m	Activase rt-PA		ADH	69b	Akineton	96b
abciximab	44m	acetazolamide		Cardiovas	49b	Adipex-P	116t	AK Tate	106b
Abelcet	20m	Cardiovas	47t	Neurology	96b	Adoxa		AK Tracin	105b
								Antimicr	21b,34b	Akarpine	107m

124 Index

t = top of page
m = middle of page
b = bottom of page

AK-Con 104b
Akineton 96t
AK-Mycin 105b
AK-Pentolate
 107b
AK-Pred 106b
AK-Sulf 105b
Alamast 105t
Alavert 69b
Albalon 50m
albendazole 22b
Albenza 22b
Albumarc 50m
albumin 50m
Albuminar 50m
albuterol
 116b, 118t
Alcaine 108m
alcohol 120m
Alcomicin 105t
Aldactazide 43t
Aldactone 37m
Aldara 55t
aldesleukin 104t
Aldomet 38m
Aldoril 43t
alefacept 54b
alemtuzumab
 104t
alendronate 58b
Alertec 116b
Alesse 98
Aleve 13b
Alferon N 104m
alfuzosin 121t
Alimta 104t
Alinia 23t
alitretinoin 56b
Alka-Seltzer 76b
Alkeran 103b
Allegra 69b
Aller-Chlor 71t
Allerdryl 71m,
 114t, 116b
Allerest 104m
Allermax
 114t,116b
Allernix
 ENT 71m
 Psych114t,116b
Aller-Relief 71t
Allium sativum
 86b
allopurinol 63m
Alluna 89m
Almora 65t

almotriptan 94b
Alocril 105t
aloe vera 84b
Alomide 105t
Aloprim 63m
Aloxi 97b
Alora 97b
alosetron 80b
Aloxi 97b
Alpha 107m
alpha-galactosi-
 dase 80b
Alphagan 107m
alprazolam 113b
alprostadil 122b
Alrex 106b
Alsoy 65b
Altace 36b
alteplase
 Cardiovas 49b
 Neurology 96b
Alternagel 76b
Altera 43t
Altocor 41t
Altoprev 41t
altretamine 103b
Alu-Cap 76b
aluminum ace-
 tate 72m
aluminum chlo-
 ride 56b
aluminum hy-
 droxide 76b
Alu-Tab 76b
Alzheimer's 92
amantadine
 Antimicr 26b
 Neurology 96t
Amaryl 63t
Amatine 49m
Ambien 114t
AmBisome 20m
Amerge 94b
Amevive 54b
Amicar 83b
Amidate 19t
amifostine 104t
Amigesic 12m
amikacin 20t
Amikin 20t
amiloride
 43m,47m

amitriptyline 108b
amlexanox 73t
amlodipine
 40b, 43m, 46t
Amnesteem 56b
amoxicillin
 Antimicr 32m
 Gastro 77b
amoxicillin-clavu-
 lanate 33t
Amoxil 32m
Amphadase 69t
amphetamine 69t
Amphojel 76b
Amphotec 20m
amphotericin B
 deoxycholate
 20m
amphotericin B
 lipid formula-
 tions 20m
ampicillin 33t
ampicillin-sulbac-
 tam 33m
Amrinone 49m
Anabolic Steroids
 58
Anacin 12m
Anafranil 108b
anagrelide 83b
anakinra 11t
Anandron 104t
Anaprox 13b
Anaspaz 121m
anastrozole 103b
Ancef 28m
Ancobon 20b
Andriol 58m
andro 58t
Androcur 104t
Androcur Depot
 104t
Androderm 58m
Androgel 58m
Androgens 58
Android 58m
androstenedione
 84b
Anectine 19b
Anesthetics &
 Sedatives 19
Anexate 120b
Anexsia 18b
Angelica sinensis
 86m
Angiomax 83m
Angiotensin
 Blockers 37
anhydrous glyc-
 erins 72b
Anorexiants 115

Ansaid 12b
Antabuse 114b
Antara 42m
antazoline 104m
Anthemis nobilis
 85b
Anthra-Derm 54b
Anthraforte 54b
anthralin 54b
Anthranol 54b
Anthrascalp 54b
Antiadrenergic
 agents 37
Antiarrheals 74
Anticoagulants 82
Anticoagulation
 goals 83
Anticonvulsants
 92
Antidepressants
 108
Antidiarrheals 74
Antidotes 120
Antidysrhythmics
 38
Antiemetics 75
Antifungals
 Antimicr 20
 Dermatol 53
Antihistamines 69
Antihyperlipidem-
 ics 40
Antihyperten-
 sives 42
Antimalarials 21
Antimanics 110
Antiminth 23m
Antimycobacteri-
 als 22
Antiparasitics
 Antimicro 22
 Dermatol 54
Antiplatelet drugs
 83
Antipsoriatics 54
Antipsychotics
 111
antipyrine 72m
Antirheumatics
 10t
Antispas 78b
Antitussives 71
Antiulcer 76
antivenin - cro-
 talidae 91t
Antivert
 Gastro 78b
 Neurology 97t
Antivirals
 Antimicro 23
 Dermatol 55
 Ophth 106
Antizol 120b

Anusol Hemor-
 rhoidal Oint-
 ment 56m
Anusol Supposi-
 tories 56b
Anusol-HC 56m
Anxiolytics 113
Anzemet 75b
APGAR score101
Aphthasol 73t
Apidra 63t
Aplisol 91b
Apo-Gain 57b
Apokyn 96t
apomorphine 96t
aprepitant 75b
Apresazide 43t
Apresoline 44t
Apri 98
aprotinin 83b
Aptivus 26m
Aquachloral Sup-
 prettes 113b
AquaMephyton
 67b
Aquasol E 68t
AraC 103b
Aralen 21m
Aranelle 98
Aranesp 83b
Arava 10t
Aredia 59t
argatroban 83m
Aricept 92t
Arimidex 104t
aripiprazole 113t
Aristocort 60m
Aristolochia 85t
aristolochic acid
 85t
Aristospan 60m
Arixtra 82b
arnica 85t
Arnica montana
 85t
Aromasin 104t
arsenic trioxide
 104m
Artane 96t
Arthrotec 12b
articaine 19m
artichoke leaf
 extract 85t
artificial tears
 108m
ASA (aspirin)
 Analgesics
 11m, 12tm,
 17mb, 18t
 Cardiovas 44m
 Gastro 76b
Asacol 81t

**125
Index**

t = top of page
m = middle of page
b = bottom of page

Asaphen
  Analgesics 12m
  Cardiovas 44m
Asarum   85t
Ascencia   62m
ascorbic acid 56b
Ascriptin   11m
Aslera   86t
Asmanex Twist-
  haler   118m
Asmavent   116b
asparaginase104m
A-spaz   121m
aspirin
  Analgesics
    11mb, 12m,
    17mb, 18t
  Cardiovas 44m
  Gastro   76b
Assailx   89m
Astelin   73b
Atasol   18b
atazanavir   25b
atenolol 43b, 45b
Atgam   91m
Ativan
  Neurology   93t
  Psych   113m
atomoxetine
              115m
atorvastatin   40b
atovaquone
          21b, 23b
atracurium   19b
AtroPen   120m
atropine
  Cardiovas   38b
  Gastro 75t, 78b
  Ophth   107b
  Toxicol   120m
Urology
          121b, 122t
Atrovent   119m
Atrovent Nasal
  Spray   74t
ATV   25b
Augmentin   33t
Auralgan   72m
Avage   52m
Avalide   43t
Avandamet   61

Avandia   61m
Avapro   37m
Avastin   104t
Avaxim   89b
Aveeno   57b
Aventyl   109t
Aviane   98
Avinza   16t
Avodart   121t
Avonex   95m
Axert   94b
Axid   91m
Axid AR   91m
Aygestin   103m
azacitidine 103b
Azactam   35t
Azasan   10m
azatadine   71t
azathioprine   10m
azelaic acid 51b
azelastine
  ENT   73b
  Ophth   104b
Azelex   51b
azithromycin   31m
Azmacort   118m
Azopt   107t
Azo-Standard
              122m
AZT   25b
aztreonam   35t
Azulfidine
  Analgesics 10b
  Gastro   81b

B

B12
  Endocrine   66b
  OB/GYN 103m
B6
  Endocrine   68t
  OB/GYN 103m
BabyBIG   91t
Bacid   88t
Bactrim   34b
Bactroban   53t
BAL in oil 120m
Balziva   98
banana bag   65b

Banophen
        114t, 116b
Baraclude   27t
Barium sulfate 51t
barium sulfate 51t
Basaljel   76b
basiliximab   91t
Bayer
  Analgesics 12m
  Cardiovas 44m
BayHep B   91t
BayRab   91t
BayRho-D   103m
BayTet   91t
BCG   104t
BCG vaccine 89b
BCNU   103b
B-D Glucose 62m
Beano   80b
becaplermin 56b
beclomethasone
  ENT   73b
  Pulm   118m
Beconase   73b
Benadryl
        114t, 116b
Benazaclin   51b
benazepril   37t
Benefix   87t
Benicar   37m
Benicar HCT 43t
Benign prostatic
  hyper.   121
Benoquin   57b
Benoxyl   51b
Bentyl   78b
Bentylol   78b
Benuryl   63b
Benylin   51b
Benzac   51b
BenzaClin   51b
Benzagel   51b
Benzamycin   51b
benzathine peni-
  cillin   31b
benzocaine
        72m, 74t
Benzodiazepines
              113
benzoic acid
        121t, 122t
benzonatate 71t
benzoyl peroxide
        51b, 52b
benztropine
  Neuro   95b

Psych   116m
benzylpenicilloyl
  polylysine 31b
Berotec   76b
Beta agonists 116
Beta blockers 45
Betagan   107t
Betaject   59b
Betaloc   45b
betamethasone
  Dermatol   56m
  Endocrine 59b
Betapace   40t
Betaseron   95m
betaxolol
  Cardiovas 45b
  Ophth   106b
Betaxon   107t
bethanechol121t
Betimol   107t
Betnesol   59b
Betoptic   106b
Betoptic S   106b
bevacizumab
              104t
bexarotene 104m
Bexxar   104m
bezafibrate   42t
Bezalip   42t
Biaxin   31m
Biaxin XL   31m
bicalutamide 104t
bicarbonate
  Cardiovas 39t
  Gastro   76b
Bicillin C-R 31b
Bicillin L-A 31b
Bicitra   123m
BiCNU   103b
BiDil   43t
Bifidobacteria
              88m
bilberry   85t
Biltricide   23m
bimatoprost107m
Biolean   86m
BioRab   90m
biotin   67t
biperiden   96t
Biquin durules40t
bisacodyl   79m
bismuth subsali-
  cylate74b, 79b
bisoprolol 43b,45t
bitter melon 85m
bitter orange 85m
bivalirudin   39m
black cohosh85m
Bladder drugs121
Blenoxane 103b

Psych   116m
Beta agonists 116
Betimol   107t
bleomycin   103b
Bleph-10   105b
Blephamide 106t
Blocadren   46t
Body mass index
              116
Bonamine
  Gastro   76t
  Neurology 97t
Bonefos   59t
Bonine
  Gastro   76t
  Neurology 97t
Boniva   59t
Boostrix   89b
boric acid   102m
bortezomib 104m
Botox   56b
Botox Cosmetic
              56b
botulinum toxin
              56b
botulism immune
  globulin   91t
Bragantia   85t
Brethine
  OB/GYN 102t
  Pulm   117b
Brevibloc   45m
Brevicon   98
Brevicon 1/35 98
Brevital   19t
Bricanyl
  OB/GYN 102t
  Pulmonary117b
brimonidine107m
brinzolamide107t
bromazepam113t
bromfenac 108t
bromocriptine
  Endocrine 68m
  Neurology 96m
budesonide
  ENT   73b
  Gastro   80b
  Pulm   118m
Bufferin   11m
bumetanide   47m
Bumex   47m
Buminate   56b
bupivacaine 19m
Buprenex   14t
buprenorphine
  Analgesics 14t
Psych
        114m,115m

126
Index

t = top of page
m = middle of page
b = bottom of page

bupropion
  110m, 117m
Burinex 47m
burn plant 84b
BuSpar 113b
buspirone 113b
busulfan 103b
Busulfex 103b
butalbital 11mb,
  12t, 17m
butenafine 53m
butoconazole
  102m
butorphanol 14t
butterbur 85m
butyl aminoben-
  zoate 74m
Byetta 87b

C

C.E.S. 99m
cabergoline 105m
Caduet 40b
Caelyx 104b
Cafergot 95t
Caffedrine 11b
caffeine
  Analgesics
    11mb, 11t
  Neurology 95t
  Psych 115b
calamine 57t
Calan 47t
Calciferol 68m
Calcijex 68b
Calcimar 68t
calcipotriene 54b
calcitonin 68m
calcitriol 66b
calcium acetate
  63b
calcium carbon-
  ate
  Analgesics 11m
  Endocrine 63b
  GI 76b, 77m
  OB/GYN 103t
Calcium channel
  blockers 46
calcium chloride
  64m
calcium citrate
  64m
calcium glucon-
  ate 64t
Calsan 63b

Caltine 68m
Caltrate 63b
Camellia sinensis
  87m
Camila 98
Campath 104t
Campral 114m
Camptosar 104t
Canasa 81t
Cancenex 89t
Cancidas 20m
candesartan
  37m, 43t
Candistatin
  Antimicr 21t
  Dermatol 53b
Canesten
  Antimicr 20m
  Dermatol 53m
Cantil 77m
capecitabine 103b
Capital with Co-
  deine suspen-
  sion 9b
Capoten 36t
Capozide 43t
capsaicin 52b
captopril 36t, 43t
Carac 52b
Carafate
  ENT 73m
  Gastro 79m
carbamazepine
  Neurology 92t
  Psych 110b
carbamide perox-
  ide 72t
Carbapenems 27
Carbatrol
  Neurology 92t
  Psych 110b
Carbex 96b
carbidopa 96mb
carbidopa-levo-
  dopa 96mb
Carbolith 113b
carboplatin 104t
carboprost 102b
Cardene 46m
Cardiac parame-
  ters 142
Cardio-Omega 3
  65b
Cardizem 46b
Cardura
  Cardiovas 38t
  Urology 121t
Carimune 91m

carisoprodol
  10b, 12t, 18t
carmustine 103b
Carnitor 65b
carteolol 106b
Cartia XT 46b
Cartilade 89t
carvedilol 45m
cascara 79m
Casodex 104t
caspofungin 20m
castor oil 79m
Cataflam 12b
Catapres
  Cardiovas 37b
  OB/GYN 103m
  Psych
    114b, 116m
Cathflo 49b
Caverject 122b
Caverject Im-
  pulse 122b
CCNU 103b
Ceclor 28b
Cedax 29b
Cedocard SR 48t
CeeNu 103b
cefaclor 28b
cefadroxil 28m
cefazolin 28m
cefdinir 29m
cefditoren 29m
cefepime 29m
cefixime 29m
Cefizox 29b
Cefobid 29m
cefoperazone
  29m
Cefotan 28b
cefotaxime 29m
cefotetan 28b
cefoxitin 29t
cefpodoxime 29m
cefprozil 29t
ceftazidime 29m
ceftibuten 29b
Ceftin 29t
ceftizoxime 29b
ceftriaxone 29b
cefuroxime 29b
Cefzil 29t
Celebrex 12t
celecoxib 12t
Celestone 59b
Celestone Solu-
  span 59b
Celexa 109m
Cellcept 91b
Cena-K 65t
Cenestin 99m
Centany 53t
cephalexin 28b

Cephalosporins
  28
Cephulac 79b
Ceptaz 29m
Cerebyx 92b
Certain Dri 56m
Cerubidine 103b
Cerumenex 72b
Cervical ripening
  100
Cervidil 100b
Cetacaine 74m
cetirizine 71t
cetrorelix acetate
  99b
Cetrotide 99b
cetuximab 104t
cevimeline 73t
chamomile 85b
chaparral 85b
CharcoAid 120m
charcoal 120m
Charcodote 120m
chasteberry 85b
Chemet 121t
Children's Nal-
  salCrom 74t
ChiRhoClin 81b
Chirocaine 19b
Chlo-Amine 71t
chloral hydrate
  113b
chlorambucil103b
chloramphenicol
  Gastro 81t
  Psych 113t
chlordiazepoxide
  Gastro 81t
  Psych 113t
chlorhexidine
  gluconate 73t
chlorodeoxy-
  adenosine 103b
Chloromycetin35t
chlorophyllin cop-
  per 57b
chloroquine 21m
chlorothiazide47b
chlorpheniramine
  71t
chlorpromazine
  112b
chlorthalidone
  43b, 47b
Chlor-Trimeton
  71t
chlorzoxazone
  10b
cholestyramine
  40m
choline magne-
  sium trisalicy-
  late 12m

chondroitin 85b
Chronovera 47t
Chronulac 79b
Chrysanthemum
  parthenium86b
Cialis 123t
ciclopirox 53m
Cidecin 35t
cidofovir 23b
cilazapril
  36m, 43b
cilostazol 50b
Ciloxan 105m
cimetidine 77m
Cimicifuga ra-
  cemosa 85m
cinacalcet 68b
Cipro 33b
Cipro Otic 72m
ciprofloxacin
  Antimicr 33b
  ENT 72m
  Opth 105m
cisatracurium 19b
cisplatin 104t
citalopram 109m
Citracal 64t
citrate
  Gastro 76b
  Urology 123b
Citri Lean 86b
Citrocarbonate
  76b
Citro-Mag 79b
Citrucel 79b
Citrus aurantium
  85m
cladribine 103b
Claforan 29m
Clarinex 69b
clarithromycin
  Antimicr 31m
  Gastro 77b
Claritin 69b
Clavulin 33t
Clear Eyes 104m
clemastine 71t
Clenia 51b
Cleocin
  Antimicr 35t
  Dermatol
    51b, 52t
  OB/GYN 102m
Cleocin T 51b
clidinium 81t
Climara 97b
Climara Pro 100t
ClindaMax 51b
clindamycin
  Antimicr 35t
  Dermatol
    51b, 52t
  OB/GYN 102m

**127
Index**

t = top of page
m = middle of page
b = bottom of page

Clindesse 102m
Clindoxyl 52t
Clinistix 62m
Clinitest 62m
Clinoril 13b
clobazam 92m
clodronate 59t
clofarabine 103b
Clolar 103b
Clomid 100b
clomiphene 100b
clomipramine
    20m
Clonapam
  Neurology 92m
  Psych 113t
clonazepam
  Neurology 92m
  Psych 113t
clonidine
  Cardiovas
    37b, 43t
  OB/GYN 103m
  Psych
    114b, 116m
clopidogrel 44t
clorazepate 113t
Clorpres 43t
Clotrimaderm
  Antimicr 20m
  Dermatol 53m
  OB/GYN 102b
clotrimazole
  Antimicr 20m
  Derm 53m,56m
  ENT 73t
  OB/GYN 102b
clozapine 111b
Clozaril 111b
coal tar 57t
cobalamin 66b
codeine 14m, 16b
    17tm, 18t
coenzyme Q10
    85b
Cogentin
  Neurology 95b
  Psych 116m
Colace
  ENT 72m
  Gastro 79m
Colazal 80b
Colbenemid 63m
colchicine 63mb
colesevelam 40m
Colestid 40m
colestipol 40m
colistin 72m
Colyte 80t
Coma scale 94t
Combantrin 21m
CombiPatch 100t

Combivent 118t
Combivir 25t
Combunox 17t
comfrey 86t
Commiphora
  mukul 85b
Commit 115t
Compazine 76t
Comtan 95b
Comvax 89b
Concerta 115b
Condylline 56t
Condylox 56t
cone flower 86b
Congest 99m
Conray 51t
Contraceptives 97
CONTRAST
  MEDIA 51
  Conversions 7
Copaxone 95m
Copegus 27b
CoQ-10 85b
Cordarone 38b
Coreg 45m
Corgard 45b
Corlopam 44t
Coronex 43t
Correctol 79m
Cortef 59b
Cortenema 59b
Corticosteroids
  Dermatol 55
  Endocrine 59
  Ophth 106
Cortifoam 59b
cortisone 59b
Cortisporin
  Dermatol 56m
  Ophth 106m
Cortisporin Otic
    72m
Cortisporin TC
  Otic 72m
Cortone 59b
Cortrosyn 68b
Corvert 39m
Corynanthe yo-
  himbe 89m
Corzide 43t
Cosamin DS 87m
Cosmegen 103b
Cosopt 107t
cosyntropin 68b
Cotazym 81m
cotrimoxazole34b
Coumadin 43m
Covera-HS 47t
Coversyl 36b
Cozaar 37b
Cranactin 86t

cranberry 86t
Crataegus laevi-
  gata 87b
creatine 86t
Creon 81m

creosote bush85b
Crestor 42t
Crinone 101m
Crixivan 26t
CroFab 55t
Crolom 105t
cromolyn 12t
cromolyn sodium
  Ophth 105t
  Pulmonary 119t
crotamiton 54m
Cryselle 98
crystalline
DMSO2 88t
Cubicin 35t
Culturelle 88m
Cuprimine 120b
Cutar 57t
cyanocobalamin
    66b, 67m
Cyclen 98
Cyclessa 98
cyclobenzaprine
    10b
Cyclogyl 107t
Cyclomen 103m
cyclopentolate
    107t
cyclophospha-
  mide 103b
Cyclogplegics 107
cyclosporine
  Immunol 91b
  Ophth 108m
  Urology 122m
Cymbalta 110m
Cynara scolymus
    85t
Cynara-SL 85t
cyproheptadine
    7t
cyproterone
  Dermatol 52t
  Oncology 104t
Cystografin 51t
Cystospaz 121m
cytarabine 103b
Cytomel 66m
Cytosar-U 103b
Cytotec
  Gastro 79t
  OB/GYN 100b
Cytovene 24t
Cytoxan 103b

D

D.H.E. 45 95t
D2T5 89b

d4T 25m
dacarbazine 103b
daclizumab 91b
dactinomycin
    103b
Dalacin 102m
Dalacin C 35t
Dalacin T 51b
dalfopristin 35b
Dalmane 113m
dalteparin 82t
danazol 103m
Danocrine 103m
Dantrium 10b
dantrolene 10b
dapiprazole 108b
dapsone 22m
Daptacel 89b
daptomycin 35t
Daraprim 23m
darbepoetin 83b
darifenacin 121m
Darvocet 17t
Darvon Com-
  pound 17t
Darvon Pulvules
    16b
Darvon-N 16b
daunorubicin
    103b
*DaunoXome*103b
Daypro 13b
Daypro Alta 13b
d-biotin 66b
DDAVP
  Endocrine 69t
  Hematology 84t
  Urology 122m
ddC 25b
ddl 25t
Debacterol 73t
Debrox 72m
Decadron
  Endocrine 59b
  Neurology 97t
  Pulm 119m
Deca-Durabolin
    58m
Declomycin 68b
Decongestants72
deferoxamine
    120m
dehydroepian-
  drosterone 86t
Delatestryl 58m
Delestrogen 59t
Delsym 71b
Delta-Cortef 59t
Deltasone 60m
Demadex 47m
demeclocycline
    68b

Demerol 14b
Demulen 98
Denavir 55t
ENT 73m
denileukin 104t
Denticare 73t
Depacon 93b
Depade 114b
Depakene
  Neurology 93b
  Psych 111m
Depen 120b
Depakote
  Neurology 93b
  Psych 111m
Depo-Cyt 103b
DepoDur 16t
Depo-Estradiol
    97b
Depo-Medrol 60t
Depo-Provera
    100m
depo-subQ pro-
  vera 101b
Depotest 58m
Depo-Testoster-
  one 58m
Deproic
  Neurology 93b
  Psych 111m
DERMATOLOGY
    51
Dermatomes 94
Dermazin 53m
desipramine 108b
desirudin 83m
Desferal 120m
desloratadine69b
desmopressin
  Endocrine 69t
  Hematology 84t
  Urology 122m
Desogen 98
desogestrel 98
Desquam 51b
Desyrel 110b
Detrol 122t
Detrol LA 122t
devil's claw 86t
dexamethasone
  Endocrine 59b
  ENT 72m
  Neurology 97t
  Ophth 106m
  Pulm 119m

128
Index

t = top of page
m = middle of page
b = bottom of page

diclofenac
 Analgesics 12b
 Dermatol 52b
 Ophth 108t
dicloxacillin 32t
dicyclomine 78b
didanosine 25t
Didronel 59b
difenoxin 75t
Differin 51b
Diflucan 37t
diflunisal 12m
Digibind
digitalis 39t
digitoxin 39t
Digitek 39t
digoxin 39t
digoxin immune
 Fab 39t
dihydrocodeine
 18t
dihydroergota-
 mine 95t
dihydrotachy-
 sterol 67t
Dilacor XR 46b
Dilantin 93m
Dilatrate-SR 48t
Dilaudid 14b
Diltia XT 46b
diltiazem 46b
Diltiazem CD 46b
dimenhydrinate
 75b
dimercaprol 120m
Dimetapp Infant
 Drops 72t
dimethyl sulfone
 88t
dinoprostone 100b
Diocarpine 107m
Diogent 105t
Diopred 106b
Dioscorea villosa
 89b
Diovan 37b
Diovan HCT 43m
Dipentum 81m
Diphen 114t, 116b
Diphenhist
 114t, 116b
diphenhydramine
 ENT 71m
 Psych114t, 116b
diphenoxylate 75t
diphtheria tet-
 anus & acellular
 pertussis 89b
diphtheria-teta-
 nus toxoid 89b
Diprivan 19t
dipyridamole 44m

Disalcid 12m
disopyramide 39t
DisperMox 32m
disulfiram 114b
Ditropan 121b
Ditropan XL 121b
Diucardin 43m
Diuretics 47
Diuril 43t
Diutensen-R 43m
divalproex
 Neurology 93b
 Psych 111m
Dixarit 37b
Dixirit 103b
dobutamine 49t
Dobutrex 49t
docetaxel 104m
docosanol 55t
 Dermatol 55t
 ENT 73m
docusate 80m
docusate calcium
 79m
docusate sodium
 ENT 73m
 Gastro 79m
dolasetron 76t
Dolobid 12m
Dolophine
 Analgesics 16t
 Psych 114b
Doloral 57t
Doloteffin 88t
Domeboro Otic
 72m
domperidone 80b
dong quai 89t
donepezil 92t
Donnatal 78b
Donnazyme 81m
dopamine 49t
dornase alfa119m
Doryx
 Antimi 21b,34b
Dostinex 98t
Dovonex 54b
doxacurium 19b
doxazosin
 Cardiovas 38t
 Urology 121t
doxepin
 Dermatol 57t
 Psych 108b
doxercalciferol
 67t
Doxil 103b
doxorubicin 103b
Doxycin
 Antimi 21b,34b

Dermatol 52t
doxycycline
 Antimi 21b,34b
 Dermatol 52t
 ENT 73m
doxylamine
 Analgesics 17m
 Gastro 75b
Dramamine 75b
Drisdol 68t
Dristan 12 Hr
 Nasal 74m
Drithocreme 54b
dronabinol 75b
droperidol 76t
drospirenone 98t
drotrecogin 35t
Droxia 104t
Drug depend-
 ence therapy
  114
Drugs in preg-
 nancy 101
Dry Eyes 108m
Drysol 56b
Dryvax 90m
DT 75b
DTaP 89b, 90m
DTIC-Dome 103b
Duac 52t
Dulcolax 79m
duloxetine 111b
Duocaine 19m
Duolube 108m
DuoNeb 118t
Duragesic 14m
Duralith 111t
Duricef 28m
dutasteride 121t
Duvoid 122m
Dyazide 43m
Dynacin 34b
DynaCirc 46m
DynaCirc CR46m
Dynapen 32t

econazole 53m
Econopred 106b
Ecostatin 53m
Ecotrin
 Analgesics 12m
 Cardiovas 44m
ED Spaz 121m
Edecrin 47m
edetate 120m
Edex 122b
edrophonium 95b
EDTA 120m
EES 31m
Efafin 65t
Effer-K 65t
Effexor 110b
Efidac/24 72t
eflornithine 57t
Efudex 52b
EFV 24b
EGb 761 87t
Egozinc-HC 56m
ELA-Max 57m
Elavil 108b
Eldepryl 96b
elderberry 86m
Eldopaque 57m
Eldoquin 57m
Electropeg 80t
Elestat 104b
eletriptan 94b
Elidel 56t
Eligard 104t
Elimite 54b
Elixophyllin 119b
Ellence 103b
Elmiron 122m
Eloxatin 104m
Elspar 104m
Eltroxin 66m
Emadine 104b
Emcyt 104t
emedastine 104b
Emend 75b

E
E Pam
 Analgesics 10b
 Neurology 92b
 Psych 113m
E. angustifolia
  86m
E. pallida 86m
E. purpurea 86m
Ear preps 72
Ebixa 92t
echinacea 86m
Echinacin Mad-
 aus 86m
EchinaGuard86m
EC-Naprosyn 13b

Dexasone
 Endocrine 59b
 Neurology 97t
Dexatrim 85m
dexchlorphenira-
 mine 71m
Dexedrine 115b
DexFerrum 64b
Dexiron 64b
dexmedetomi-
 dine 19t
dexmethylpheni-
 date 115b
Dexone 59b
Dexpak 59b
dexrazoxane 104t
dextran 50m
dextroampheta-
 mine 115mb
dextromethor-
 phan 71b
dextrose 62m
Dextrostat 115b
DHEA 86t
DHPG 24t
DHT 67t
DiaBeta 62t
Diabetes num-
 bers 60
Diabetes-related
 agents 60
Diamicron 61b
Diamox
 Cardiovas 47t
 Ophth 107t
Diane-35 52t
Diarr-eze 75t
Diastat
 Analgesics 10b
 Neurology 92m
Diastix 62m
diatrizoate 51t
Diatx 66b
Diazemuls
 Neurology 92m
 Psych 113m
diazepam
 Analgesics 10b
 Neurology 92m
 Psych 113m
diazoxide 62m
dibucaine 56m
Dicetel 81m
dichloralphena-
 zone 95m
Diclectin 75b

Dermatol 51t
Econazole

Dexamethasone

Emerg contra-
 ception 99
Emergency
 DRUGS 141
Emetrol 76t
EMLA 57t
Empirin 45t
Empirin with Co-
 deine 17t
Emtec 18t
emtricitabine
  25mb
Emtriva 25m
E-mycin 31m
Enablex 121m
enalapril
  36m, 43mb

129 Index

t = top of page
m = middle of page
b = bottom of page

enalaprilat 36m
Enbrel 10t
Endantadine
  Antimicr 26b
  Neurology 96t
Endocet 17b
Endocodone 16m
ENDOCRINE 58
Endodan 17b
Endrate 120m
Enduronyl 43m
Enemol 80m
Enfamil 65b
enfuvirtide 24m
Engerix-B 91m
Enjuvia 99m
Enlon 95b
enoxaparin 82m
Enpresse 98
ENT
ENT combinations 70
entacapone 96b
entecavir 27t
Entocort EC 80b
Entozyme 81m
Entrophen
  Analgesics 12m
  Cardiovas 44b
Epaxal 89b
ephedra 86m
Ephedra sinica 86m
ephedrine 49t
Epiject
  Neurology 93b
  Psych 111m
epinastine 105b
epinephrine 49t
epinephrine racemic 119m
EpiPen 49m
EpiPen Jr 49m
EpiQuin Micro 57t
epirubicin 103b
Epitol
  Neurology 92m
  Psych 110b
Epival
  Neurology 93b
  Psych 111m
Epivir 27b
eplerenone 37t
epoetin 84t
Epogen 84t
epoprostenol 44t
Eprex 84t
eprosartan 37m, 43b
eptifibatide 44b
Epzicom 25m

Equalactin 80t
Equetro 110b
Erbitux 104t
Erectile dysfunction 122
Ergamisol 104m
ergocalciferol 68m
ergotamine 95t
erlotinib 104t
Errin 98
Ertaczo 54t
ertapenem 27b
Erybid 31m
Eryc 31m
Erycette 52t
Eryderm 52t
Erygel 52t
Eryped 31m
Erysol 52t
Ery-Tab 31m
Erythromid 31m
erythromycin
  Derm 51b, 52t
erythromycin
  Ophth 105b
erythromycin
  base 31m
erythromycin
  ethyl suc 31mb
erythromycin lactobionate 31m
erythropoietin 84t
escitalopram 109m
Esclim 97b
Esgic 11m
Esidrix 43b
Eskalith 111t
esmolol 45b
esomeprazole 78t
Esoterica 57m
Estalis 100t
estazolam 113m
esterified estrogens 97m, 100tm
Estrace 97m, 99m
Estraderm 97b
estradiol 97m, 100t
estradiol acetate 97m
estradiol acetate vag ring 97m
estradiol cypionate 97b
estradiol gel 97b
estradiol topical 97b
estradiol emulsion 97b
estradiol transdermal 97b
estradiol vaginal ring 99t

estradiol vaginal tab 99t
estradiol valerate 99t
Estradot 97b
estramustine 104t
Estrasorb 97b
Estratest 100t
Estring 99t
Estrogel 97b
estrogen cream 99m
Estrogens 97
estrogens conju 99m, 100m
estrogens synthetic 99m
estropipate 99m
Estrostep Fe 98
eszopiclone 114t
etanercept 10t
ethacrynic acid 47m
ethambutol 22m
ethanol 120m
ethinyl estradiol
  Dermatol 52t
  OB/GYN 97m, 98, 100t
ethosuximide 92b
ethynodiol 98
Ethyol 104t
Etibi 22m
etidronate 59t
etodolac 12b
etomidate 95t
etonogestrel 97m
Etopophos 104m
etoposide 104t
Euflex 104t
Euglucon 62t
Eulexin 104t
Eurax 54m
evening primrose oil 86m
Everone 200 58m
Evista 101b
Evoclin 51b
Evoxac 73t
Evra 97m
Excedrin Migraine 11b
Exelon 111m
exemestane 104t
exenatide 62m
Ex-Lax 80m
Exsel 58t
ezetimibe 42t
Ezetrol 42t

F

Factive 34m
factor VIIa 84t
factor VIII 84m
factor IX 84t
famciclovir 27b
famotidine 77m
Famvir 27b
Fansidar 21b
Fareston 104t
Faslodex 104t
fat emulsion 65b
FazaClo 111b
Feba-Nam 79m
felbamate 92b
Felbatol 92b
Feldene 12b
felodipine 43m, 46t
Femaprin 85b
Femara 104t
FemHRT 100t
Femizol-M 102b
FemPatch 97b
Femring 97b
Femtrace 97b
fenofibrate 42m
fenoldopam 44t
fenoterol 117m
fentanyl 14m
fenugreek 86b
FeoSol Tabs 64m
Fergon 64b
Fer-in-Sol 64b
Ferodan 64b
Fero-Grad 64b
Ferlecit 65m
ferrous fumarate 64m
ferrous gluconate 64b
ferrous sulfate 64b
Fexicam 13b
fexofenadine 69b
feverfew 86b
FiberCon 80t
Fiberall 80m
Fibelin 86t
filgrastim 84t
Finacea 51b
finasteride
  Dermatol 57m
  Urology 121t
Finevin 51b
Fioricet 11b
Fiorinal 11b
Fioricet with Codeine 17m
Fiorinal-C 1/2 17m
FiorinalC-1/4 17m
Fiorinal with Codeine 17m

fish oil 65b
FK 506 91b
Flagyl
  Antimi 23t, 35m
  OB/GYN 102b
Flamazine 53m
Flarex 102b
flavoxate 121b
Flebogamma 91m
flecainide 39m
Fleet enema 80t
Fleet Flavored Castor Oil 79m
Fleet Mineral Oil Enema 79b
Fleet Pain Relief 56m
Fleet Phospho-Soda 79b
Fletcher's Castoria 80m
Flexeril 10b
Flexium 88b
Flextend 87m
Flolan 44t
Flomax 121t
Flonase 74t
Florazole ER 23t, 35m
Florinef 59b
FloventHFA 118m
Floxin 33b
Floxin Otic 72b
floxuridine 103b
fluconazole 20m
flucytosine 20b
Fludara 103b
fludarabine 103b
fludrocortisone 59b
Flumadine 120b
flumazenil 120b
FluMist 90t
flunarizine 95m
flunisolide
  ENT 74t
  Pulm 118m
fluocinolone 58m
Fluor-A-Day 64b
fluoride 64b
Fluoride dose 64
fluorometholone 106b
Fluor-Op 106b
Fluoroplex 52b
fluorouracil

**130
Index**

t = top of page
m = middle of page
b = bottom of page

Dermatol 52b
Oncology 104t
Fluotic 64b
fluoxetine
109m, 114m
fluphenazine
112m
flurazepam 113m
flurbiprofen 12b
flutamide 104t
fluticasone
ENT 74t
Pulm 118bm
fluvastatin 41t
Fluviral 90t
Fluvirin 90t
fluvoxamine 109b
Fluzone 90t
FML 106b
FML Forte 106b
FML-S Liquifilm
106m
Focalin 115b
folate 67t
Folgard 67t
folic acid
Endocrine
66b, 67tm
OB/GYN 103m
folinic acid 104m
**Follistim-Antagon
Kit** 99b
Foltx 67t
Folvite 67t
fomepizole 120b
fondaparinux 82b
Foradil 117m
formoterol
117m,118t
Formulas 8
formulas – infant
65b
Formulex 78b
Fortamet 61m
Fortaz 29m
Forteo 69t
Fortovase 26m
Fosamax 68t
fosamprenavir26t
foscarnet 23b
Foscavir 23b
fosfomycin 35t
fosinopril
36m, 43m
fosphenytoin 92b
Fosrenol 69m

Fragmin 82t
FreeStyle 62m
French maritime
pine tree 88m
Frisium 92m
Froben 12b
Frova 94b
frovatriptan 94b
FTC 25m
FTV 26m
Fucidin 52b
Fucidin H 56m
FUDR 103b
Fulvicin 20b
Fungizone 20m
Furadantin 35m
furosemide 47t
fusidic acid
52b, 56m
Fuzeon 25t

G

G115 87t
gabapentin 92b
Gabitril 93m
gadodiamide 51t
gadopentetate 51t
galantamine 112t
Gamimune 91m
gamma hydroxy-
butyrate 97t
Gammagard 91m
Gamunex 91m
ganciclovir 24t
ganirelix 99b
Garamycin
Antimicr 20t
Dermatol 52b
Ophth 105t
garcinia 86b
**Garcinia cambo-
gia** 86b
garlic supple-
ments 86b
Gastrocrom 119t
Gastrografin 51t
Gas-X 79t
gatifloxacin
Antimicr 34t
Ophth 105m
Gaviscon 77t
G-CSF 84m
gefitinib 104t
Gelclair 73m
gemcitabine 104t
gemfibrozil 43m
gemifloxacin 34m
gemtuzumab
104m
Gemzar 104t
Gengraf 91b

Genisoy 89t
Genoptic 105t
Genotropin 69t
Gentak 105t
gentamicin
Antimicr 20t
Dermatol 52b
Oph 105t, 106m
GenTeal 108m
Gentran 50m
Genxene 113t
Geodon 112t
GHB 97t
GI cocktail 78b
ginger 86b
ginkgo biloba 87t
Ginkgold 87t
Ginkoba 87t
Ginsai 87t
Ginsana 87t
ginseng 87t
glatiramer 95m
Glaucoma 107
Gleevec 104m
Gliadel 103b
gliclazide 61b
glimepiride 61b
glipizide 61t, 62t
GlucaGen 62m
glucagon 62m
Gluconorm 61b
Glucophage 61b
glucosamine 87m
glucose home
testing 62b
Glucotrol 62t
Glucovance 61b
GlucoWatch 62b
Glumetza 61b
Glutose 62t
glyburide 61t, 62t
glycerin 79b
GlycoLax 80t
glycopyrrolate80b
**Glycyrrhiza gla-
bra** 88t
**Glycyrrhiza ura-
lensis** 88t
Glynase PresTab
62t
Glyquin 57b
Glysennid 80t
Glyset 60m
GM-CSF 84m
GnRH Agonists
99
goldenseal 87t
GoLytely 80t
**Goody's Extra
Strength
Headache
Powder** 78b

goserelin
OB/GYN 99b
Oncology 104t
Gout-Related 63
gramicidin 105b
granisetron 75b
grape seed ex-
tract 87b
Gravol 75b
green goddess
78b
green tea 88t
Grifulvin V 20b
Grisactin 500 20b
griseofulvin 20b
growth hormone
human 69t
guaifenesin 72t
guanfacine 38t
guarana 87b
guggul 87b
guggulipid 87b
Guiatuss 72t
Gynazole 102m
Gyne-Lotrimin
102b
Gynodiol 97m

H

H pylori Rx 78
Habitrol 115t
haemophilus b
89b, 90b
Halcion 113b
Haldol 112m
HalfLytely 80t
Halfprin 44m
haloperidol 112m
Harpadol 86t
**Harpagophytum
procumben** 86t
Havrix 89b
hawthorn 87b
H-BIG 91b
HCE50 87b
HCTZ 43b
Healthy Woman
89t
HeartCare 87b
Hectorol 67t
Helidac 77b
Hemabate 102m
Hemcort HC 56m
Hemofil M 84m
Hemorrhoid care
56
Hepalean 83t
heparin 83t
hepatitis A inacti-
vated 90m
hepatitis A vac-
cine 89b

hepatitis B
89b, 90tm
Hepsera 26b
Heptovir 25m
HERBALS 84
Herceptin 104m
Hespan 50m
hetastarch 50m
Hexabrix 51m
Hexalen 103b
Hexit 54m
Hextend 50m
HibTITER 89b
histrelin 104t
Hivid 25b
homatropine107b
Hormone Re-
placement
combos 100
horse chestnut
seed extract
87b
HP-Pac 77b
huang qi 85t
huckleberry 85t
Humalog 63t
Humatin 23m
Humatrope 69t
Humulin 63t
hyaluronic acid
57m
hyaluronidase 69t
Hycamtin 104m
hydralazine
43b, 44t
HydraSense 74m
**Hydrastis cana-
densis** 87t
Hydrea 104t
hydrochlorothi-
azide
43tmb, 47b
Hydrocil 80m
hydrocodone 15b,
17mb, 18m
hydrocortisone
Derm 56m, 58t
Endocrine 59b
ENT 72mb
Ophth 106m
Hydrocortone 59b
**Hydromorph
Contin** 14b
hydromorphone
14b
hydroquinone
57m, 58m
hydroxychloro-
quine 10m
hydroxyproges-
terone 100b
hydroxyurea 104t

**131
Index**

t = top of page
m = middle of page
b = bottom of page

hydroxyzine 71m
hyoscyamine
  Gastro 78b, 79t
  Urology 121mb
      122t
Hyosol 121m
Hyospaz 121m
Hypaque 51t
Hypericum perfo-
  ratum 88b
Hypnotics 113
Hypotears 108m
Hytrin
  Cardiovas 38m
  Urology 121m
Hytuss 72t
Hyzaar 43m

I

ibandronate 59t
ibritumomab104m
ibuprofen
  13t, 17t, 18m
ibutilide 39m
Idamycin 103b
idarubicin 103b
IDV 26t
Ifex 103b
ifosfamide 103b
Ilotycin 105b
Imagent 51m
imatinib 103b
Imdur 48t
imipenem-
  cilastatin 27b
imipramine
  Psych 108b
  Urology 122m
imiquimod 55t
Imitrex 95t
Immucyst
  Immunol 89b
  Oncology 104t
immune globulin
      91m
Immunine VH 84t
Immunizations 89
Immunoglobulins
      91
Immunoprin 10m
Immunosuppres-
  sion 92
Imodium 75t
Imodium Advan-
  ced 74b
Imogam 91m
Imovane 114t
Imovax Rabies
     90m
Imuran 91m
inamrinone 49m
Inapsine 76t

indapamide 47b
Inderal 46t
Inderal LA 46t
Inderide 43m
indinavir 26t
Indocid 102t
Indocin
  Analgesics 13t
  OB/GYN 102t
Indocin SR 13t
indomethacin
  Analgesics 13t
  OB/GYN 102t
Infanrix 89b
InFed 27t
Infergen 27t
Inflamase 106b
infliximab
  Analgesics 10t
  Gastro 81t
influenza vaccine
     90t
Infufer 64b
INH 22m
Inhaled steroids
     118
Inhaler colors 117
Inhibace 36m
InhibacePlus 43m
Innohep 83t
InnoPran XL 46t
Inspra 37t
Insta-Glucose
     62m
insulin 63t
Intal 119t
Integrilin 44b
interferon alfa-2
    104m
interferon alfa-2b
    104t
  Antimicr 27m
  Oncology 104m
interferon alfa-
  con-1 27t
interferon alfa-n3
    104m
interferon beta-
  1A 95m
interferon beta-
  1B 95m
interleukin-2 104t
IntestiFlora 89b
Intralipid 65b
Intron A
  Antimicr 27t
  Oncology 104m
Intropin 49t
Invanz 27b
Invirase 26b
iodixanol 51t
Iodotope 66m
iohexol 51t

Ionamin 116t
iopamidol 51m
iothalamate 51m
ioversol 51t
ioxaglate 51m
ipecac syrup120b
IPOL 90m
ipratropium
  ENT 74t
  Pulm118t,119m
Iquix 105m
irbesartan
    37m, 43t
Iressa 104m
irinotecan 104m
iron dextran 64b
iron polysaccha-
  ride 64b
iron sucrose 64b
ISMO 48t
isocarboxazid
    109t
isometheptene
    95m
Isomil 75t
isoniazid 22mb
isopropyl alcohol
    72b
isoproterenol 39m
Isoptin 47t
Isopto Atropine
    107b
Isopto Carpine
    107m
Isopto Cetamide
    105b
Isopto Homatro-
  pine 107b
Isordil 48t
isosorbide 43t
isosorbide dini-
  trate 48t
isosorbide mono-
  nitrate 48t
Isotamine 22m
isotretinoin 52t
Isotrex 52t
Isovue 51m
isradipine 46m
Istalol 107t
Isuprel 39m
itraconazole 20b
IV solutions 64
Iveegam 91m
ivermectin 23t

J

Jantoven 83m
Japanese en-
  cephalitis 90t
JE-Vax 90t
Jolivette 98

Junel 98
Junel Fe 98

K

K+10 65t
K+8 65t
K+Care 65t
K+Care ET 65t
Kabikinase 50m
Kadian 16t
Kaletra 26t
Kaochlor 65t
Kaon 65t
Kaon Cl 65t
Kaopectate 74b
Kaopectate Stool
  Softener 79m
karela 85m
Kariva 98
Kay Ciel 65t
Kayexalate 69m
K-Dur 65t
Keflex 28b
Keftab 28b
Kefurox 29t
Kefzol 28m
Kelnor 98
Kenalog 60m
Kenalog in Ora-
  base 73b
Kepivance 104t
Keppra 93t
Kerlone 45t
Ketalar 19t
ketamine 19t
Ketek 31t
ketoconazole
  Antimicr 21t
  Dermatol 53b
ketoprofen 13t
ketorolac
  Analgesics 13m
  Ophth 108t
ketotifen
  Ophth 105t
  Pulm 119m
K-G Elixir 65t
Kidrolase 104t
Kineret 10t
Kira 88b
Klaron 52m
Klean-Prep 80t
K-Lease 65t
Klonopin
  Neurology 92m
  Psych 113t
K-Lor 65t
Klor-con 65t
Klorvess 65t

K+10 65t
Klorvess Effer-
  vescent 65
Klotrix 65
K-Lyte 65t
K-Lyte Cl 65
K-Norm 65
Kogenate 84m
Kolyum 65
kombucha tea87b
Kondremul 79b
Konsyl 80m
Konsyl Fiber 80t
Korean red gin-
  seng 87t
K-Phos 65t
Kristalose 79b
K-Tab 65
Ku-Zyme 81m
Ku-Zyme HP81m
K-vescent 65
Kwai 85m
Kwellada-P 54m
Kyolic 86b
Kytril 75m

L

labetalol 45m
Labor induction
    100
Lac-Hydrin 57m
Lacrilube 108m
Lactaid 81t
lactase 81t
lactic acid 57m
Lactinex 88m
Lactobacillus 88m
lactulose 79b
Lamictal
  Neurology 93t
  Psych 111t
Lamisil
  Antimicr 21t
  Dermatol 54t
Lamisil AT 54t
lamivudine 25m
lamotrigine
  Neurology 93t
  Psych 111t
Lanoxicaps 39t
Lanoxin 39t
lansoprazole
    77t, 79b
Lansoyl 79b
lanthanum car-
  bonate 69m
Lantus 63t

132
Index

t = top of page
m = middle of page
b = bottom of page

Lanvis 104t
Largactil 112b
Lariam 21b
Larrea divaricata 85b
Lasix 47m
latanoprost 107m
Laxatives 79
LDL goals 41
Lectopam 113t
leflunomide 10t
Legalon 88t
Lenoltec 18t
leopard's bane 85t
lepirudin 83m
Lescol 41t
Lessina 98
letrozole 104t
leucovorin 104m
Leukeran 103b
Leukine 84m
Leukotriene in-
hibitors 118
leuprolide
OB/GYN 99b
Oncology 104t
Leustatin 103b
levalbuterol 117m
levamisole 104m
Levaquin 34t
Levatol 45b
Levbid 121m
Levemir 63t
levetiracetam 93t
Levitra 123t
Levlen 98
Levlite 98
levobetaxolol 107t
levobunolol 107t
levobupivacaine 19b
levocabastine
ENT 74t
Ophth 104b
levocarnitine 65b
levodopa 96b
levofloxacin
Antimicr 34t
Ophth 105m
Levolet 66m
levonorgestrel 97m, 98, 100t
Levophed 49b
Levora 98
levorphanol 14b

Levo-T 66m
Levothroid 66m
levothyroxine 66m
Levoxyl 66m
Levsin
Gastro 79t
Urology 121m
Levsinex 121m
Lexapro 61t
Lexiva 26t
Lexxel 43m
LI-160 88b
Librax 81t
Librium 113t
licorice 85t
lidocaine
Anesth 19mb
Cardiovas 39m
Derm 57tm, 58t
lidocaine viscous 73m
Lidoderm 57m
lindane 54m
linezolid 35b
Lioresal 10b
liothyronine 66b
Lipidil Micro 42m
Lipidil Supra 42m
Lipitor 40b
Liposyn 65b
lisinopril 36b, 43b
Lithane 111t
lithium 111t
Lithobid 111t
Lithostat 123m
LiveBac 88m
Livostin 104b
Livostin Nasal Spray 74t
Lo/Ovral 98
Locals 19
LoCHOLEST 40m
Lodine 12b
Lodosyn 96m
lodoxamide 105t
Loestrin 98
Loestrin Fe 98
Lofibra 42m
lomefloxacin 33b
Lomine 78b
Lomotil 75t
lomustine 103b
Loperacap 75t
loperamide 74b, 75t
Lopid 42m
lopinavir-ritonavir 26t
Lopressor 45b
Lopressor HCT 43m
Loprox 53m

Lorabid 29t
loracarbef 29t
loratadine 69b
lorazepam
Neurology 93t
Psych 113t
Lorcet 17m
Lortab 17m
losartan 37b,43m
Losec 80t
Lotemax 106b
Lotensin 36t
Lotensin HCT 43m
loteprednol 106mb
Lotrel 43m
Lotriderm 56m
Lotrimin 53mb
Lotrimin Ultra 53m
Lotrisone 56m
Lotronex 80b
lovastatin 40b,41t
Lovenox 82m
Low-Ogestrel 98
Loxapac 112b
loxapine 112b
Loxitane 112b
Lozide 47b
Lozol 47b
LPV/r 26t
LS spine 94
L-Thyroxine 66m
Lumigan 107m
Luminal 93m
Lunesta 114t
Lupron
OB/GYN 99b
Oncology 104t
Lupron Depot 99b
Luride 64b
Lustra 57m
Lutera 98
Luvox 109b
lymphocyte im-
mune glob 91m
Lyrica 93t
Lysodren 104m

M

M.O.S. 16t
ma huang 84b
Maalox 77t
Macrobid 35m
Macrodantin 35m
Macrodex 50m
Macrolides 31
mafenide 52b
magaldrate 77t
Maganate 65t
magic mouth-
wash 73m

Maglucate 65t
magnesium car-
bonate
Analgesics 11m
Gastro 77t
mag chloride 64b
mag citrate 79b
mag gluconat 65t
mag hydroxide
Analgesics 11m
GI 77m,79b
mag oxide 65t
mag sulfate
Analgesics 11m
Endocrine 65t
Magnevist 51t
Mag-Ox 400 65t
Magtrate 65t
Malarone 21b
malathion 54m
maltodextrin 73m
Manchurian or
Kargasok 87b
mannitol 37t
Mantoux 91b
Marcaine 19b
Marine Lipid
Concentrat 65b
Marinol 75b
Marplan 109t
Marvelon 98
Matricaria recu-
tita - German
chamomile 85b
Matulane 103b
Mavik 37t
MAX EPA 65b
Maxair 117b
Maxalt 94b
Maxaquin 33b
Maxdex 76t
Maxidex 105t
Maxidone 17m
Max Strength
Pepcid 77m
Maxipime 29b
Maxitrol 106m
Maxzide 43m
MD-Gastroview 51t
measles mumps
& rubella 90t
measles mumps 90t
mechlorethamine 103b
Meclicot
Gastro 76t
Neurology 97t

meclizine
Gastro 76t
Neurology 97t
Medispaz 121m
Medivert
Gastro 76t
Neurology 97t
Medrol 60t
medroxyproges 100m, 101m
mefenamic acid 13m
mefloquine 21b
Mefoxin 29t
Megace 101m
Megacillin 31b
megestrol 101m
Melaleuca alter-
nifolia 89m
melaleuca oil 89m
Melanex 57m
melatonin 88t
Mellaril 112b
meloxicam 13m
melphalan 103b
memantine 92t
Menactra 90t
Menest 97m
Meni-D
Gastro 76t
Neurology 97t
meningococcal
vaccine 90t
Menjugate 90t
Menofem 85m
Menomune-
A/C/Y/W 90t
Menostar 97b
Mentax 53m
mepenzolate 79t
meperidine 14b
Mephyton 67t
mepivacaine 19b
Mepron 23t
mequinol 58t
mercaptopurine 104t
Meridia 116m
Meritate 120m
meropenem 28m
Merrem IV 28m
Mersyndol with
Codeine 17m
mesalamine 81t
Mesasal 81t
M-Eslon 16t
mesna 104t
Mesnex 104t
Mestinon 95b
mestranol 98
Metabolife 86m
Metadate 115b

133
Index

t = top of page
m = middle of page
b = bottom of page

Metadol
  Analgesics 16t
  Psych 114b
Metaglip 61t
Metamucil 80m
Metaprel 117m
metaproterenol
  117m
Metastron 104m
metaxalone 11t
metformin 61m
methadone
  Analgesics 16t
  Psych 114b
Methadose
  Analgesics 16t
  Psych 114b
methazolamide
  107t
Methblue 122m
methenamine
  121b, 122t
Methergine 100m
methimazole 66m
Methitest 58m
methocarbamol
  11t
methohexital 19t
methotrexate
  Analgesics 10m
  Oncology 103m
methyclothiazide
  43m
methyldopa
  38m, 43t
methylene blue
  Toxicol 120b
  Urology
  121b, 122m
methylergono-
vine 100m
Methylin 115b
methylphenidate
  115b
methylprednis-
olone 60t
methylsulfometh-
ane 88t
methyltestoster-
one
  Endocrine 58m
  OB/GYN 60m
Meticorten 60t
metipranolol 107t
metoclopramide
  76t
metolazone 48t
metoprolol

43m, 45b
Metrika A1CNow
  62m
MetroCream 53t
MetroGel 53t
MetroGel-Vaginal
  102b
MetroLotion 53t
metronidazole
  Antimic 23t,35m
  Dermatol 53t
  Gastro 77b
  OB/GYN 102b
Mevacor 41t
mexiletine 39b
Mexitil 39b
Miacalcin 68m
micafungin 21t
Micardis 37b
MicardisHCT 43b
MicardisPlus 43m
Micatin 53b
miconazole
  Dermatol 53b
  OB/GYN 102b
Micozole 102b
MICRhoGAM
  103m
Microgestin Fe 98
Micro-K 65
Micronase 60m
MicroNefrin 119m
Micronor 98
Microzide 47t
Midamor 47t
midazolam 19t
midodrine 49m
Midrin 95t
Mifeprex 103m
mifepristone
  103m
miglitol 60m
Migraine 94
Migra-Lief 86b
Migral 95t
MigraSpray 86b
mild & strong
  silver 89t
Milk of Magnesia
  79b
milk thistle 88t
milrinone 49b
mineral oil 79b
Minerals 63
Minestrin 1/20 98
Minipress 38m
Minirin
  Endocrine 69t
  Urology 122b
Minitran 48b
Minizide 43m
Minocin 34b

minocycline 34b
Min-Ovral 98
Minox 57b
minoxidil 57b
Mintezol 23b
MiraLax 79b
Mirapex 96m
Mircette 98
mirtazapine 110m
misoprostol
  Analgesics 12b
  Gastro 77b
  OB/GYN 100b
mitomycin 103b
Mitomycin-C 103b
mitotane 104m
mitoxantrone
  103b
Mivacron 19b
mivacurium 19b
M-M-R II 93t
Moban 112b
Mobic 13m
Mobicox 13m
moclobemide
  110m
modafinil 116t
Modecate 112m
Modeten 112m
Modicon 98
Modulon 81b
Moduret 47t
Moduretic 47t
moexipril 36b,43b
molindone 112b
mometasone
  ENT 74t
  Pulm 118m
Momordica cha-
rantia 85m
Monarc-M 84m
Monazole 102b
Monistat 102b
Monistat 1-Day
  103t
Monistat-Derm
  53b
Monistat 45t
Monitan 45t
Monoclate P 84m
Monocor 45t
Monodox 21b,34b
monogyna 85t
Monoket 48t
Mononine 84m
Monopril 36m
Monopril HCT
  43m
montelukast 118b

Morinda citrifolia
  88t
morphine 16t
Motofen 75t
Motrin 13t
Mouth and Lip
  preps 73
Movana 88b
moxifloxacin
  Antimic 34m
  Ophth 105m
MRI contrast 11t
MS Contin 16t
MSIR 16t
MSM 88t
Mucaine 76b
Mucinex 72t
Mucomyst
  Contrast 56m
  Pulmonary 119t
Mucosil 119t
Multiple sclerosis
  94
multivitamins 67t
mupirocin 53t
Murine Ear 72m
Muscle relaxants
  10b
Muse 122b
Mustargen 103b
Mutamycin 103b
MVI 67t
Myambutol 22m
Mycamine 21t
Mycelex
  Antimic 22m
  Dermatol 53b
  ENT 73t
Mycelex 7 102b
Mycelex-3 102b
Mycifradin 81t
Mycobutin 22t
Mycolog II 56m
mycophenolate
  mofetil 91b
Mycostatin
  Antimic 21t
  Dermatol 53b
  ENT 73t
  OB/GYN 103t
Mydfrin 108t
Mydriacyl 108t
Mydriatics 107
Myfortic 91b
Mylanta 73m
Mylanta Chil-
dren's 76b
Mylanta susp 73t
Myleran 103b
Mylicon 79t
Mylotarg 104m

Myocet 103b
Myotonachol
  122m
Mysoline 93m
M-Zole 102b

N

NABI-HB 91t
Nadopen-V 32t
nafarelin 99b
nafcillin 32m
naftifine 53b
Naftin 53b
nalbuphine 14t
Nalcrom 119t
nalidixic acid 33m
nalmefene 18b
naloxone
  Analgesics 18b
  Psych 115m
naltrexone 114b
Namenda 92t
nandrolone 58m
naphazoline 104m
Naphcon 104m
Naprelan 13b
Napron 13b
Naprosyn 13b
naproxen 13b
naratriptan 94b
Narcan 18b
Nardil 109t
Nasacort 74m
NaSal 74m
Nasal prepara-
tions 73
NasalCrom 74t
Nasalide 74t
Nasarel 74t
Nascobal 66b
Nasonex 74t
nateglinide 61b
Natrecor 50b
Navane 112m
Navelbine 104m
Nebcin 20t
NebuPent 23m
Necon 98
Necon 98
nedocromil
  Ophth 105t
  Pulmonary 119b
nefazodone 110m

t = top of page
m = middle of page
b = bottom of page

NegGram 33m
nelfinavir 26m
Nembutal 19m
neomycin
  Derm 53t, 56m
  ENT 72mb
  Gastro 81t
  Ophth 105b, 106m
Neoral 91b
Neosar 103b
Neosporin cream 53t
Neosporin ointment
  Dermatol 53t
  Ophth 105b
Neosporin solution 105b
neostigmine 95b
Neostrata 57m
Neo-Synephrine
  Cardiovas 49b
  ENT 74m
  Ophth 108t
Nephrocap 67t
Nephrolithiasis 123
Nephron 119m
Nephrovite 67t
Neptazane 107t
Nerve roots 94
nesiritide 50b
NESP 83b
Neulasta 84m
Neumega 84m
Neupogen 84m
Neuromuscular blockers 19
Neurontin 92b
Neutra-Phos 67t
Neutrexin 23b
nevirapine 24b
Nexium 78t
NFV 26m
niacin
  Cardio 40b, 42b
  Endocrine 67m
niacinamide 66b
Niacor
  Cardiovas 42b
  Endocrine 67m
Niaspan
  Cardiovas 42b
  Endocrine 67m

Niastase 84t
nicardipine 46m
Nicoderm 115t
Nicolar 42b
Nicorette 114b
Nicorette inhaler 115t
nicotine gum 115t
nicotine inhalation 115t
nicotine lozenge 115t
nicotine nasal spray 115t
nicotine patches 115t
nicotinic acid 42b
Nicotrol 115t
Nidazol 23t, 35m
nifedipine
  Cardiovas 46m
  OB/GYN 102t
Niferex 64b
Nilandron 104t
Nilstat
  Antimicr 21t
  Dermatol 53b
  ENT 73m
nilutamide 104t
Nimbex 19b
nimodipine 47m
Nimotop 47m
Nipent 104t
Nipride 44t
nisoldipine 46m
nitazoxanide 23t
Nitrates 48
Nitro-BID 48b
Nitro-Dur 48b
nitrofurantoin 35m
nitroglycerin IV infusion 48m
nitroglycerin ointment 48m
nitroglycerin spray 48m
nitroglycerin sublingual 48b
nitroglycerin sus release 48b
nitroglycerin transderm 48b
nitroglycerin transmucosal 48b
Nitroguard 48b
Nitrol 48m
Nitrolingual 48b
Nitropress 44t
nitroprusside 44t
NitroQuick 48b

Nitrostat 48m
Nix 54m
nizatidine 77m
Nizoral
  Antimicr 21t
  Dermatol 53b
NoDoz 115b
Nolvadex 101b
noni 88t
Nonsteroidals table 13
Nora-BE 98
Norco 17b
Norcuron 19b
Nordette 98
Norditropin 69t
norelgestromin 97m
norepinephrine 49b
norethindrone 98, 100tm
Norflex 11t
norfloxacin 33b
Norgesic 11b
norgestimate 98, 100m
norgestrel 98
Norinyl 98
Noritate 53t
Noroxin 33b
Norpace 39t
Norpramin 108b
Nor-Q.D. 98
Nortrel 98
nortriptyline 109t
Norvasc 46m
Norvir 26m
Nostril 74m
Nostrilla 74m
Novamoxin 32m
Novantrone 103b
Novasen
  Analgesics 12b
  Cardiovas 44m
Novasoy 89t
Novolin 63t
NovoLog 63t
NovoRapid 63t
NovoSeven 84t
Novothyrox 66m
NSAIDs 12, 13
Nubain 14t
Nu-Iron 64b
Nu-Iron 150 64b
NuLev
  Gastro 79t
  Urology 121m
NuLytely 80t
Numby Stuff 57m
Numorphan 16m
Nupercainal 56m

Nuprin 13t
Nuromax 19b
Nursoy 65b
Nutramigen Lipil 65b
Nutritionals 65b
Nutropin 69t
NuvaRing 97m
NVP 24b
Nyaderm
  Antimicr 21t
  Dermatol 53b
  OB/GYN 103t
nystatin
  Antimicr 21t
  Derm 53b, 56m
  ENT 73m
  OB/GYN 103t
Nytol
  ENT 71m
  Psych 114t

O

Oaklide 104t
oatmeal 57b
Ocean 74m
Octagam 91m
Octostim 84t
octreotide 84t
OcuCarpine 107t
Ocuflox 105m
Ocupress 106b
Ocusert 107t
Oenothera biennis 86m
Oesclim 97b
Oesctrol 97m
ofloxacin
  Antimicr 33b
  ENT 72b
  Ophth 105m
Ogen 99t
Ogestrel 98
olanzapine 111b, 114m
olmesartan 37b, 43b
olopatadine 104b
olsalazine 81m
Omacor 65b
omega-3 fatty acid 65b
omeprazole 78t
Omnicef 29m
Omnipaque 51t
Omniscan 51t
Oncaspar 104m
Oncotice Immunol 89b
Oncology 104t
Oncovin 104t
ondansetron 75m
One-a-day 87b, 88b, 89m
OneTouch 62m
Ontak 104t
Onxol 104m
Ophthaine 108m
Ophthetic 108m
Opioid equival 15
Opioids 14
opium tincture 75t
oprelvekin 84m
Oprisine 10m
Opticrom 105t
Optimine 71t
Optipranolol 107t
Optiray 51m
Optivar 104b
Oracit 123m
Oracort 73b
OraDisc A 73t
Oral contraceptives 98
Oramorph SR 16t
Orap 112m
Orapred 60t
orciprenaline 117m
ORDERING INFO 143
Oretic 47b
Orgalutran 99b
Orimune 90m
orlistat 81b
orphenadrine 11b
Ortho Evra 97m
Ortho Novum 98
Ortho-Cept 98
Ortho-Cyclen 98
Ortho-Est 99m
Ortho-Novum 98
Orudis 13m
Oruvail 13m
Orvaten 49m
Os-Cal 63b
oseltamivir 26b
Osmitrol 97t
Ostac 59t
Osteoforte 68m
Outpatient peds drugs 6
Ovcon 98
Ovide 54m
Ovol 79t
Ovral 98
Ovrette 98
Ovulation Stimulants 100
oxacillin 32m
oxaliplatin 104m
Oxandin 58m
oxandrolone 58m
oxaprozin 13b
oxazepam 113b

oxcarbazepine93t	Parcopa 96t	pentazocine	PhosLo 63b	**135** **Index** t = top of page m = middle of page b = bottom of page
Oxeze 117m	paregoric 75t	14m, 18t	phosphorated	
oxiconazole 54t	paricalcitol 67b	pentobarbital 19m	carbohydrates	
Oxistat 54t	Pariet 73t	Pentolair 107b	76t	
Oxizole 54t	Parkinsons 94	pentosan 122m	phosphorus 65t	
oxprenolol 45b	Parlodel	pentostatin 104t	Photofrin 104m	
oxyaxantha	Endocrine 68m	Pentothal 19m	Phrenilin 12t	polyethylene
oxybate 97t	Neurology 89m	pentoxifylline 50b	Phyllocontin 119t	glycol 80b
Oxybutyn 121b	Parnate 109m	Pen-Vee K 32t	Phyto Joint 86t	polyethylene gly-
oxybutynin 121b	paromomycin23m	Pepcid 77m	phytonadione 67b	col w lytes 80t
Oxycocet 17b	paroxetine 109b	Peptic Relief 77b	Phytosoya 89t	Polygam 91m
Oxycodan 17b	Parvolex	Pepto-Bismol 74b	Pilocar 107m	Polymox 32m
oxycodone	Contrast 51m	Percocet 17b	pilocarpine	polymyxin
16m, 17tb, 18t	Pulmonary 121t	Percodan 17b	ENT 73b	Derm 53t, 56m
OxyContin 16m	Toxicology119b	Percolone 16m	Ophth 107m	ENT 72mb
Oxyderm 51b	Patanol 108b	perflexane 51m	Pilopine HS107m	Ophth
OxyFAST 16m	Paullinia cupana	pergolide 96m	pimecrolimus 56t	105b, 106m
OxyIR 16m	87b	Periactin 127t	pimozide 112m	polymyxin B 105b
oxymetazoline	Pausinystalia	Peri-Colace 80t	pinaverium 81m	Polysporin
74m	yohimbe 89m	Peridex 73t	pindolol 45b	Dermatol 53t
oxymorphone	Pavulon 19b	perindopril 36b	Pinworm 23m	Ophth 105b
16m	Paxil 109b	Periogard 73t	Pin-X 23m	Polytar 57t
oxytocin 100b	Paxil CR 109b	Periostat	pioglitazone 61m	polythiazide43mb
Oxytrol 121b	PCO 87m	Antimic 34b	Piper methysti-	Polytopic 53t
	Peak flow 117t	ENT 73m	cum 87b	Polytrim 105b
P	PediaCare 72t	Permax 96m	piperacillin 33t	Pondocillin 33m
	Pediapred 60t	permethrin 54m	piperacillin-tazo-	Ponstan 13m
P.C.E. 31m	Pediarix 90t	perphenazine	bactam 33m	Ponstel 13m
Pacerone 38b	Pediatrix 18b	112b	piperonyl butox-	Pontocaine 19b
Pacis	Pediazole 31b	Persantine 44m	ide 54m	porfimer 104m
Immunol 89b	Pediotic 72b	Petadolex 85m	pirbuterol 117b	Portia 98
Oncology 104t	Peds immuniza-	Petaforce 85m	piroxicam 13m	potassium 65t
paclitaxel 104t	tions 90	Petasites hybri-	Pitocin 100b	potassium forms
palifermin 104t	Peds rehydrat 66	dus 85m	Pitressin 69b	65
palivizumab 85b	Peds vitals drug 7	pethidine 14t	pivampicillin 33t	Potent V 89m
palonosetron75m	PedvaxHIB 89b	petrolatum 108m	plague 90t	Power-Dophilus
pamabrom	pegaspargase	Pexeva 109b	Plan B 97m	91b
Pamelor 109t	104t	PGE1,PGE2100b	Plaquenil 10m	PPD 91b
pamidronate 59t	Pegasys 27m	Pharmorubicin	Plasbumin 50b	pralidoxime 120b
Panadol 18b	pegfilgrastim 84m	103b	plasma protein	pramipexole 96m
Panafil 57b	peginterferon	Phazyme 79t	fraction 50b	pramlintide 63m
Panax ginseng	alfa-2a 27m	Phenazo 122m	Plasmanate 50b	Pramosone 58t
87t	peginterferon	phenazopyridine	Plasmatein 50b	Pramox HC 58t
Panax quinque-	alfa-2b 27m	122m	Platinol-AQ 104m	pramoxine
folius L. 87t	PEG-Intron 27m	phenelzine 109t	Plavix 44m	56m, 58t
Pancrease 81m	Peg-Lyte 80t	Phenergan	Plenaxis 104t	Prandase 60m
pancreatin 81m	pemetrexed 104t	ENT 73m	Plendil 46t	Prandin 61b
Pancrecarb 81m	pemirolast 109b	Gastro 76m	Pletal 50b	Prasterone 85t
pancrelipase 81m	Penbritin 33t	pheniramine104m	Pneumo 23 90t	Pravachol 41t
pancuronium 19b	penbutolol 45b	phenobarbital	pneumococcal	pravastatin 41t
Panglobulin 91m	penciclovir	Gastro 78b	vaccine 90t	praziquantel 23m
Panixine Disper-	Dermatol 57b	Neurology 93m	Pneumovax 90t	prazosin
Dose 28b	ENT 73m	phentermine 116t	Pnu-Imune 90t	38m, 43b
Panretin 57b	penicillamine120b	phentolamine 44t	Podocon-25 54t	Precedex 19m
Pantoloc 78b	penicillin G 33t	phenyl salicylate	Podofilm 54t	Precision 62m
pantoprazole78m	penicillin V 33t	121b, 122t	podofilox 54t	Precose 60m
pantothenic acid	Penicillins 31	phenylephrine	Podofin 54t	Pred Forte 106b
66b, 87b	Penlac 57b	Cardiovas 49b	podophyllin 54t	Pred G 106m
papain 57b	Pentacarinat 23m	ENT 72t, 74m	Polaramine 71m	Pred Mild 106b
paracetamol 18t	Pentam 23m	Ophth 108t	polio vacci 90t	prednisolone
Parafon Forte	pentamidine 23m	Phenytek 93t	Polocaine 19b	Endocrine 60t
DSC 10b	Pentasa 81t	phenytoin 93t	polycarbophil 80t	Ophth 106tmb
Paraplatin 104m			Polycitra 123m	

**136
Index**

t = top of page
m = middle of page
b = bottom of page

prednisone 60m
Pred-Pak 60t
Prefest 100m
pregabalin 97b
Prelone 60t
Premarin 99m
Premesis 103m
Premphase 100m
PremPlus 100m
Prempro 100m
Pre-Pen 31b
Prepidil 100b
Pressors 49
Pressyn AR 69b
Pretz 74m
Prevacid 78t
Prevalite 40m
Previfem 98
Prevnar 90m
PrevPac 77b
Priftin 22b
prilocaine 57t
Prilosec 78m
Primacor 49b
　88m
Primadophilus
　88m
primaquine 22t
Primaxin 27b
primidone 93m
Primsol 35b
Principen 33t
Prinivil 36b
Prinzide 43b
Priorix 90t
ProAmatine 49m
Pro-Banthine 79t
probenecid 63mb
Probiotica 88b
probiotics 88m
procainamide 39b
procaine penicil-
lin 31b, 32t
Procanbid 39b
procarbazine103b
Procardia
　Cardiovas 43m
　OB/GYN 102t
Prochieve 101m
prochlorperazine
　76t
Procrit 84t
Proctofoam 56b
procyanidolic oli-
gomers 87b
Prodium 122m
ProdiumPlain80m

Pro-Fast 116t
progesterone gel
　101t
progesterone mi-
cronized 101b
Progestins 100
Proglycem 62m
Prograf 91b
proguanil 21b
Proleukin 104t
Prolixin 112m
Proloprim 35b
Promega 65b
Promensil 88b
Pro-Meta 117m
promethazine
　ENT 71m
　Gastro 76m
Prometrium 101b
Promotion 87m
Pronestyl 39b
Propacet 17b
propafenone 39b
Propanthel 79t
propantheline 79t
proparacaine
　108m
Propecia 57m
propofol 19m
propoxyphene
　16b, 17b, 18m
propranolol
　43m, 46t
Propyl Thyracil
　　　　22b, 35m
Propylene glycol
　72b, 73m
propylthiouracil
　66m
Proquin XR 33b
Proscar 121t
Prosed/DS 121b
Prosobee 65b
ProSom 113m
Prostata 88b
Prostatonin 88m
Prostep 115t
Prostigmin 95b
Prostin E2 100b
Prostin VR 52m
protamine 84m
Protenate 50b
Protonix 78m
Protopam 120b
Protopic 56t
protriptyline 109t
Protropin 69t
Protylol 78b
Proventil 116b
Provera 101m
Provigil 116t
Provol 88m

Prozac 109m
pseudoephedrine
　72t
Pseudofrin 72t
psyllium 80m
PTU 66m
Pulmicort 118m
Pulmozyme119m
Purge 79m
Purinethol 104t
Purinol 63m
PVF-K 32t
pycnogenol 88b
pygeum african-
um 88b
pyrantel 23m
pyrazinamide
　22m
Pyridiate 122m
Pyridium 122m
pyridostigmine95b
pyridoxine
　Endocrine 66b,
　67m, 68t
　Gastro 75b
pyrimethamine
　21b, 23m
PZA 22m

Q

QT interval drugs
　9
Quadramet 104m
Quanterra 88b
Quanterra Mental
　Sharpness 87t
Quelicin 19b
Questran 40m
quetiapine 111b
Quick-Pep 115b
quinapril 36b, 43t
quinidine
　Antimicr 12t
　Cardiovas 40t
quinine 11t, 22t
Quinolones 11
quinupristin 35b
Quixin 105m
QVAR 118m

R

R&C 54m
RabAvert 90m
rabeprazole 78t
rabies immune
　globulin 91m
rabies vaccine
　90m
Radiography
　contrast 51
rally pack 65b

raloxifene 101b
ramelteon 114t
ramipril 36b
Raniclor 28b
ranitidine 77b
Rapamune 91b
Rapinex 78m
Raptiva 92b
rauwolfia 43b
Rauzide 43b
Razadyne 92t
Reactine 71t
Rebetol 27b
Rebetron 27m
Rebif 95m
Reclipsen 98
Recombinate84m
Recombivax HB
　90t
red clover isofla-
vone 88b
Redoxon 66b
ReFacto 84m
Refludan 83m
Refresh 108m
Regitine 44t
Reglan 76t
Regonal 95b
Regranex 56b
Rejuva-A 52m
Relafen 13m
Relenza 26b
Relief 108t
Relpax 94b
Remeron 110m
Remicade
　Analgesics 10t
　Gastro 81t
Remifemin 85m
Renagel 69b
Renedil 46t
Renese-R 43b
Renocal 51t
Renografin 51t
ReoPro 84t
repaglinide 61b
Requip 96b
Rescula 107m
Resectisol 51t
RespiGam 91m
Restasis 108t
Restoril 113m
Restylane 52m
Retavase 50m
reteplase 50m
Retin-A 52m
Retisol-A 52m
Retrovir 25b
Revatio 122b
Reversol 95b

Revex 18m
Rev-Eyes 108m
ReVia 114b
Reyataz 25b
Rheomacrodx 50m
Rheumatrex
　Analgesics 10m
　Oncology 104t
Rhinalar 74t
Rhinocort Aqua
　73b
RHO immune
　globulin 103m
Rhodacine 13t
Rhodis 13m
RhoGAM 103m
Rhotral 45t
Rhovail 13m
ribavirin 27mb
riboflavin
　66b, 67m, 68t
RID 54m
Rideril 112b
rifabutin 22m
Rifadin 22b, 35m
rifampin 22b,35m
rifapentine 22b
Rifater 22b
rifaximin 35b
Rilutek 97t
riluzole 97t
Rimactane
　22b, 35m
rimantadine 26b
rimexolone 106b
Rimostil 88b
Riomet 61m
Riopan 77t
Ripped Fuel 88b
risedronate 59m
Risperdal 112t
risperidone 112t
Ritalin 115b
ritonavir 26m
Rituxan 104m
rivastigmine 92t
Rivotril
　Neurology 92m
　Psych 113t
rizatriptan 94b
Robaxin 11t
Robinul 80b
Robitussin 72t
Rocaltrol 66b
Rocephin 29b
rocuronium 19b
Rofact 22b, 35m
Roferon-A 104m
Rogaine 57b
Rogitine 44t

137
Index

t = top of page
m = middle of page
b = bottom of page

Rolaids 77t
Rolaids Calcium
Rich 76b
Romazicon 120b
ropinirole 96b
Rosasol 53t
rosiglitazone61tb
Rosula 52t
rosuvastatin 42t
Rowasa 81t
Roxanol 16t
Roxicet 17b
Roxicodone 16m
Rozerem 114t
RSV immune
globulin 91m
RTV 26m
RU-486 103m
Rubex 103b
Rubini 86m
Rufen 13t
Rylosol 40t
Rythmodan 39b
Rythmol 39b

S

S.A.S.
Analgesics 10m
Gastro 81b
S-2 119m
Saccharomyces
boulardii 88b
s-adenosylmeth-
ionine 88b
Saint John's wort
88b
Saizen 69t
Salagen 73b
Salazopyrin
Analgesics 10m
Gastro 81b
salbutamol 118t
Salflex 12m
salicin 89m
Salicis cortex89m
saline nasal
spray 74m
Salix alba 89m
salmeterol
117b, 118t
Salofalk 81t
salsalate 12m
samarium 153
104m
Sambucas nigra
86m
Sambucol 86m
SAM-e 88b
sammy 88b
Sanctura 122t
Sandimmune 91b
Sandoglobul 91m

Sandostatin 81m
Sans-Acne 52t
saquinavir 26m
Sarafem 109m
sargramostim
84m
saw palmetto 88b
SBE prophylaxis
32
scopolamine
76m, 78b
SeaMist 74m
Sea-Omega 65b
Seasonale 98
SecreMax 81b
secretin 81b
Sectral 45t
Sedapap 12t
Select 1/35 98
Selective Estro-
gen Receptor
Modulators101
selegiline 96b
selenium sulfide
58
Selpak 96b
Selsun 58t
senna 80m
sennosides 80t
Senokot 80t
Sensipar 68b
Sensorcaine 19m
Septocaine 19m
Septra 50m
Ser-Ap-Es 43b
Serax 113b
Serenoa repens
88b
Serevent Diskus
117b
Serophene 100b
Seroquel 115b
Serostim LQ 69t
sertaconazole54t
sertraline 110t
sevelamer 69m
Seville orange
85m
shark cartilage
89t
Sibelium 95m
sibutramine 116m
Siladryl
114t, 116b
sildenafil 122b
Silvadene 53m
silver-colloidal 89t
silver ion 89t
silver sulfadiaz-
ine 53m
Silybum mari-
anum 88t

silymarin 88t
simethicone
74b, 77t, 79t
Similac 65b
Simulect 91b
simvastatin 42t
Sinemet 96m
Sinequan 108b
Sinex 74m
Singulair 118b
Sinupret 86m
sirolimus 91b
Skelaxin 11t
Slo-Fe 64m
Slow-Fe 64m
Slow-K 65
Slow-Mag 64b
Slow-Niacin 67m
Slow-Trasicor45b
smallpox 90m
sodium ferric glu-
conate 65m
sodium iodide I-
131 66m
sodium phosphat
Gastro 80m
Urology 122t
sodium polysty-
rene 69m
sodium sulfacet-
amide
Derm 51b, 52m
Ophth 106tm
Solag 58t
Solagé 58t
Solaquin 59m
Solaraze 52b
solifenacin 121b
Solu-Cortef 59b
Solugel 51b
Solu-Medrol 60t
Soma 11t
Soma Comp 12t
Soma Compound
w Codeine 18t
Somatropin 69t
Sominex
114t, 116b
Somnote 113b
Sonata 114t
sorbitol 80m
Soriatane 54b
Sotacor 40t
sotalol 40t
Sotamol 40t
Sotret 52t
soy 89t
Soyalac 65b
Spacol 121m
Spasdel 121m
Spectazole 53m

Spectracef 29m
Spiriva 117b
spironolactone
37m, 43t
Sporanox 20b
Sprintec 98
SQV 26m
SSD 53m
St John's wort
88b
Stadol 14t
Stalevo 96b
starch 56b
Starlix 61b
Starnoc 114t
Statex 16t
stavudine 25m
Stay Awake 115b
Stelazine 112m
Stemetil 76t
Sterapred 60m
stevia 89t
Stevia rebaudi-
ana 89t
Stieprox sham-
poo 53m
Stieva-A 52t
Stimate
Endocrine 69t
Hematology 84t
Stimulants 115
stinging nettle 88t
Strattera 110t
Streptase 50m
streptokinase50m
streptomycin 20t
streptozocin 103b
Striant 58m
Stromectol 23t
strontium-89104m
Sublimaze 14m
Suboxone 115m
Subutex 114m
succimer 121t
succinylcholine
19b
sucralfate 79m
Sudafed 72t
Sulamyd 105b
Sular 46m
Sulcrate 79m
Sulf-10 105b
sulfacetamide
Sulfacet-R 52m
sulfadiazine 34m
sulfadoxine 21b
Sulfamylon 52b
sulfasalazine
Analgesics 10m
Gastro 81b

Sulfatrim 34b
sulfisoxazole 31b
sulfonated phe-
nolics 73t
sulfur 51b, 52m
sulfuric acid 73t
sulindac 13b
sumatriptan 95t
Sumycin 34b
SuperEPA 65b
Supeudol 16m
Supplifem88b,89t
Suprax 29m
Supro 89t
Surgam 14t
Surpass 76b
Sustiva 25b
Swim-Ear 72b
Symax 121m
Symbicort 118t
Symbyax 114m
Symlin 63m
Symmetrel
Antimicr 26b
Neurology 96t
Sympathomim115
Symphytum 86t
Synacthen 68b
Synagis 27t
Synalgos-DC 18t
Synarel 99b
Synera 58t
Synercid 35b
Synphasic 98
Syntest 100m
Synthroid 66m

T

T-20 24m
T3, T4 66m
Tabloid 104t
tacrolimus
Dermatol 56t
Immunol 91b
tadalafil 122t
Tagamet 77m
Talacen 18t
Talwin 14m
Tambocor 39m
Tamiflu 26b
Tamofen 101b
Tamone 101b
tamoxifen 101b
tamsulosin 121t
Tanacetum par-
thenium L. 86b

t = top of page
m = middle of page
b = bottom of page

Tapazole 66m
Tarabine 104m
Tarceva 104t
Targretin 104m
Tarka 43b
Tarsum 57t
Tasmar 96t
Tavist 71t
Tavist ND 69b
Taxol 104m
Taxotere 104m
tazarotene 52m
Tazicef 29m
Tazocin 33m
Tazorac 52t
Taztia XT 46b
Td 25t
TDF 25m
tea tree oil 89m
Tears Naturale
  108m
Tebrazid 25t
Tecnal 11b
Tecnal C 17m
tegaserod 81b
Tegens 85t
Tegretol
  Neurology 92m
  Psych 110b
Tegrin 57t
telithromycin 35t
telmisartan
  37b, 43m
temazepam 113m
Temodal 103b
Temodar 103b
temozolomide
  103b
Tempra 18b
tenecteplase 50m
Tenex 38t
teniposide 104m
Ten-K 65
tenofovir 25b
Tenoretic 43b
Tenormin 45t
Tensilon 48t
Tequin 34t
Terazol 103t
terazosin
  Cardiovas 38t
  Urology 121m
terbinafine
  Antimicr 21t
  Dermatol 54t
terbutaline

OB/GYN 102t
Pulmonary117b
terconazole 103t
teriparatide 58m
Tesalin 85m
Teslac 104t
Tessalon 71b
Testim 58t
testolactone 104t
Testopel 58b
testosterone 58m
tetanus immune
  globulin 87m
tetanus toxoid 90m
tetracaine
  Dermatol 58t
  ENT 74m
  Ophth 108m
tetracycline
  Antimicr 34b
  Gastro 75b
Tetracyclines 34
Teveten 37b
Teveten HCT 43b
Tev-Tropin 69t
Thalitone 47b
Theo-24 119b
Theo-Dur 119b
Theolair 119b
theophylline 119b
TheraCys 104t
Therapeutic drug
  levels 5
Theroxidil Extra
  Strength 57b
thiabendazole23b
thiamine
  66b, 67m, 68t
thiethylperazi76m
thioguanine 104t
thiopental 19m
Thioplex 103t
thioridazine 112b
thiotepa 103t
thiothixene 112m
Thisylin 88t
thonzonium 72m
Thorazine 112b
Thrombolysis in
  MI 50
Thrombolytics 49
Thyroid agents 66
Thyro-Tabs 66t
tiagabine 93m
tiaprofenicacid14t
Tiazac 46b
Ticar 33m
ticarcillin 33m
ticarcillin-clavu-
  lanate 33t

Tice BCG
  Immunol 89b
  Oncology 104t
Ticlid 44b
ticlopidine 44b
Tigan 76m
tigecycline 35b
Tilade 119b
Timentin 33m
Timolide 43b
timolol
  Cardio 43b, 46t
  Ophth 107b
Timoptic 107t
Tinactin 54t
Tindamax 23b
tinidazole 23b
tinzaparin 83t
tioconazole 103t
tiotropium 119b
tipranavir 26m
tirofiban 44b
Titralac 76b
tizanidine 11m
TNKase 50m
TOBI 20t
TobraDex 106m
tobramycin
  Antimicr 20t
  Oph 105t, 106m
Tobrex 105t
Tocolytics 102
tocopherol 68t
Tofranil
  Psych 108b
tolcapone 96t
Tolectin 14t
tolmetin 14t
tolnaftate 54t
tolterodine 122t
topical steroids55
Topamax
  Neurology 93b
  Psych 111m
Toposar 104m
topotecan 104m
Toprol-XL 45t
Toradol 13m
Torecan 76m
toremifene 104t
torsemide 47m
tositumomab
  104m

Tracrium 19b
tramadol 12t, 18b
Trandate 45m
trandolapril
  37t, 43b
Transderm-Scop
  76m
Tranxene 113b
tranylcypromine
  109m
Trasicor 45b
trastuzumab104m
Trasylol 83b
Travatan 107m
travoprost 107m
trazodone 110b
trefoil 88b
tretinoin
  Derm52m, 58b
  Oncology 104m
Trexall
  Analgesics 10m
  Oncology 104t
triamcinolone
  Dermatol 56m
  Endocrine 62b
  ENT 73b, 74m
  Pulm 118m
Triaminic Infant
  Drops 72t
triamterene 43m
Trianal 11b
Triatec 18t
Triazide 43m
triazolam 113b
Tricor 42m
Tri-Cyclen 98
triethanolamine
  72b
trifluoperazine
  112m
trifluridine 106t
Trifolium prat-
  ense 86m
Triglide 42m
Trigonella 86m
trihexyphenidy96t
TriHIbit 90b
Tri-K 65
Trikacide23t,35m
Trilafon 112m
Trileptal 93t
Tri-Levlen 98
Trilisate 14t
Tri-Luma 58m
TriLyte 80t
trimebutine 76m
trimethobenza-
  mide 76m

trimethoprim
  Antimicr 35t
  Ophth 105t
trimethoprim-sul-
  famethox 34b
trimetrexate 23b
Trimox 32t
Tri-Nasal 74m
Trinessa 98
Trinipatch 48b
Tri-Norinyl 98
Trinovin 88b
Tripacel 89b
Tripedia 89b
Triphasil 98
Tri-Previfem 98
triptorelin 104t
Triquilar 98
Trisenox 104m
Tri-Sprintec 98
Trivora-28 98
Trizivir 25m
tropicamide 108t
trospium 122t
True Track Smart
  System 62m
Trusopt 107t
Truvada 25b
tuberculin PPD
  91b
Tubersol 91b
Tucks 56b
Tums
  Endocrine 63b
  Gastro 76b
Twinject 49m
Twinrix 90m
Tygacil 35b
Tylenol 18b
Tylenol with Co-
  deine 18t
Tylox 18t
Typherix 90b
Typhim Vi 90b
typhoid vaccine
  90b

U

ubiquinone 85b
Ultracet 18t
Ultradol 12b
Ultram 12b
Ultraquin 57t
Ultrasound con-
  trast 51
Unasyn 33m
Unidet 122t
Uniphyl 119b
Uniretic 43b
Unisom Night-
  time Sleep 75b
Unithroid 66m

**139
Index**

t = top of page
m = middle of page
b = bottom of page

Univasc 36b
unoprostone 107m
urea 57b
Urecholine 122t
Urised 122t
Unispas 121t
Urocit-K 123t
Urodol 122t
Urogesic 122t
urokinase 91m
Urolene blue
  Toxicology 120b
Urology 122m
Uromitexan 104t
UroXatral 121t
URSO 81b
ursodiol 81b
Ursofalk 81b
Urtica dioica
  radix 88t
Usept 122t
UTA 122t
Uterotonics 122t
UTI Relief 122m

V

Vaccinium mac-
  rocarpon 86t
Vaccinium myrtil-
  lus 85t
Vagifem 99t
Vaginitis 30, 102
Vagistat-1 103t
valacyclovir 24m
Valcyte 24t
valerian 89m
Valeriana offici-
  nalis 89m
valganciclovir 24t
Valium
  Analgesics 10b
  Neurology 92m
  Psych 113m
valproic acid
  Neurology 93b
  Psych 113m
valrubicin 103b
valsartan
  37b, 43m
Valstar 103b
Valtaxin 103b
Valtrex 24m
Vancenase 73b
Vancocin 35b
vancomycin 35b
Vaniqa 57t
Vanspar 113b
Vantas 104t
Vantin 29m
Vaponefrin 119m
Vaqta 89b
vardenafil 123t

varicella vaccine
  90b
varicella-zoster
  imm glob 91m
Varilrix 90b
Varivax 90b
Vascon-A 104m
Vascoray 51m
Vaseretic 43b
Vasocidin 106m
Vasocon 104m
Vasotec 35b
Vaxigrip 90t
VCR 104m
vecuronium 19b
Veetids 32t
Velban 104m
Velcade 104m
Velivet 98
Venastat 47t
venlafaxine 110b
Venofer 65b
Venoglobulin 91m
Ventodisk 116b
Ventolin 116b
VePesid 104m
Veramil 47t
verapamil 43b,47t
Verelan 47t
Vermox 23t
Versed 19m
Versel 58t
Vesanoid 104m
VEScare 121b
vetch 85t
Vexol 106b
Vfend 21m
Viactiv 63b
Viadur 104t
Viagra 122b
Vibramycin
  Antimi 21b,34b
  Dermatol 52t
Vibra-Tabs 21b
Vick's 71b
Vicodin 18m
Vicoprofen 18m
vidarabine 106t
Vidaza 103b
Videx 25t
Vigamox 105m
vinblastine 104m
Vincasar 104m
vincristine 104m
vinorelbine 104m
Viokase 81m
Vira-A 106t
Viracept 26m
Viramune 24b
Virazole 27m
Viread 25m

Virilon 58m
Virilon IM 58m
Viroptic 106t
Visicol 80m
Visine-A 104m
Visipaque 51t
Visken 45b
Vistaril 71m
Vistide 23b
vitamin A 68t
Vitamin A Acid
  Cream 52t
vitamin B1 68t
vitamin B2 68t
vitamin B3
  Cardiovas 42b
  Endocrine 67m
vitamin B6 68t
vitamin B12 66b
vitamin C
  66b, 67b
vitamin D
  67t, 68m
vitamin D2 68b
vitamin E 68t
vitamin K 67b
Vitamins 66t
Vitex agnus 85b
Vitus vinifera 87m
Vivactil 109t
Vivarin 115b
Vivelle 97b
Vivol
  Analgesics 10b
  Neurology 92m
  Psych 113m
Vivotif Berna 90b
VLB 104m
VM-26 104m
VMA extract 85t
Volmax 116b
Voltaren
  Analgesics 12b
  Ophth 108t
Voltaren Ophtha
  108t
Voltaren Rapide
  12b
Voltaren XR 12b
Volume expand-
  ers 92t
voriconazole 21m
VoSol otic 72b
VoSpire ER 116b
VP-16 104m
Vumon 104m
Vytorin 42t
VZIG 91m

W

warfarin 83m
Wartec 54t

websites 8
Welchol 40m
Wellbutrin 110m
Wellcovorin 104t
Wellcovorin Uni-
  tract 89m
wild yam 89b
willow bark ex-
  tract 89m
witch hazel 56b
wolf's bane 85b
Women's Tylenol
  Menstrual
  Relief 19t
Wycillin 32t
Wygesic 18m

X

Xalatan 107m
Xanax 113b
Xatral 121t
Xeloda 103b
Xenadrine 84m
Xenical 81m
Xibrom 108t
Xifaxan 35b
Xigris 35m
Xopenex 117m
Xylocaine
  Anesthesia 19b
  Cardiovas 38b
  Dermatol 57m
  ENT 73m
Xylocard 39m
Xyrem 97t

Y

Yasmin 98
yellow fever vac-
  cine 90b
YF-Vax 90b
Yocon 123t
yohimbe 89m
yohimbine 123t
Yohimex 123t

Z

Zaditen 119m
Zaditor 104b
zafirlukast 119t
zalcitabine 25b
zaleplon 114t
Zanaflex 92t
zanamivir 26b
Zanosar 103b
Zantac 77b
Zarontin 92t
Zaroxolyn 48t
ZDV 25t
ZE 139 85t
ZeaSorb AF 54t

Zebeta 45t
Zegerid 78b
Zelnorm 81b
Zemplar 67b
Zemuron 19b
Zenapax 91t
Zerit 25m
Zestoretic 43b
Zestril 35b
Zetia 42t
Zevalin 104m
Ziac 43b
Ziagen 25t
zidovudine 25mb
zileuton 119t
Zinacef 29b
Zinecard 104t
Zingiber offici-
  nale 86b
ziprasidone 112t
Zithromax 31t
Zmax 31t
Zocor 41t
Zofran 75m
Zoladex
  OB/GYN 99b
  Oncology 104t
zoledronic acid
  59m
zolmitriptan 95t
Zoloft 110t
zolpidem 114t
Zometa 59m
Zomig 95t
Zonalon 57t
Zonegran 94b
zonisamide 94b
zopiclone 114t
Zorbtive 69t
Zorcaine 19m
Zostrix 57t
Zosyn 33m
Zovia 98
Zovirax
  Antimicr 24t
  Dermatol 55t
Zyban 114m
Zydone 18m
Zyflo 119t
Zylet 106m
Zyloprim 63t
Zymar 105m
Zyprexa 111b
Zyrtec 71t
Zyvox 35m
Zyvoxam 35m

Page left blank for notes

Page left blank for notes

ADULT EMERGENCY DRUGS (selected)

ALLERGY	diphenhydramine (*Benadryl*): 50 mg IV/IM. epinephrine: 0.1-0.5 mg IM/SC (1:1000 solution), may repeat after 20 mins. methylprednisolone (*Solu-Medrol*): 125 mg IV/IM.
HYPERTENSION	esmolol (*Brevibloc*): 500 mcg/kg IV over 1 minute, then titrate 50-200 mcg/kg/minute fenoldopam (*Corlopam*): Start 0.1 mcg/kg/min, titrate up to 1.6 mcg/kg/min labetalol (*Normodyne*): Start 20 mg slow IV, then 40-80 mg IV q10 min prn up to 300 mg total cumulative dose nitroglycerin (*Tridil*): Start 10-20 mcg/min IV infusion, then titrate prn up to 100 mcg/minute nitroprusside (*Nipride*): Start 0.3 mcg/kg/min IV infusion, then titrate prn up to 10 mcg/kg/minute
DYSRHYTHMIAS / ARREST	adenosine (*Adenocard*): PSVT (not A-fib): 6 mg rapid IV & flush, preferably through a central line or proximal IV. If no response after 1-2 minutes then 12 mg. A third dose of 12 mg may be given prn. amiodarone (*Cordarone, Pacerone*): Life-threatening ventricular arrhythmia: Load 150 mg IV over 10 min, then 1 mg/min x 6h, then 0.5 mg/min x 18h. atropine: 0.5-1.0 mg IV/ET, repeat q 5 min to maximum of 0.04 mg/kg. diltiazem (*Cardizem*): Rapid atrial fibrillation: bolus 0.25 mg/kg or 20 mg IV over 2 min. May repeat 0.35 mg/kg or 25 mg IV 15 min after first dose. Infusion 5-15 mg/h. epinephrine: 1 mg IV/ET for cardiac arrest. [1:10,000 solution] lidocaine (*Xylocaine*): Load 1 mg/kg IV, then 0.5 mg/kg q8-10min prn to max 3 mg/kg. Maintenance 2g in 250ml D5W (8 mg/ml) at 1-4 mg/min drip (7-30 ml/h).
PRESSORS	dobutamine (*Dobutrex*): 2-20 mcg/kg/min. 70 kg: 5 mcg/kg/min with 1 mg/mL concentration (eg, 250 mg in 250 mL D5W) = 21 mL/h. dopamine (*Intropin*): Pressor: Start at 5 mcg/kg/min, increase prn by 5-10 mcg/kg/min increments at 10 min intervals, max 50 mcg/kg/min. 70 kg: 5 mcg/kg/min with 1600 mcg/mL concentration (eg, 400 mg in 250 ml D5W) = 13 mL/h. Doses at mcg/kg/min: 2-4 = (traditional renal dose, apparently ineffective) dopaminergic receptors; 5-10 = (cardiac dose) dopaminergic and beta1 receptors; >10 = dopaminergic, beta1, and alpha1 receptors. norepinephrine (*Levophed*): 4 mg in 500 ml D5W (8 mcg/ml) at 2-4 mcg/min. 22.5 ml/h = 3 mcg/min. phenylephrine (*Neo-Synephrine*): 50 mcg boluses IV. Infusion for hypotension: 20 mg in 250ml D5W (80 mcg/ml) at 40-180 mcg/min (35-160ml/h).
INTUBATION	etomidate (*Amidate*): 0.3 mg/kg IV. methohexital (*Brevital*): 1-1.5 mg/kg IV. rocuronium (*Zemuron*): 0.6-1.2 mg/kg IV. succinylcholine (*Anectine*): 1 mg/kg IV. Peds (<5 yo): 2 mg/kg IV; consider preceding with atropine 0.02 mg/kg. thiopental (*Pentothal*): 3-5 mg/kg IV.
SEIZURES	diazepam (*Valium*): 5-10 mg IV, or 0.2-0.5 mg/kg rectal gel up to 20 mg PR. fosphenytoin (*Cerebyx*): Load 15-20 "phenytoin equivalents" per kg either IM, or IV no faster than 100-150 mg/min. lorazepam (*Ativan*): 0.05-0.15 mg/kg up to 3-4 mg IV/IM. phenobarbital: 200-600 mg IV at rate ≤60 mg/min; titrate prn up to 20 mg/kg. phenytoin (*Dilantin*): 15-20 mg/kg up to 1000 mg IV no faster than 50 mg/min.

CARDIAC DYSRHYTHMIA PROTOCOLS (*Circulation* 2000; 102, suppl I)

For adults and children >8 years old. Alter dosing & Joules based on child's weight.

Basic Life Support

All cases: Two initial breaths, then compressions 100 per minute
One or two rescuer: 15:2 ratio of compressions to ventilations

V-Fib, Pulseless V-Tach

CPR until defibrillator ready
Defibrillate 200 J
Defibrillate 200-300 J
Defibrillate 360 J
Intubate, IV, then *options*:
- Epinephrine 1 mg IV q3-5 minutes
- Vasopressin 40 units IV once only; no epi if no response in 5-10 min
- Defibrillate 360J after each drug dose

Options:
- Amiodarone 300 mg IV; repeat doses 150 mg
- Lidocaine 1.0-1.5 mg/kg IV q3-5 minutes to max 3 mg/kg
- Magnesium 1-2 g IV
- Procainamide 30-50 mg/min IV to max 17 mg/kg
- Bicarbonate 1 mEq/kg IV
Defibrillate 360 J after each drug dose

Pulseless Electrical Activity (PEA)

CPR, intubate, IV.
- Consider 5 H's: hypovolemia, hypoxia, H+ acidosis, hyper / hypokalemia, hypothermia
- Consider 5 T's: "tablets"-drug OD, tamponade-cardiac, tension pneumothorax, thrombosis-coronary, thrombosis-pulmonary embolism
Epinephrine 1 mg IV q3-5 minutes
If bradycardia, atropine 1 mg IV q3-5 min to max 0.04 mg/kg
Consider bicarbonate 1 mEq/kg IV if ↑K+ or tricyclic/ASA overdose

Asystole

CPR, intubate, IV, assess code status
Confirm asystole in >1 lead
Search for and treat reversible causes
Consider early transcutaneous pacing
Epinephrine 1 mg IV q3-5 minutes
Atropine 1 mg IV q3-5 min to max 0.04 mg/kg

Bradycardia (<60 bpm), symptomatic

Airway, oxygen, IV
Atropine 0.5-1 mg IV q3-5 min to max 0.04 mg/kg
Transcutaneous pacemaker
Options:
- Dopamine 5-20 mcg/kg/min
- Epinephrine 2-10 mcg/min

Unstable Tachycardia (>150 bpm)

Airway, oxygen, IV
Consider brief trial of medications
Premedicate whenever possible
Synchronized cardioversion 100 J
Synchronized cardioversion 200 J
Synchronized cardioversion 300 J
Synchronized cardioversion 360 J

Stable Monomorphic V-Tach

Airway, oxygen, IV
If no CHF, then choose just one top agent (procainamide, sotalol) or other agent (amiodarone, lidocaine)
If CHF (EF<40%), then DC cardioversion after pretreatment with either:
- Amiodarone 150 mg IV over 10 min; repeat q10-15 min prn
- Lidocaine 0.5-0.75 mg/kg IV; repeat q5-10 min prn to max 3 mg/kg

Stable Wide-Complex Tachycardia

Airway, oxygen, IV
If no CHF, then *options*:
- DC cardioversion
- Procainamide 20-30 mg/min IV to max 20 mg/kg
- Amiodarone (see stable V-tach dose)
If CHF (EF<40%), then *options*:
- DC cardioversion
- Amiodarone

Stable Narrow-Complex SVT

Airway, oxygen, IV
Vagal stimulation
Adenosine 6mg IV, then 12 mg prn.
Further treatment based on specific rhythm (junctional tachycardia, PSVT, multifocal atrial tachycardia) and presence or absence of CHF.

Tarascon Publishing Order Form on Next Page

Price per Copy by Number of Copies Ordered				
Total # of each ordered →	1–9	10–49	50–99	≥100
Tarascon Pocket Pharmacopoeia				
• Classic shirt pocket edition	$11.95	$10.95	$9.95	$8.95
• Deluxe lab coat pocket edition	$19.95	$16.95	$14.95	$13.95
• PDA edition on CD, 12 month subscription	$29.95	$25.46	$23.96	$22.46
• PDA edition on CD, 3 month subscription	$8.97	$7.62	$7.18	$6.73
Other Tarascon Pocketbooks				
• *Tarascon Primary Care Pocketbook*	$14.95	$13.45	$11.94	$10.44
• *Tarascon Internal Med & Crit Care Pocketbook*	$14.95	$13.45	$11.94	$10.44
• *Tarascon Pocket Orthopaedica*	$14.95	$13.45	$11.94	$10.44
• *Tarascon Adult Emergency Pocketbook*	$14.95	$13.45	$11.94	$10.44
• *Tarascon Peds Emergency Pocketbook*	$11.95	$9.90	$8.95	$8.35
• *How to be a Truly Excellent Junior Med Student*	$9.95	$8.25	$7.45	$6.95
Tarascon Rapid Reference Cards & Magnifier				
• *Tarascon Quick P450 Enzyme Reference Card*	$1.95	$1.85	$1.75	$1.65
• *Tarascon Quick Pediatric Reference Card*	$1.95	$1.85	$1.75	$1.65
• *Tarascon Quick HTN/LDL Reference Card*	$1.95	$1.85	$1.75	$1.65
• *Tarascon Fresnel Magnifying Lens and Ruler*	$1.00	$0.89	$0.78	$0.66
Other Recommended Pocketbooks				
• *Managing Contraception*	$10.00	$9.75	$9.50	$9.25
• *OB/GYN & Infertility*	$14.95	$14.55	$14.25	$13.80
• *Airway Cam Pocket Guide to Intubation*	$14.95	$14.55	$14.25	$13.80
• *Reproductive Endocrinology/Infertility-Pocket*	$14.95	$14.55	$14.25	$13.80
• *Reproductive Endocrinology/Infertility-Desk*	$24.95	$24.55	$24.20	$23.80

Shipping & Handling (based on subtotal on next page order form)					
If subtotal is →	≤$12	$13-29.99	$30-75.99	$76-200	$201-700
Standard shipping	$1.00	$2.50	$6.00	$8.00	$15.00
UPS 2-day air *(no PO boxes)*	$12.00	$14.00	$16.00	$18.00	$35.00

Tarascon Pocket Pharmacopoeia® Deluxe PDA Edition

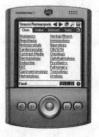

Features
- Palm OS® and Pocket PC® versions
- Meticulously peer-reviewed drug information
- Multiple drug interaction checking
- Continuous internet auto-updates
- Extended memory card support
- Multiple tables & formulas
- Complete customer privacy

Download a FREE 30-day trial version at www.tarascon.com

Subscriptions thereafter priced at $2.29/month

Ordering Books From Tarascon Publishing

INTERNET	**MAIL**	**FAX**	**PHONE**
Order through our OnLine store with your credit card at www.tarascon.com	Mail order & check to: **Tarascon Publishing** PO Box 517 Lompoc, CA 93438	Fax credit card orders 24 hrs/day toll free to **877.929.9926**	For phone orders or customer service, call **800.929.9926**

Name				
Address				
City	State	Zip		Residential ☐ Business ☐
Phone		Email		

TARASCON POCKET PHARMACOPOEIA®	Quantity	Price*
Classic Shirt-Pocket Edition		$
Deluxe Labcoat Pocket Edition		$
PDA software on CD-ROM, 3 month subscription‡		$
PDA software on CD-ROM, 12 month subscription‡		$
OTHER TARASCON POCKETBOOKS		
Tarascon Primary Care Pocketbook		$
Tarascon Internal Medicine & Critical Care Pocketbook		$
Tarascon Pocket Orthopaedica®		$
Tarascon Adult Emergency Pocketbook		$
Tarascon Pediatric Emergency Pocketbook		$
How to be a Truly Excellent Junior Medical Student		$
TARASCON RAPID REFERENCE CARDS & MAGNIFIER		
Tarascon Quick P450 Enzyme Reference Card		$
Tarascon Quick Pediatric Reference Card		$
Tarascon Quick HTN & LDL Reference Card		$
Tarascon Fresnel Magnifying Lens and Ruler		$
OTHER RECOMMENDED POCKETBOOKS		
Managing Contraception		$
OB/GYN & Infertility		$
Airway Cam Pocket Guide to Intubation		$
Reproductive Endocrinology/Infertility Pocket edition		$
Reproductive Endocrinology/Infertility Desk edition		$

*See prior page for prices / shipping. ‡Download at tarascon.com for ~10% discount!

☐ VISA ☐ Mastercard ☐ American Express ☐ Discover		**Subtotal**	$
Card number		CA only add 7.75% sales tax	$
Exp date	CID number (if available)	Shipping / handling*	$
Signature		**TOTAL**	$